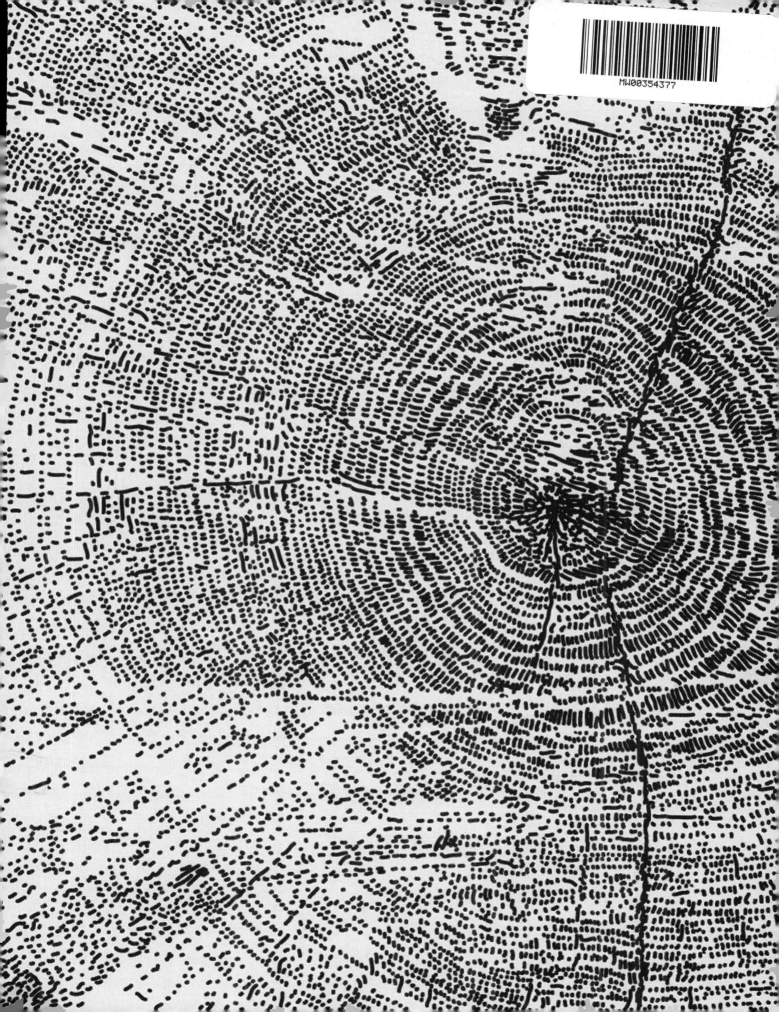

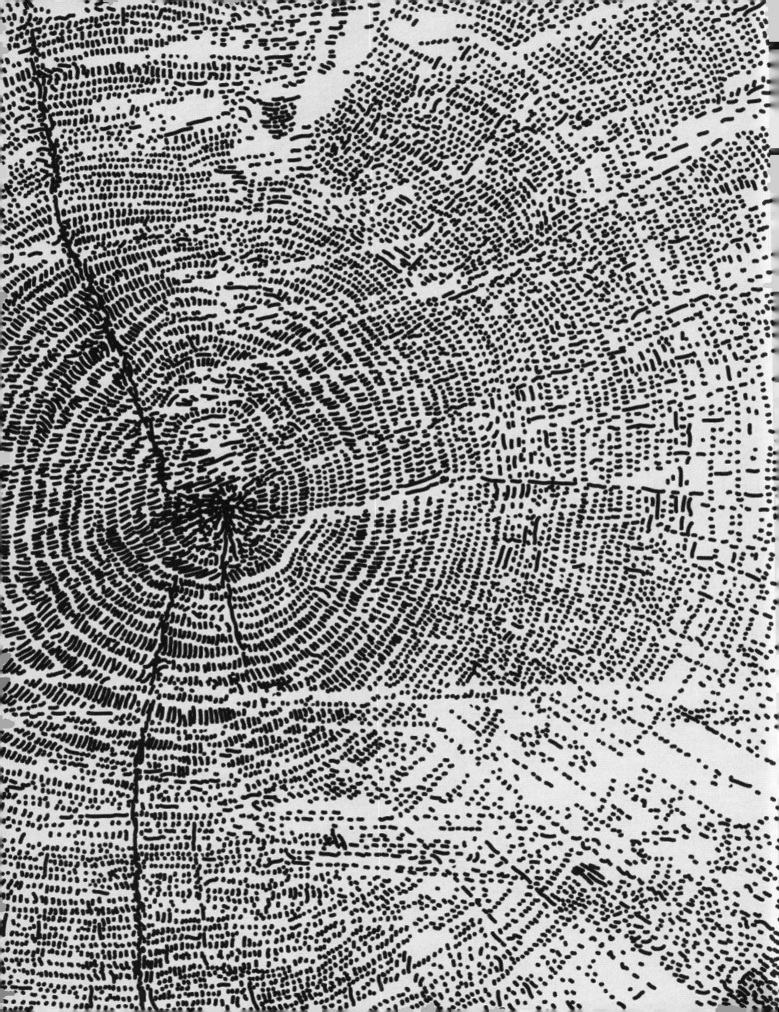

REIKI
PLUS PLUS

ALSO BY DANY LYNE

Riding the Wave:
Tales of Transformation
2014

ME TOO LOUD & CLEAR:
How I Walked the Talk from Silence to Active Hope
2019

Sacred Tree for All Seasons:
Reclaiming Your Capacity to Heal • The Guidebook and Oracle Cards
2019

REIKI
PLUS PLUS

EMBRACE YOUR
SACRED TREE
TO TRANSCEND TRAUMA

DANY LYNE

UNLEASH, Toronto, Canada

Excerpts from pp. 225-6 from THE TIBETAN BOOK OF LIVING AND DYING by RIGPA FELLOWSHIP and EDITED BY PATRICK GAFFNEY & ANDREW HARVEY. Copyright © 1993 by Rigpa Fellowship. Reprinted by permission of HarperCollins Publishers.

Lyne, Dany, 1962-, author
    Reiki Plus Plus / Dany Lyne.

ISBN 978-0-9939204-4-8

Copy editing and proofreading: Strong Finish Editorial Design
Art direction: Dany Lyne
Cover and front matter design: Candice Craig
Design and layout: Candice Craig alchemydesign.ca
Layout revisions: Carlos Gouveia cgmultimedia.ca
Photoshop art: Sharon Switzer

Printed and bound in Canada.

For Bee Stevens

Dearest Bee,

In you, I see the journey clearly. I see myself and I see so many friends, clients, and students. Your bold and transformational trek is a blessing and a most precious grace you bestow to our community and the world. This book is my prayer for you and for all living beings.

CONTENTS

PART ONE: SACRED TREE APPRENTICESHIP

PART TWO: REIKI PLUS PLUS

LEVEL ONE

LEVEL THREE

PART THREE: REIKI PLUS PLUS IN ACTION

AUTHOR'S NOTE

The women who share their stories in Part Three all read, edited, and approved several drafts of the text pertaining to their respective histories. To protect their privacy, pseudonyms are used throughout and traits, events, and locations are often shifted to equivalents.

Reiki Plus Plus is a compilation of my thoughts, opinions, and conclusions. The information presented here is believed to be accurate and sound, based on my knowledge and experience. How you decide to use it is up to you. Using the techniques herein is acknowledging that you have read, understand, and agree to this disclaimer and therefore that informed consent has been established.

ACKNOWLEDGEMENTS

I am grateful to all the clients and students who invited me to join their healing and transformational journeys. Without their trust and generosity, I would not have had the honour of being a compassionate witness often enough to observe the magnificent competence of the human organism in self-healing action. The proficiency of their energy bodies (including their physical body) to transcend trauma (including sexual abuse trauma) speaks to the power and manifestation of innate harmony in action. Initially discovering, and later uncovering, their built-in high-frequency resources and self-healing capacity motivates me to share the enchanting magic of our innate alchemical vigour: our Sacred Tree.

I thank Damian Rogers for reading the mega-manuscript I dropped off on her porch in the spring of 2018. I'm forever grateful for her perspicacity and involvement in the early stages of what I refer to as "The Sacred Tree Trilogy." Her spirit and enthusiasm permeate all the content that under her guidance transformed into several books, including *Sacred Tree for All Seasons: Reclaiming Your Capacity to Heal • The Guidebook and Oracle Cards*.

I am also indebted to Allyson Taché, the beautiful woman I was introduced to in a yoga class who, after spending two hours together in a coffee house reminiscing about our mutual journeys in Burkina Faso, offered me her loft in a secluded fifteenth-century tower in a small town in Corsica, France. The bulk of these manuscripts were channelled and chiselled on the rooftop of this ancient tower held tightly by the windswept mountains and Mediterranean Sea as well as the robust and magical Maquis shrubland of Le Cap Corse. I also thank Allyson and my beloved neighbours— Deirdre Newman, Roy Pelletier, and Evelyne Desutter—for their spirit, laughter, and joyful car rides into town for groceries and supplies, not to mention exquisite afternoons on the beach and the trails. My spirit soared on their welcoming wings, and these pages are imbued with their generosity.

Thank you, Katherine Dynes, for being a stalwart ally and friend regardless of the velocity of my enthusiasm and tenacity when manifesting creative projects!

INTRODUCTION

I devise a delicious plan to regroup at the Sivananda Ashram in the Bahamas in February 2017: three wonderful weeks of a Swami Vishnudevananda Saraswati–infused atmosphere, Sivananda yoga twice a day, meditation umpteen times a day, delightful catnaps in my tiny baby-leaf-green tent, and lots of lazing around on the white sand beach. While there, Eva, one of the inspiring women and healers with whom I shared most meals, unexpectedly encourages me to write a book about my work with clients. We are sitting on the beach, the wind and waves uncharacteristically rambunctious on our last morning together. Her precipitous gaze punctuates her statement as dramatically as the roar of the Atlantic.

I return to Toronto a writing machine. Although the thought of a book temporarily morphs into an inflamed urgency to update the manuals I had produced seven years earlier to support my Reiki Level One, Two, and Three workshops, I find myself getting more and more impassioned, to the point of generating just as much new material as I am rewriting. Six weeks into this frenzied undertaking, I catch my flight to Yelapa, Mexico, and settle into a quaint palapa on a hill. In my mind, I'm finishing the Reiki manuals and then writing a book about my journey with ancestors in Ghana and Burkina Faso in 2016. By week three, forget about Africa for the time being, as I am fully aware that these so-called manuals have become *the book* I am writing now.

In the meantime, the Canadian Reiki Association has an empty folder in their cabinets where the requisite documentation supporting my renewed membership as a practitioner and teacher should be. The troublesome prospect of reapplying to be a certified member propelled me into a pertinent debate about whether I wanted to remain not only affiliated with the association but also with the Reiki practice itself. Had my work veered away from this modality in the past decade? After all, so many colleagues, students, and clients were now referring to my practice as "Reiki Plus Plus"—the *plus plus* their charming acknowledgement of the other modalities and intuitive guidance informing my sessions. So, is it still Reiki?

In my opinion, the potential for healing, self-healing, and clearing the path for innate wisdom to flow via Reiki and self-Reiki has been watered down by professional associations in an effort to standardize guidelines.

Unfortunately, in their aim to validate Reiki within the professional healthcare arena, regulatory bodies often steer away from aspects of the Reiki practice that skeptics could refer to as "woo-woo." Yet the ancient, intuitive, and alchemical capacity to self-heal and heal that Dr. Mikao Usui tapped into when he created the Reiki system in the early twentieth century is a celebration of our innate power and wisdom. Our spirit is everything *but* woo-woo or airy-fairy. To cut our Reiki or self-Reiki practice off from this precious resource is akin to saying that only book knowledge exists and that innate wisdom and ancestral guidance is not "official" enough.

Meanwhile, Reiki practitioners are rarely asked to study anatomy and are not encouraged to consciously interact with the energetic signatures of specific organs and tissues. It dawned on me while training as a craniosacral therapist that Usui studied medicine. I now teach self-Reiki and Reiki with this in mind. He knew the human form intimately, not just as a Buddhist monk and spiritual practitioner but as a practitioner schooled in the Western allopathic tradition. In his notebooks, Usui links the hand positions with the organs and specifies the energy vortexes and chakras they control and stimulate. To practise self-Reiki and Reiki with this level of clarity creates a dynamic force field between your physical body, all energy bodies, and the power you hold in your hands to receive a multitude of minute signals and information. In the end, I haven't left Reiki behind at all. Rather, I celebrate the "invisible" force field within us and acknowledge its less easily detectable treasures.

Reiki Plus Plus exemplifies the approach I initiate in my meditative explorations to self-heal alongside hundreds of clients and students who also want to devote themselves to self-healing. It is my goal to support this community, and others like us who want to self-heal and thrive, by sharing the guidance I intuit in sessions when my hands read my body or that of others. My requisite (if at times excruciating) journey of witnessing, deciphering, and comprehending my past is the foundation of my intuitive and meditative Reiki Plus Plus self-healing practice. While the fifteen years of brutal sexual abuse by my maternal grandfather and father, and my mother's betrayal, and the decades of mayhem in my twenties and thirties fuel my determination, my steadfast journey of self-inquiry and self-Reiki continue to inspire my impetus to compassionately witness and hold sacred space for myself and others.

PART ONE: SACRED TREE APPRENTICESHIP

In these chapters, I include revised sections from my memoir, *Riding the Wave: Tales of Transformation*, about the unanticipated ancestral visitation of my great-aunt and the spontaneous Reiki initiation I experienced in the week before my maternal grandmother's death. I then describe the life-changing impact of my Reiki training, self-Reiki practice, and exploration within the Sacred Tree realm I encountered when my biological eyes were closed. I also describe the pivotal insights I gained when I studied craniosacral therapy and medical Qigong; namely, our innate vertical axis connecting us to the earth and the sun and the influence of Nature's cyclical rhythms on our evolution and well-being. Furthermore, I introduce you to the quintessential journey back to love and compassion and the interplay of our "traumatized astronauts" and our "architects of survival" trapped in capsules of unlove.

PART TWO: REIKI PLUS PLUS

LEVELS ONE, TWO, AND THREE

These chapters amalgamate basic Reiki training with Reiki Plus Plus Sacred Tree training. While I set the stage for you to explore the foundation of Reiki, I also highlight the power of developing a self-Reiki practice and encourage you to discover a more intuitive and creative engagement with your innate power to self-heal and alchemically transform trauma into wisdom.

For instance, in Level One, while I present the foundational information about Reiki, its uses, history, Usui's five principles, and the introductory sequence of hand positions, I also include information about the anatomy of your Sacred Tree, including the seven chakras, the Sun and Earth Star Chakras, and the three dantians. Throughout, I emphasize the significance of your Sacred Tree's powerful vertical axis and its fundamental orientation to the earth and the sun.

In Level Two, while I include the foundational Reiki symbols and distance Reiki method, I also encourage you to develop your intuitive perception and to consciously practise engaging with specific organs and their cyclical wisdom.

I familiarize you with the energetic organ groupings called elemental orbs, an ancient map of health and healing laid out by Chinese sages, traditional Chinese medicine (TCM) doctors, and medical Qigong practitioners. Their elemental medicine wheel is an infinite source of inspiration revealing the interplay among the organs, their yin–yang groupings, and the dynamic relationships among the physical, emotional, mental, and spiritual dimensions of their functioning. Although I merely introduce this vast body of knowledge in this book, I continue to delve into this cycle's insightfulness in the self-Reiki meditation tool and divination platform I have created: *Sacred Tree for All Seasons: Reclaiming Your Capacity to Heal • The Guidebook and Oracle Cards.*

In Level Three, I emphasize the seemingly simple yet often most daunting enterprise of all: practise, self-practise, and then practise and self-practise some more, ad infinitum. To inform this essential and substantive personal practicum, Part Three follows as a helping hand.

PART THREE: REIKI PLUS PLUS IN ACTION

These chapters are a second edition, if you will, of Part Three of my first book, *Riding the Wave: Tales of Transformation.* Using my notes, memory, and observations during Reiki sessions, I created dialogue inspired by the experience my clients and I shared in my healing studio. The reconstituted sessions document the rebellion, collapse, hope, courage, and healing of nine women, ranging in age from seventeen to sixty, from different socioeconomic and cultural backgrounds. In particular, I present to you the therapeutic journeys of women who in one or many aspects of their histories and healing have travelled through the same tumultuous and muddy waters of sexual violation and intergenerational trauma as I have.

At some point,
someone has to
really show up with a
generous open heart!

Someone has to transcend
the blame and shame
and whatever else
to smother the cycle of violence
with love by the bushelful.

No one is more qualified
for this enterprise
than you are.

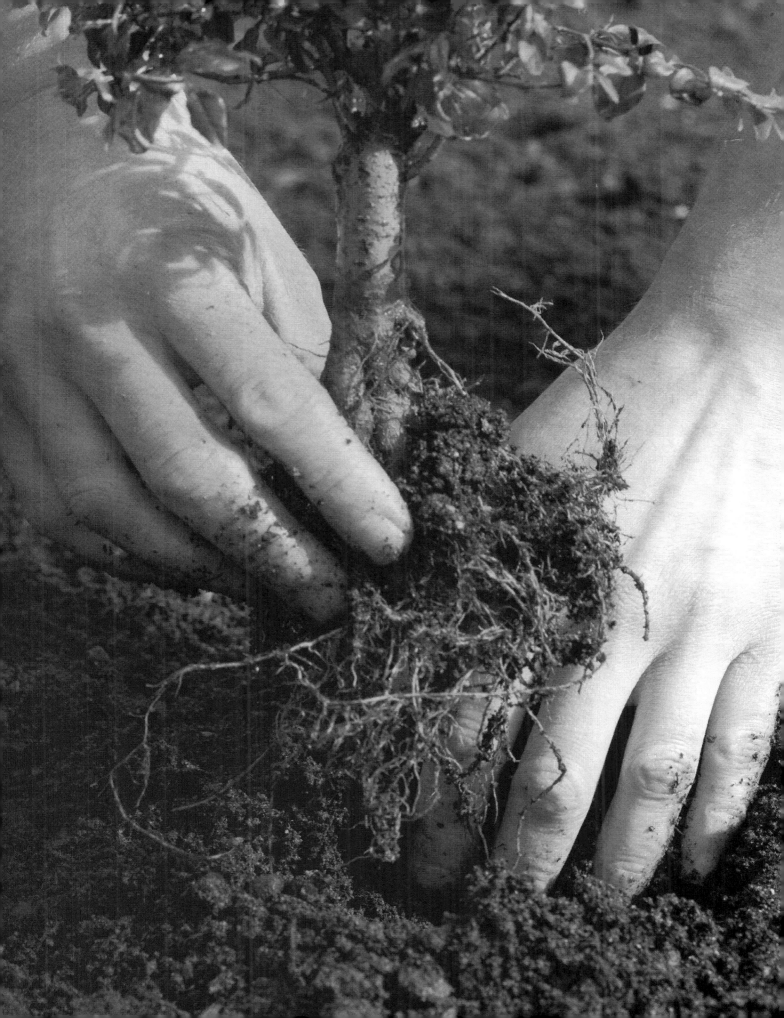

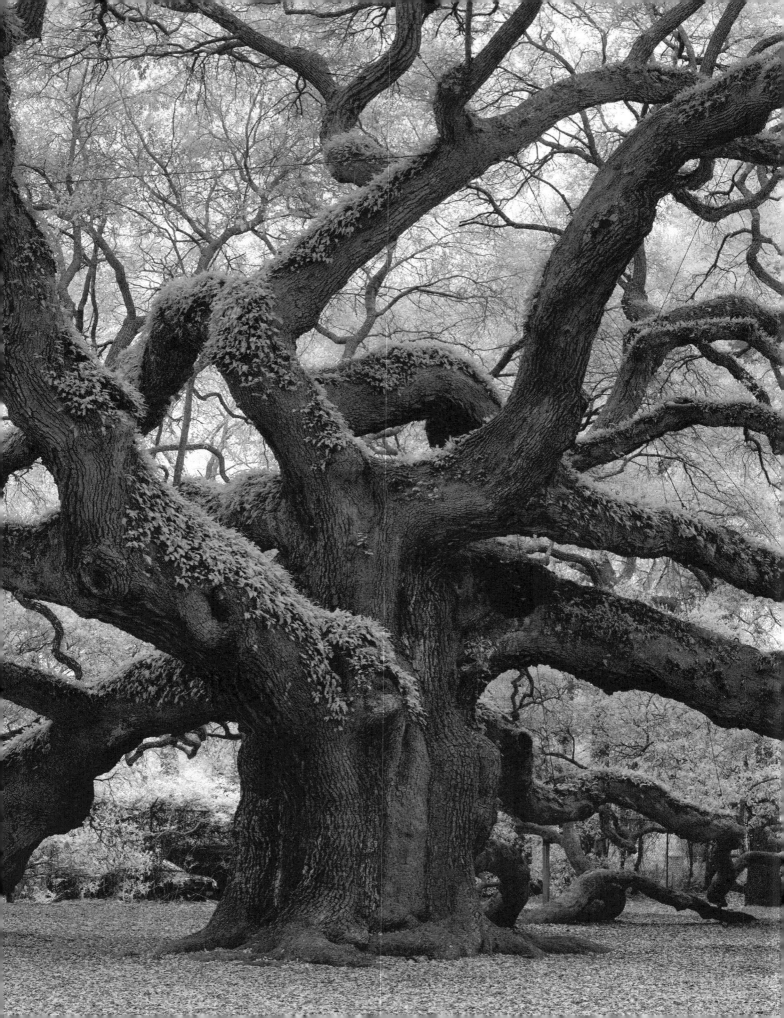

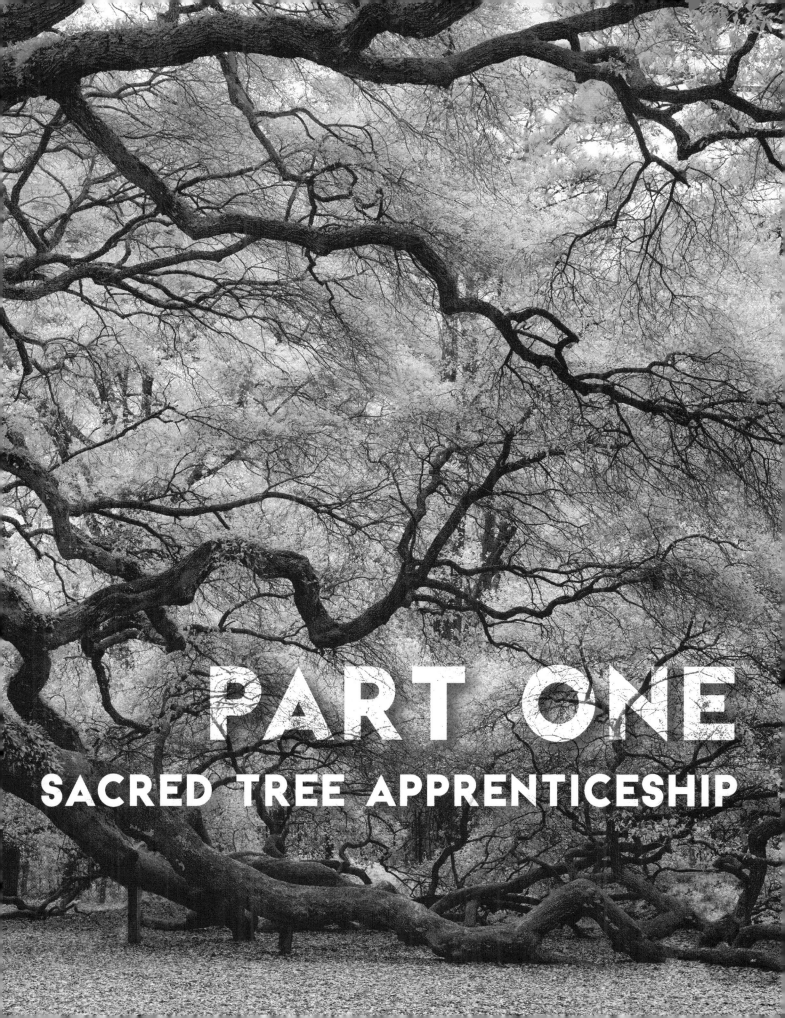

PART ONE
SACRED TREE APPRENTICESHIP

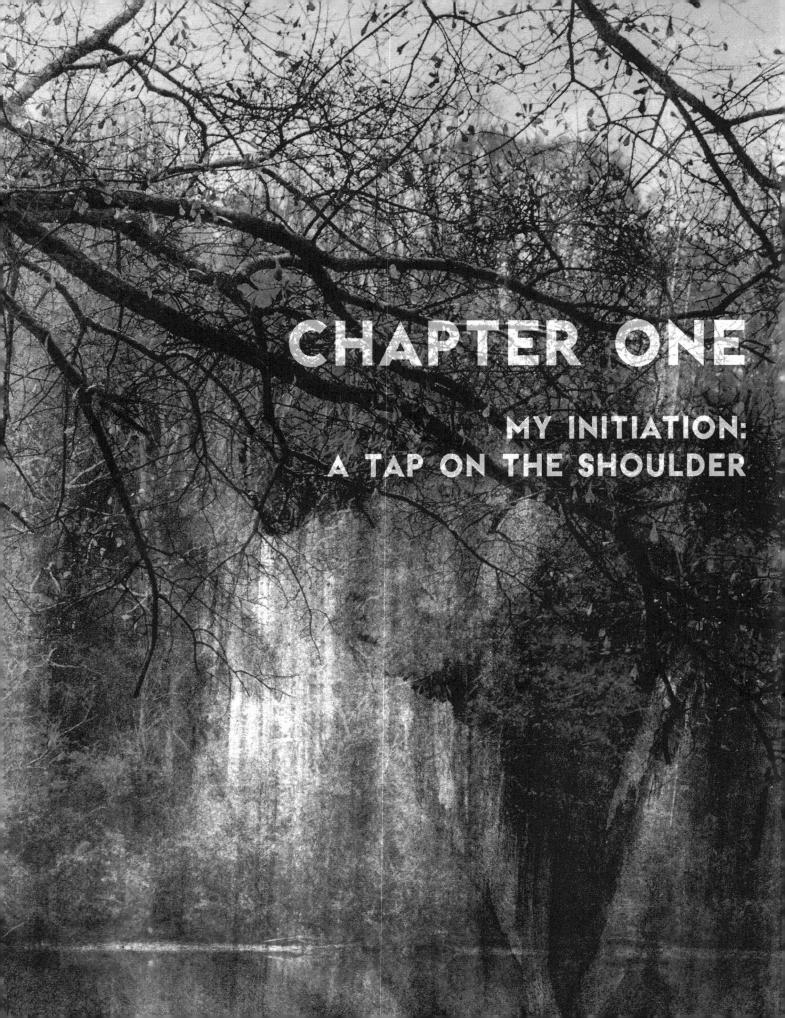

CHAPTER ONE

MY INITIATION:
A TAP ON THE SHOULDER

My life has changed many times. It changed when I completed my master's degree in 1993. Before that it changed when I was almost killed in a hunk of metal in the heart of Nevada's Valley of Fire in the late 1980s. And after that it changed when I encountered my true self shining back at me in the darkness of the moon eclipsing the sun in mid-afternoon in 1993 when I was thirty-one years old. That moment marked my first compassionate look into myself, which unearthed my first memories of being sexually assaulted by my maternal grandfather and father more times than you can count. This awakening irrevocably plunged me into the depths of my being-ness in a family wrought with transgenerational wounds and trauma. I could also say that my induction into the world of theatre and opera design by Dr. Paul Baker most changed my life. And I could also say that my thirteen-year relationship with K and the friendships that matured during that era healed me and changed the course of my life dramatically.

Although all of that is true, what really changed my life was the day my great-aunt, *ma tante* Blanche, tapped me on the shoulder to let me know that my maternal grandmother, her sister, my beloved Mamy, was dying. I'm sitting at my desk in the fall of 2003 with several design assistants plugging away at the mountains of drafting, model-making, and organizing associated with the many opera productions I am designing simultaneously. As per usual, after designing for a few hours in the early morning, I am now ensconced at my desk managing rather than designing my projects. I am ploughing my way through my daily diet of emails from directors, production managers, technical directors, lighting designers, cutters, tailors, prop masters, and God knows who else—someone who is facing yet another roadblock or having a eureka moment they'd like to pass by me—when I feel a *tap-tap-tap* on my right shoulder.

I turn around to find nothing but the usual: design assistants with their heads tucked in a model box, or their eyes transfixed by a computer screen, or bent over a miniscule divan to recreate in three-eighths-of-an-inch scale the magnificence we envision for Act 2. I turn my attention back to the all-consuming emails when again I feel a *tap-tap-tap* on my right shoulder. Again I see nothing. No one seems to need my immediate attention, and you could cut the level of concentration in the air at the various workstations in my studio with a knife. Again *tap-tap-tap*. I pivot my whole body to face the emergency. Nothing. Silence. Yet I feel a presence. I feel something. The air is thicker over my right shoulder. In fact, turning around seems useless because the presence or sensation pivots with me. I spend the next two days turning around whenever I feel this mysterious and urgent request for my attention. Sometimes I even turn around when I feel nothing, hoping to catch the presence by surprise.

Just last week, Lionel, my chiropractor, had announced that he was welcoming Rose A. Weinberg, a Reiki master, homeopath, energy intuitive, nutritionist, and author, to his practice: "She is giving fifteen-minute trial sessions for a week to encourage my clients to try it out." I was vaguely interested, but the only slot she had available was for an hour after my treatment with Lionel so I raced home to my looming deadlines rather than wait. However, another day of *tap-tapping* and I am on the phone booking a session, hoping Rose can tell me what the commotion is all about. At the clinic she greets me with a smile, and just as I walk through the door to her office she asks, "So who's your friend?" "Huh? That's exactly why I'm here. I have no idea. I keep feeling a presence." *Ma tante* Blanche graciously identifies herself and speaks to Rose, who relays the message to my untrained ears. "Your great-aunt is trying to be in touch with you. Your grandmother is dying and needs your help. She, too, will help, but your grandmother needs you to be there when she dies."

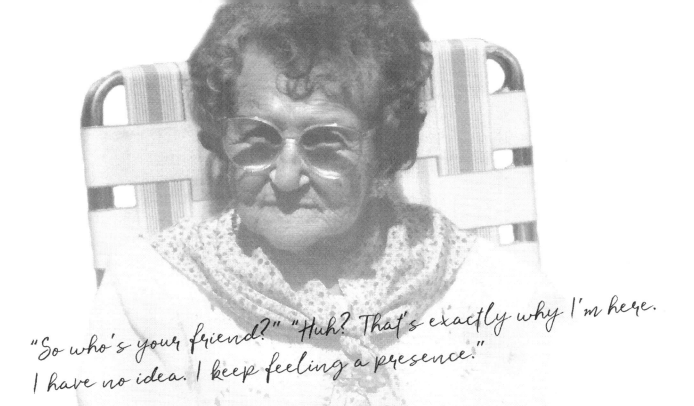

"So who's your friend?" "Huh? That's exactly why I'm here. I have no idea. I keep feeling a presence."

By the time I start breathing again, I am so focused on the fact that Mamy is dying that I do not stop for a second to wonder at the marvel that my invisible, dead great-aunt is here, communicating with silent words a most prescient message. I have things to do and places to go. I drive home as fast as I can and breathlessly run into the studio to announce to all my assistants that I am going out of town in half an hour. They need to leave now but should come back in the morning to carry on. I holler like a fishwife to K: "Mamy is dying! I have to leave now!" Just then, the phone rings. "What the hell? It's my mother! She never calls!" "Mamy is in the hospital; I think you should come," she says. Too abruptly I respond, "I'm on it. I'm leaving now. What hospital is she in?" "She's at the hospital in Ste-Agathe," my stunned mother replies. "OK. À demain." I pack, K and I hug, and as I jump in the car, I state rather cryptically, "I'll be back with her in a week!" Who knows what I mean.

If the most surreal moment is not the felt-sense of my great-aunt's presence over my shoulder or Rose sensing her presence right off the bat, then it's the fact that now I do not feel myself driving the car. I feel the momentum of the car slicing through the darkness on the TransCanada without actually registering that I am steering it or pressing on the gas pedal. Even stranger is the fact that I feel safe, loved, and urgently needed, more than sad, stressed out, or overwhelmed, which is what one might expect to feel under the circumstances.

"Whoops! Yikes, I'm veering right! What the hell? The car is taking the exit ramp!" As I consider my options to avoid going off the 401, my new, improved ears hear my invisible travelling companion loud and clear: "T'as faim. T'as besoin d'manger. Y'a un Swiss Chalet sur l'autre côté de l'autoroute. Mange une cuisse pis tu vas t'sentir mieux!" "OMG, she's right! There it is on the other side of the highway! I hadn't seen it. That's so her!" *Ma tante* was Mamy's oldest ally when it came to chicken dinner at St-Hubert. Swiss Chalet will have to do in an emergency. And it did! I was the only customer. Unrushed, the server was most touched by my story—the grandmother dying part, that is; I did not let her in on my dead aunt's mission to help me get there, or the fact that she was probably digging into a transparent but nonetheless deeply appreciated quarter-chicken dinner as we spoke.

Seven hours later, we cruise into the parking lot of the Centre Hospitalier Laurentien in Ste-Agathe-des-Monts, Québec. "Two a.m. We made record time! OK! Park the car, tuck the keys in your pocket, and find Mamy." Visiting hours are not on, to say the least, but that poses no problem with Blanche in charge of the operation. Legalities are clearly the least of her concerns. I walk and she floats right through security and up the stairs. A friendly nurse welcomes us without batting an eyelash. It seems perfectly sensible to her that I wish to see my grandmother at this hour. "Son nom s'il vous plaît?" "Emelia Tremblay." "Ah oui, c'est la p'tite madame dans la chambre 324. Elle va être contente de vous voir. C'est par là."

There she is: *Mamy! Ma Mamy, maintenant mourante, assise dans son lit hospitalier.* "Allô, Mamy! Me voilà!" "Bonsoir," she replies politely. She hesitantly reaches out for my hand. She is visibly relieved that I welcome her touch. I feel a disconcerting distance. "J'ai une p'tite fille comme vous," she tells me. "Elle vit à Toronto." My heart pinches in reaction to her confusion. She doesn't recognize me! Am I too late? Is her mind so far gone that I will not really connect with her? I yell as quietly as possible to avoid waking up her roommate. "Mamy, c'est moi! Mamy! C'est moi, Lyne. Je suis ici avec toi." Her teary, weakened eyes blink behind her gold-rimmed glasses. In the eerie glow of the fluorescent light, my face thankfully becomes intelligible. Her eyes open wide and her beautiful, familiar face cracks into a thousand lines of love, recognition, and gratefulness. Her heart reaches mine with breathtaking force. It is so clear that I am the answer to all her prayers. "Ah ben là! Lyne? C'est toi?" "Oui, Mamy, c'est moi, Lyne." "Ah mon Dieu! Ma p'tite! Ah ma belle p'tite! Ma cocotte!"

It is an embrace I will never forget and a most precious gift from beyond the grave. *Ma tante*'s love infuses our hug with timeless peace, allowing us both to feel the depth of our intimacy. I feel reassured that nothing has been lost in the years of meagre annual visits. We are both immensely grateful to feel each other's love and touch one more time, at least one more time. Mamy's laugh pulls me out of infinity. She is flabbergasted by her initial mistake and apologizes for being old and sometimes confused. She is ninety-nine years and ten days old, to be precise.

I sit for long, delicious hours by her bed, blissfully and hungrily savouring her being. My parents are not early birds, so we are graced with many hours of private time, free to express our love and devotion, something we both crave after the mean years of monitored closeness and stolen hugs and kisses. Our hands are entwined in silence while my head rests on her belly. She lovingly combs my hair with her trembling, arthritic fingers—something I never thought I would re-experience as an adult. And we bask in *ma tante* Blanche's unconditional love. Everything and everyone is unmistakably touched by her other-worldly guidance. It's like the staff is on the best happy pills ever devised; their attitude is so over the top in terms of kindness, service, willingness, and competence. Her peacefulness, love, and gentleness bathe our embraces with a timeless beauty, while Mamy's room, the whole floor, and everyone on it are graced by a sacred sense of purpose.

I am keenly aware of *ma tante*'s presence around Mamy and around me at all times, sometimes with both of us, somehow in two places at once. She is the production manager, conductor, and director of her sister's death, or so it appears. She seems to be in charge of how it plays out on the earthly plane, or at the very least she is in on the plot and shares its intricacies with me. In the silence, when my grandmother slips into sleep, I hear *ma tante*, imparting what seems like divine advice. With holy guidance I am granted the power to create living peace for Mamy in her last days on Earth, a gift I am honoured to bestow.

Ma tante tells me when to make phone calls, what arrangements to make, when to excuse myself to eat or go to the washroom, and when to rush back to my grandmother, who sometimes needs immediate help with her dentures, food, water, bed, blankets, morphine drip, or whatever. She instructs me precisely and concisely so that I can facilitate and implement every practicality for death and dying. My sense is that she, too, is rather busy doing the same thing on the other side. I am raised out of the mire of my bereavement and taught the way of the heart and of the now. I am honoured and guided to perform my sacred task with a confidence, grace, expertise, and gusto that are not really accessible to little old me in the normal sense of what I think of as me.

I could never have guessed that my grandmother's sister, my shrivelled little great-aunt, in death no less, would be the one to swoop into my life to make sure in one grand gesture that her sister died with dignity and that I lived the rest of my life aware that I, too, was touched by grace and could live consciously guided by it. A massive door was pushed open by the tiniest of women, barely four-feet, six-inches high the last time I saw her. Yet now she appears to be rather tall, her see-through head floating close to the ceiling. And it's more like a photograph than a film. Her mouth does not move as she speaks, yet I hear her voice, vaguely familiar, in the sense that I recognize her intonations, but the information flows faster and lighter than her actual voice did on the earthly plane. The sounds she produces do not slice through the silence but rather amplify it. I am never more aware of the silence in myself or in the room than when she speaks.

In those quiet moments, *ma tante* fills me in on the backstory. For instance, unbeknownst to me, she herself had died alone, scared, sad and abandoned in this very hospital a few years ago. Her dying wish was that her beloved sister should not experience this horror when it was her time. It's clear she is fulfilling her promise in spades. It's also evident that she heard Mamy's prayers to see me before she died and thus ensured her dying wish was fulfilled. My female ancestors shared their precious bond and wisdom with me. It is with them, in these extraordinary circumstances, that I was introduced to compassion in action and with it to paranormal hearing, seeing, feeling, and understanding. We were a victorious team of women joined by blood, history, and love, whether dead, dying, or alive; we were expressing unconditional love while our shared violence lay like a deflated balloon by the side of the road.

I learn that *ma tante*'s love for me is boundless and that my presence in her life, though manifest in the flesh only a few times a year for a few hours, was the highlight of her heart-life. Although she was said to be childless, I now know that taking a child in your heart is truly to be with child. I am her child more so than I ever was to my biological mother. Her love is so strong and her commitment to her sister and me so great that it cuts through all my previous notions of family, of divine grace, and of reality itself. Her love is the bridge on which I travel to transcend the limitations of everyday consciousness. Her generosity is the energy that I have been yearning for my whole life. To witness her commitment to Mamy, for whom she had been like a mother, is a balm that blesses my soul.

As we communicate, our focus is unearthly. Nothing interrupts the flow of our presence and love for each other, not even the midmorning arrival of my controlling and anxious mother and stunned father. Their anticipated plan of attack—that's the only way they know how to deal—is pre-empted before the first strike. Nor do the nurses, roommates, family feuds, our shared history, other patients' emergencies, hospital rules, or the limitations of Western medicine interfere with our newfound sense of the sacred. My parents (especially my mother, who had not permitted us to ever be alone together since I was kicked out of the house) danced around us like the ballroom champions they once were. They gracefully respected our needs. It was the first time that my mother could not or would not be the commanding officer dictating the terms of engagement.

Ma tante not only supervised all matters of death but all matters of the heart in the past, present, and future. Miraculously, my parents witnessed me for the first time as a capable, autonomous, competent, intelligent, and responsible adult. The bubble of horror burst and out of it emerged my whole being at least twenty feet taller. It was remarkable how tiny my parents were and how easily they could be pushed aside. Their ignorance hung around their neck like the noose it actually was. All their power collapsed in a dull heap of ash. My breath alone scattered it.

Nothing and no one could interfere or act on Mamy's behalf unless their love and attention was wholly devoted to her highest and greatest good. My parents' lives and choices had hardly prepared them for such a simple and honest act of presence. It was astounding to see their mouths open to utter their usual vile nonsense, only to shut again with not so much as one syllable pronounced. *Ma tante* seemed to silence them. Their startled eyes and the strange slackness of their jaws and lips attested to the involuntary gag order that yielded a pause long enough to let them absorb the wisdom imparted by our transparent companion. Only then could they talk, barely sounding like the people we had come to know.

The blessed pause broke their spell. It's like all artifice or illusion was dispelled and all the violence and its wounds were soothed enough for compassion to emerge. Rather than look down upon us, they looked up, not in subservience, which would simply reverse our roles, but beyond the duality of power or powerlessness: they looked and actually saw. My parents were granted sacred lenses that allowed them to see me, Mamy, the hospital staff, and perhaps even themselves. It's like the world came into focus and the strange, three-dimensional puzzle they had been trapped in disintegrated. All that was left was the true energy of life itself.

During that one week before Mamy's death, my parents actually witnessed me, whether at the hospital, at a restaurant, or in their home. They even witnessed me at work because some urgent opera business pressed in on our miraculous family transformation. Nicolas Muni and I talked for hours, comparing notes on all the various one-act operas that could be paired with *The Maids* at the Cincinnati Opera in the upcoming summer season. Of all times and of all places for me to listen to *The Emperor of Atlantis*! Viktor Ullman, the composer and librettist, wrote the opera while interned in Theresienstadt, a Nazi ghetto, before he was killed at Auschwitz-Birkenau in 1944.

My father, a staunch Holocaust denier, sat in flabbergasted awe as the opera, sung in German and undeniably a testament to Jewish suffering, invaded his living room. I luxuriated in Ullman's artistry, knowing it alone was proving my father wrong. My mother rattled dishes in her habitual briskness yet in unusual deferral to my purpose. Now huddled on the couch, he in stunned silence and she in excruciating pain, the singing voices having cracked their heads open, they listen to my side of the conversation with Nic. Later, they asked how old Nic was and confirmed that they understood correctly that he was the director and artistic director of the opera house. Neither of them could fathom why a man of his age and stature would discuss with their daughter, at length, so many aspects of the opera and, by the sounds of it, actually respect and value her opinion as much as she did his. The two artists' collaboration, mutual respect, and shared artistic passion were clearly big news for *les Laportes* that night. They talked about it often in the following days and even mentioned it to family members and friends, though less as a source of pride than one of astonishment.

Rather than marching in with vengeful pride and conquering my despotic tyrants, I glided in on the wings of my ancestors' love and Ullman's art, effortlessly navigating the tattered fabric of our family dynamic and structure. Although a shift of great magnitude was occurring, on many levels, I was not willing it as much as I was undergoing and observing it. In other words, I was not creating it; rather, I was being created by it. Ullman's music infused me with compassion for the dead and dying, and my grandmother's death infused me with life. The fundamental energy of life expressed itself through me with such force that I transformed without even considering all the implications. I felt more alive and more grateful to be alive than ever before. The grace that touched my life became three-dimensional, and my parents' ethos shattered.

My hands embraced my grandmother's being to soothe her aches and pains. I caressed her soul with mine; I saw her and she saw me far beyond physical reality. We spoke in silence more than we had ever spoken audibly. We said everything and said absolutely nothing. We loved, that's all we did: we loved each other, life, death, and the world, all the living beings in it and all the suffering that comes with it. Our love transcended the physical suffering that the present circumstances imposed. Intestinal cancer is painful. Like most deaths, hers did present suffering. Yet I know that when we joined our energies together while guided by *ma chère tante*, we transcended her pain and on some level death itself. I sensed that we three were going through a gateway together and that it was a grand beginning of a new chapter rather than the painful ending of the only chapter we would share. Mamy, too, felt big; if I was twenty feet high, she was forty, and my aunt was eighty, and the other beings and energies with her were one hundred and eight feet, a thousand—who can count and what does it matter anyway?

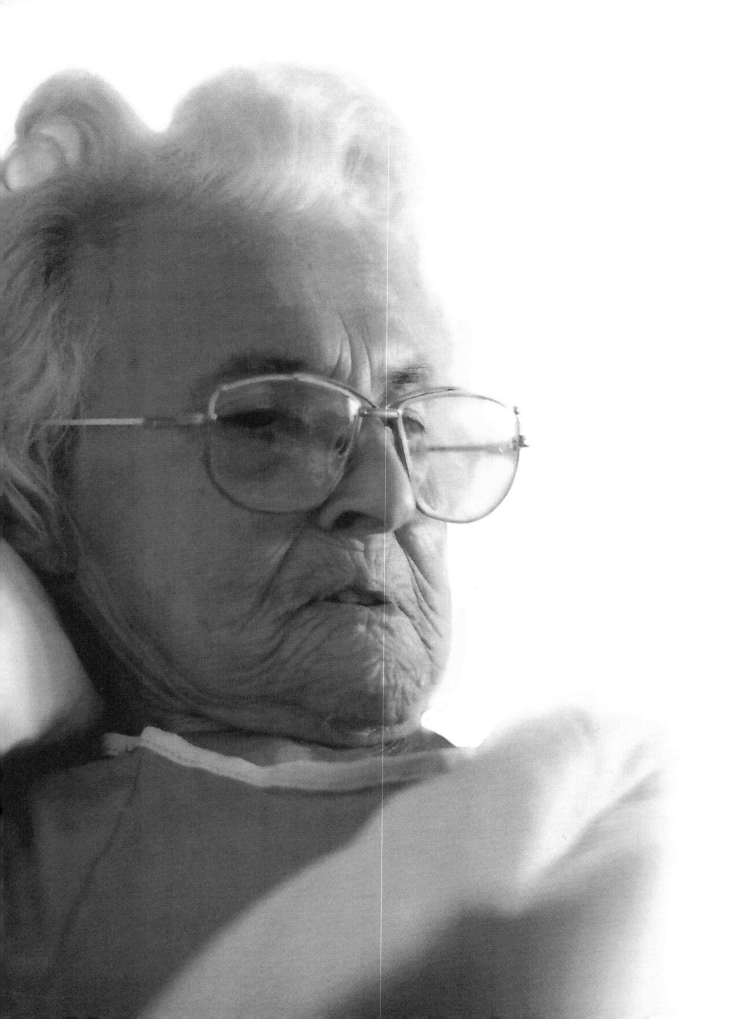

At the height of our ecstatic experience of unconditional love, I hit a wall. I had slept only two hours a day and had barely experienced drowsiness, yet suddenly I was dropping to the floor with bone-deep exhaustion. I was sitting by my grandmother's side, holding on to every precious moment, when intense nausea overcame me and I heard *ma tante* say, "Go home. Get some sleep. You have to sleep." "Sleep? Go to my parents' house? Leave Mamy? No." I couldn't tear myself away. I hung on for as long as I could, until the din of my discomfort and stubbornness yielded to my heart's painful song. I ran out of the room for fear of breaking down in Mamy's presence. All the sadness that I had not expressed in the past few days assailed me like a frenzy of starved sharks. I wailed and pounded on the steering wheel, keenly aware of the precious time my parents had blithely pillaged and destroyed. My accumulated anguish gnawed the marrow right out of me. Hopelessness attacked me. Eventually, a resigned silence overcame me, and like an automaton I fired up the engine and drove to my parents' townhouse, took a shower, and crashed into a deep, dreamless sleep.

Thirteen hours later, I bolted upright, aware that I had to get to the hospital. Minutes later, with car keys in hand and one foot already through the front door, I am stopped mid-flight by a phone call. "It's the head nurse. She thinks we need to come to the hospital," my stunned mother tells me. I am so out of there and already en route that I do not think to organize anything with my parents. When I arrive, Mamy's roommate tells me that Mamy has had a terrible morning. She uncharacteristically swore at the nurse who was cleaning her and then succumbed to a fit of rage. I am wracked with guilt. "While I was sleeping, Mamy had felt utterly alone, abandoned, and overwhelmed." *Ma tante* hollers through the drama overcoming me: "Mamy is terrified of death. That's why she's holding on. She is also holding on to be with you. She needed to be alone to let go. It is time. You need to get through to her that you will be with her without fail and that I, too, will be there, on the other side. The message you need to get through to her is that she will not be alone for a second. We've got her covered."

My grandmother is in such a state that she cannot comprehend a thing I am saying. Mind you, in terms of her everyday consciousness, what I'm saying is pretty far-fetched. Interspersed with many *Je t'aime*s, I continue my attempts at delivering her sister's message. "Les mûres vont être bonnes c't'année!" Oh dear, she's officiously informing me that the blackberries are going to be really good this year. I'm really not getting through; she's now smacking her lips, already tasting the sweet juiciness of her childhood. Then suddenly Mamy opens her eyes and mouth wide, and the light goes on just before it goes out. In a stroke of recognition, she succumbs to trust. She holds on to my hand and lets go of consciousness. My parents arrive and soon the doctor comes in, having been summoned as well. He lifts Mamy's nightgown, exposing her wispy grey pubic hair. He presses on her belly. We all witness her flesh failing to bounce back. No words are needed to convey the significance of this moment. The end approaches.

Mamy is transferred to a tiny private room with a fabulously large square window overlooking a climbing forest in the foothills. Snowflakes flutter in the late afternoon light, covering the ground with an early whiteness. My grandmother's clacking sounds pull me out of my poetic reverie. Her dentures interfere with her breath. I reach into her mouth to remove them, and as I do so, Mamy's face caves in and shockingly presents the mask of death. My mother can't bear it and so thankfully leaves me alone with my beloved love-mother. I lay my head on her belly and breathe with her. We peacefully glide through her breathing when the head of the bed unbiddenly hikes up, then just as jarringly dips back down. The foot of the bed then elevates, raising Mamy's feet above her head. I now have visions of her being served for lunch doubled up in a mattress sandwich. "What the hell? The buttons are useless—the damn thing is going berserk!" By now the foot of the bed is going down but the head is going even farther up than previously. The whole damn thing is so tilted that I need to hold on to my precious elder in her pre-death coma for fear that the bed will send her flying into the stratosphere before her time.

I scream at the top of my lungs. "Help! None of the buttons are responding." My mother hears my cries, runs in, and then runs out to get a nurse. He flies in, assesses the situation in a fraction of a second, dives under the bed, and pulls the plug out of the wall. He gets up, combs the hair off his forehead, and blandly says, "Ah … she's close. There are visitors! The electricity often goes wacky when they're here." With these cryptic words, he reaches for the door and walks out of the room.

My nerves are shot and so are my mother's. I send her down to get a Styrofoam cup of tea. I sit in silence. I settle into love again, cradling Mamy in my arms, reiterating that I am here and so is *ma tante*, that she has nothing to worry about, that Blanche has everything covered, electric beds notwithstanding. It's all under control, the bed is unplugged, so no more of that anyway, and she will not be alone for a second. Mamy's breathing is now laboured and slow. An unforgettable guttural rattling sound tells me that she is going. I call out, "Mamy!" Overcoming her pre-death coma, she turns her head toward me, opens her eyes, shines her last bright ray of earthly love straight into mine, breathes her last, long, laborious breath, and drops lifeless into my loving arms.

I invite my parents to light a candle. We pray together: mother, father, and daughter joined for a few instants in the magnitude of the moment. I ask to be left alone with her. Relieved, my mother says a quick goodbye to her own mother while my father awkwardly fumbles for his car keys. Although they welcomed her in their home and cared for her for years, their relief—and their fear of death—overrides the depth of their loss in that moment. Alone at last, my hands reach for my dear Mamy's body. I touch her feet and then settle on her shins. "She's still here! Her flesh is still thick with her presence. When I close my eyes, I feel her even more!" I feel our souls intertwine in our familiar embrace of timeless love. My hands feel the heat of her presence and my heart sings my devotion.

A nurse comes in, unobtrusively assessing my state of mind. She immediately turns to leave, assuring me that I can stay with my grandmother a while longer. She's not kidding! Even though beds are at a premium and the official hospital protocol states otherwise, we remain undisturbed for five hours. The only disruptions are my own breaks at the sink to soak my hands in cold water to soothe them. The heat building between Mamy's cold body and my hands is so strong that I feel painful burning sensations.

Ma tante hovers above, her smile comforting me and her presence guiding me still. On one level, I have no idea what I am doing, yet I know deep in my heart that this is exactly what I am supposed to be doing to help Mamy transition into the next expression of her spirit. The energy that runs in her body also climbs up my arms and runs through my body. I have never felt this level of rushing movement and intensity without fear. Soothed by *ma tante*'s compassionate presence, I soften into the intensely powerful energy in order to absorb its life-affirming and loving gifts.

Celebration and victory transport me. We are together! All three of us! We are finally together! It's been a long haul! We made it through! Instead of a departure, this is a reunion, theirs with each other after years of daunting geographical distance and mine with both of them after years of imposed estrangement… We are no longer trapped in my parents' framework; our lives are nourished rather than choked. We are free! Oh thank God, Mamy is making it out and so is *ma tante*. I can only imagine the personal power *ma tante* is presently savouring. She now has the power to be with us, love us, take care of us, and really, really help us. She's not just worrying about us and loving us from afar; we are now really a part of one another's lives! We are together forever. I might not have a family, but I have ancestors! Unconditional love is forever.

I run to the sink to cool my hands one last time. I settle in again. My grandmother's energy is shifting. I feel a huge rush of energy akin to Niagara Falls running through my being. While I am surrounded, inundated, and nourished with love, my body jolts. Translucent white moving shapes outside the window catch my eye. Two young girls, Mamy and Blanche, are running up the snow-covered hill, hand in hand. Their laughter is a welcome indicator that Mamy has joined her sister on the other side. Oh my God, she is finally experiencing safety again! She's running with her sister through the forest behind their childhood home. Mamy will savour the delicious blackberries after all, along with her innocent joy and freedom! She is transported back in time, before my grandfather ever laid his hands on her, my mother, or me!

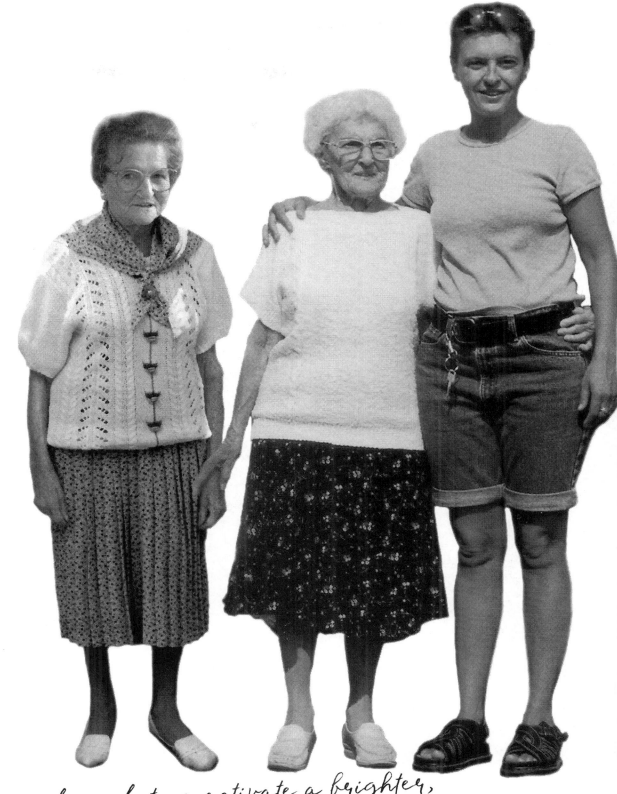

Reunited in love, let us activate a brighter, softer, and more potent expression of life for all living beings.

CHAPTER TWO

MY REIKI PATH: PROGRESSING FROM CLIENT TO STUDENT

I pull up to the curb in front of our place in Toronto and climb the steps with my grandmother's ashes under my arm. K is stunned. She remarks that when I left, I had enigmatically said, "I will be back with her in a week!" And here I am! All I know is that everything feels different and everything will change. I do not know what or how, but the week was transformational on all levels, there is no question. Actually, there are many. I recount the whole story, stumbling on the biggest mystery of all. What was the heat in her cold, defunct body? How could I feel it? What was I doing? Can I do it again on living bodies? One thing is for sure, I definitely have to book another Reiki session with Rose. A few days later, I describe everything I experienced to Rose and welcome the soothing energetic release she facilitates. Rose suggests that the heat was Reiki energy and that I should consider signing up for her Level One workshop in Richmond Hill the following weekend. "It's perfect timing! I'll be there with bells on!"

It's already a huge snowstorm at 7 a.m. that weekend, never mind by 4 p.m., when I'll be travelling back downtown. I am undeterred by the low visibility and slippery roads. Unsurprisingly, everyone arrives late and slightly unhinged, which sets us up for a good Reiki day. Our long, treacherous treks to get there heighten the sense that we are signed up for an adventure.

Mamy and *ma tante*, by now the dynamic duo more than ever before, are certainly not fooling around. After receiving my attunement, I place my hands on the student with whom I have been paired. The energy current climbs up my arms instantly and I burst into tears. "It's the same thing! It was Reiki!" I regroup and settle my hands on the student's body again. Straightaway upon contact I *sense* peril. Everything in my body tells me that this woman is in great danger. Oh! I mysteriously *see* in my mind's eye a man flailing his arms and throwing his weight around. I *sense* that he is hitting someone. Oh my God, he's hitting her! He is hitting the woman whose body I am now touching! I am in way over my head here!

Is this real? Oh, it's real. I can feel it. Shit. What do I do? She's really in danger. She has to get out of there! "Rose! Rose! I need to talk to you in the kitchen." I'm in a total panic. Rose listens and calms me down. She has *sensed* something too. She will finish the session on my behalf to assess the student's situation. Sure enough, Rose confirms my findings. She talks gently to her student, who then bursts into tears. It is the first time that her fear is validated. She feels in danger, but her family and friends like her guy. "They don't know the half of it!" She feels frightened, confused, and helpless. She confirms that she feels utterly trapped.

Well! I virtually need to be peeled off the ceiling to drive home. My concern for the student, not to mention my inside view of her predicament, overwhelms me. I join a few friends at the Café Diplomatico on College Street. I can barely sit still. I feel like I am floating—or rather I'm sitting and everyone else is floating. I'm demolished by the memory of my grandmother's passing, the student's threatening boyfriend, and yet I'm thrilled to pieces to have felt the energy again.

Later that night in bed, I remember falling apart the previous winter while watching *Imagining Argentina*, a film directed by Christopher Hampton. The movie is set during the "dirty war" in 1970s Buenos Aires, Argentina, when the military government was abducting those opposed to its rule. The protagonist is theatre director Carlos Rueda (Antonio Banderas), whose journalist wife, Cecilia (Emma Thompson), has "disappeared." Throughout the film, he recognizes that he has a unique gift that helps him *see* the disappeared and their fate. Carlos is clairvoyant: if he places his hands on a distraught family member, scenes of their beloved's torture and demise play themselves out in his mind's eye.

I cried through the whole movie. The premise of the film offers the director the opportunity to show many scenes of the torture that the Argentinean government denied. Granted, the film is disturbing. However, I not only cried during the film; I sobbed *comme une madeleine* for hours after. I have watched most anti-war films of value produced in the past twenty-five years, so my reaction to this particular movie stood out as unique and baffling. I now realize that what disturbed me most was the precise way in which the protagonist opens up to the intuitive flow of visual information. I was—and am—rattled to the core by a strange feeling of familiarity and recognition. It is exactly this aspect of me that Mamy and *ma tante* are now stirring. Yep, they're not messing around.

I soon decided—or rather the dynamic duo prompted me—to study with Rose again. Although I was still an opera design fiend, I completed my Reiki Level Two training, and with it committed to a daily regimen of Reiki self-practice, usually before sleep, and a session with Rose every two or three weeks. It was now clear to me that I had lost my capacity to consciously interact with the life force and my energy body to spark self-healing. Western medicine and its advocates had taught me to be passive. For most of my life, I had placed all my hope, faith, and trust in others to give me the right pills and chemicals to cure me, or to alter my physical body through procedures meant to eradicate my health problems. I had been erroneously encouraged to neglect the emotional, mental, and spiritual aspects of my physical dis-eases. Now I was learning that healing was an act of self-transformation that involved every layer and level of my life: physical, emotional, mental, and spiritual.

Long before Reiki, back in the early days of my healing journey and having memories of sexual abuse, I reacted to this call to action as an additional burden to my dis-ease: "I'm sick and hurt and now I have to heal myself too?"

I interpreted the message as one of blame and responsibility rather than a key to personal power. Sorrow, victimization, and abandonment choked my heart and thwarted my connection to the beauty and bounty of self-healing. In time, I realized that healing was an act I performed, that I could really make it happen rather than wait for it to come as a result of an outside force. Talk about empowerment! It turns the whole thing on its head.

The more I practised self-Reiki, the clearer it became that I was not just a physical structure made of molecules. I experienced more and more tangibly the fact that I am composed of dynamic energy fields that surround and penetrate my material body. I experienced my being, whether it be the strength of a muscle I exercised yesterday or a gnashing pain in my third rib as my *physical energy body*, my joy or torrential emotions as my *emotional energy body*, my binding and all too often crippling belief systems as my *mental energy body*, and my existential misgivings or devotion as my *spiritual energy body*. Although startling at first, I eventually delighted in the possibility of interacting and shifting these malleable energy fields for the better. It was impossible to deny that the pulsing and flowing webs of light transformed under my hands.

In meditation and self-Reiki practice (most often in bed and most profoundly while in the bathtub), I observed that my dis-eases and physical pain were initiated by blocks or disturbances in these energy fields much like rocks in a stream collecting sticks and leaves. I learned that these disruptions were then transmitted to my material body, sometimes becoming serious illness or excruciating pain that interfered with, well, everything. I then realized that my "annoying" symptoms and discomfort were a kind of guidance that reliably called for my attention to prompt action, change, and healing. If I welcomed and listened to the sensations, their messages generously conveyed which aspects of my life were out of alignment. In time, self-Reiki helped me let go of impatient frustration and fear and taught me to soften into a state of grateful awareness. Accepting these voices not only empowered me by awakening my self-healing potential, but it simultaneously awakened the paramount movers and shakers: self-love and compassion. Talk about another dynamic duo to welcome, embrace, and integrate.

I explored my energy fields with the gusto of a prospector at the height of the gold rush. As you can imagine, it was rather satisfying because I had treasures stored just about everywhere. My energy fields, currents, chakras, and

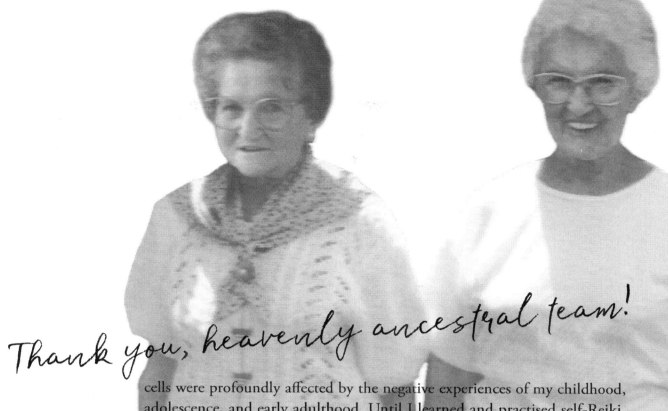

Thank you, heavenly ancestral team!

cells were profoundly affected by the negative experiences of my childhood, adolescence, and early adulthood. Until I learned and practised self-Reiki, and received energy healing, most of the shock, trauma, physical and emotional injuries, sexual abuse, social and cultural programming, limiting belief systems, colonization, misinformation, and indoctrination had lain static. I acknowledged, to my dismay at first and eventually to my delight, that the whole damn thing, every minute detail of my ordeal, was truly etched in my energy bodies, including all the cells of my physical body—but thankfully with non-permanent ink. So off I went to the races, with Mamy and *ma tante* blowing wind in my sails.

It's one thing to do all of this; it's quite another to really ride the wave of transformation. Let me lay down my pom-poms for a minute to delve into the more challenging aspects of my growth and healing. Because Reiki energy and all the love also created confusing, seemingly counterproductive cross-currents in my life. Initially, it unlocked my creative energy; I was on fire.

From 2003 to 2006, I worked from 5:30 a.m. to 9:30 p.m. six days a week, producing drawings and ideas effortlessly. I was undeniably plugged into generous muses and as much artistic curiosity and passion as a day could hold. I lived in a delightful vortex of collaborative creativity with Nic Muni, Tim Albery, and Peter Hinton at the Canadian Opera Company, the

Stratford Festival, the Cincinnati Opera, De Vlaamse Opera, Opera North, and the National Reis Opera. Together we soared on a magic carpet ride of artistic exploration and expression. On the other hand, I was starved. Producing art around the clock took its toll. I was an inspired stress ball at best and all too often a sopping mess, sprawled out on the floor in yet another fit of despair and fatigue. While artistic freedom sparked my desire to create, technical and financial challenges dragged me down.

Reiki energy fostered a new relationship between my true self and me. The *me* I knew produced art diligently and indefatigably. The *me* I knew less sent smoke signals letting me know that the house was burning down fast. The blazing trail of projects I left in my wake was becoming more and more flamboyantly creative and less and less soul-nourishing. My highs were higher but extremely short-lived; the higher they got, the lower they dropped me. The ritual practice of self-Reiki lifted the veil. The life force running through me at a greater velocity supported me brilliantly on one obvious level; and though it seemed like it was letting me down on another level by allowing a burnout to take root, it was also pushing me to face what I needed to change in order to grow into a more gentle and wiser person. Self-Reiki created a space for truth and love to enter my life. I could no longer fool myself into believing that opera or theatre design were still the most rewarding, beneficial, and fulfilling expressions of my life force.

The Reiki sessions also dug deep into my being, unearthing sorrow that needed a lot of space and time to be felt, healed, and cleared. Again, it appeared there were two seemingly contradictory currents. Although I still kept some distance from my parents in the three years before confronting them, only phoning them once a week and seeing them twice a year, I nonetheless forged a newfound honesty. For example, my great-aunt helped me figure out why I should come out to them. Previously, I hadn't been able to justify the turmoil and effort that such an act would entail. When truth became the prime motivator in my life, it became clear to me that I gained nothing by hiding my relationship with K. By virtue of hiding my relationship, I was hiding my joy. My parents embraced delightful K and welcomed her into the family, hoping that this would indeed be the beginning of a more expansive closeness.

Only a few months before confronting my parents, after a seemingly agreeable and groundbreaking four days in the Laurentians celebrating Christmas and New Year's at my parents' home with K and my whole extended family, the truth grabbed me by the balls and said, "Enough." Victoriously smiling ear to ear, K climbed into the Subaru station wagon pointing west only to hear me say, "Never again! I'm never doing this again." I had now just crashed into the underbelly of the familial glacier. I was painfully aware that I was not honouring myself by pretending that the joy in my life had anything to do with my parents or family. That they now accepted K and embraced this aspect of my life did not change the fact that they were still denying my truth by not acknowledging the violence in my childhood home.

So, on the one hand, I was cooking with propane, artistically thriving and removing emotional roadblocks right, left, and centre; on the other hand, I was really, truly growing. But I did not yet fully understand the extent to which my life was going to have to change in order to align with the benefits of the healing life force. The more I tapped into the energy of Universal Love, the more I harnessed inner strength and personal power. The more I manifested my personal power, the more my life seemed to fall apart.

First, I closed down my design studio. Then, I officially divorced my family. And then even my relationship with K looked like a thing of the past. I found myself facing the undeniable fact that *everything* was on the line. Throw menopause and shifting hormones into the mix and I had the life force on steroids manifesting chaos and collapse through me and despite me. It literally all came down like a house of cards in the space of two years. Universal Love in action is not a tear-jerking Bell commercial. From what I could gather, there was absolutely nothing warm and fuzzy about it. I have come to conclude that self-Reiki, Reiki treatments, and any practice that calls in the earth, the sun, and Universal Love should come with a flashing "put on your seat belt" warning.

Regardless of the obvious discomfort and fear, I kept doing self-Reiki and consistently tried to get out of the way of the transformational power blessing my life. Once I said yes to Reiki, yes to Universal Love, yes to the earth, and yes to the sun, I was signed up for a thorough shakedown of all the structures that were not in alignment with my highest and greatest good. Opera and theatre design had long been in alignment with my life purpose, but now they weren't. The sexual abuse and my mother's betrayal I experienced were integral to my journey, but now walking away from my parents and their insistent denial was essential. Although K and I had shared thirteen beautiful years, the relationship no longer aligned with our life paths.

Truth, though painful when it set in,
melted the icebergs above and below the surface
and paved the way to a
life-affirming and sustainable
expression of my essence.

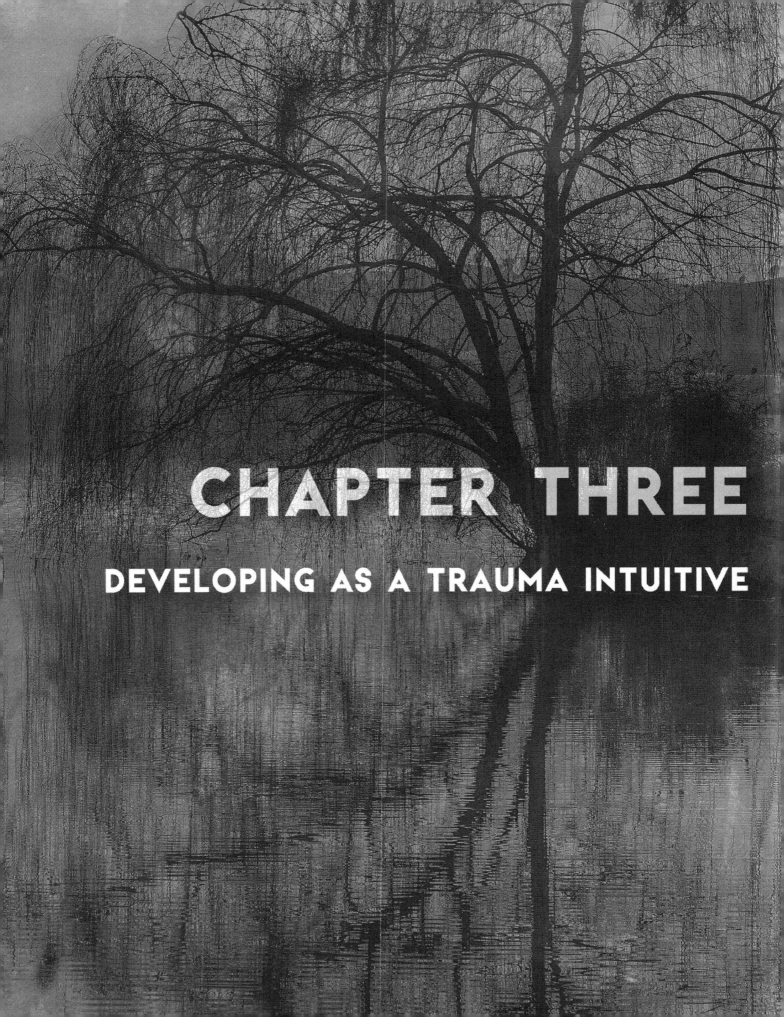

CHAPTER THREE

DEVELOPING AS A TRAUMA INTUITIVE

OPENING UP MY INNATE INTUITION

The summer before winning the Siminovitch Prize in Theatre, I completed my Reiki Level Three training with Rose and transformed my design studio into a Reiki room. I then launched into the daunting process of attracting enough volunteers to fulfill the Canadian Reiki Association's mandate for my Level Three practicum. My close friend Katherine Dynes and her partner, Nan Shepherd, encouraged me by consistently booking sessions for at least two years. Their openness and honesty and that of many others facilitated the wild process of integrating the knowledge and skills I intuitively developed. Wild because my official Reiki training essentially consisted of only a few days. The unofficial training included lots of private Reiki sessions (and the integration process that that entails) and self-Reiki.

Aside from studying and reading, most of the learning actually happened in the formless darkness once my eyes were closed. Whether alone in my bedroom before sleep, in the tub, or in a session with a practicum client, it was when I closed my eyes and settled into a meditative state that the action began. I soon found that I could *sense, see, hear,* and *know* not only my own energy fields but those of my practicum clients. To my surprise, I was perceiving traumatic events in their lives too. Beyond helping me remember and heal my own traumas, my hands seemed to be clear conduits that conveyed messages even when I hadn't experienced the events myself. I intuitively *sensed* with my reawakened innate clairsentience, I *saw* events with my innate clairvoyance, I *heard* with my innate clairaudience, and I *knew* with my innate claircognizance (more on these intuitive perceptions in Chapter 9).

The far-reaching implications of opening up my innate and intuitive conduits to access vast amounts of information simply dazzled me. With practice, I started recognizing the energy signatures of shock and trauma and all the emotions that come with that territory: terror, horror, fear, powerlessness, hopelessness, shame, self-loathing or humiliation. *Recognize* is the key word; most of what I initially *sensed, saw, heard*, and *knew* were events and emotional states linked to adversity and abuse that I myself was familiar with. Very convenient. I could smell trauma and abuse, especially sexual abuse, a mile away and reliably recognized the lingering presence of the perpetrators' energy and the impact of their violence on my client.

Add all those years of vigorous and rigorous textual analysis in theatre and opera into the mix and I promptly grasped the narrative my intuition revealed to my heart. Although I felt utterly depleted by my design career, I recognized how my knowledge, expertise, and creativity were nourishing and informing me in a very different yet bizarrely similar context. In a sense, I had simply left fiction behind and instead embraced reality, both mine, in terms of the collapse of my old denial structures, and that of my clients' abuse histories. Rather than investigate and analyze the motives of fictional characters, I unexpectedly found myself using the same skills to navigate the complex narratives of people's lives. I embraced their stories and their hurt past selves with the same verve and gusto I had once dedicated to theatrical and operatic characters.

I felt honoured to be an advocate for their younger, scared selves. It was a thrill to march into the room where they were trapped, help them vanquish their perpetrators, and swoop their helpless selves out of the misery and into their loving hearts. Early on, when I studied and practised self-reiki and Reiki, I recognized I had signed up for perceiving my own trauma, but by now it was clear that I was eagerly signing up to help others perceive what they are scared to acknowledge or deterred from accepting. As my practice evolved and I further developed my Sacred Tree and its intuitive *sensing, seeing, hearing,* and *knowing,* I surrendered more and more to what my innate clairsentience, clairvoyance, clairaudience, and claircognizance were unveiling in sessions (not dissimilar to the protagonist in *Imagining Argentina*). I then stepped into the ethos of a *trauma intuitive*, a term I created to better describe my work and experience.

A compassionate witness volunteers to view the "home movies" too few aspire to see!

RECOGNIZING THE SACRED TREE

Yet another big piece of the puzzle had to sizzle in my fingers before I could really land in the connection between human beings and all other living beings, including the earth and the sun. In addition to self-Reiki and Reiki treatments with Rose, I booked many sessions with a registered massage therapist who had studied craniosacral therapy techniques. Craniosacral therapy was not her main focus, yet even the most basic techniques she introduced in our massage sessions set the stage for a major breakthrough in my healing journey. Theatre and opera were no longer all-consuming, so I had enough time to process and assimilate the information pouring from the gates that craniosacral therapy had opened, allowing me to finally acknowledge, witness, and integrate the scope of my maternal grandfather's and father's treachery, violence, and sexual abuse.

Later, in my own craniosacral training, I encountered the awesome power of the mystical yet tangible force of the body's innate interconnectedness with the earth and the sun directly under my fingers. In a flash of insight in a class one day, I *sensed* that the bones, organs, and tissues I lightly manipulated knew exactly where they should be and how to calibrate to the earth and sun energies. I was utterly awed by the wisdom that I had the honour of working with. *They know, they know!* I kept telling myself. *They are out of alignment because they can't get to where they know they should be. They are trapped by trauma and adversity—it's not that they don't know where they should be.*

I humbly realized that I had no real news to share with the bones and tissues. I recognized that as a practitioner I was far from in charge and that I had to honour the physical manifestation of ancient forces in my colleague's body. I tuned in much more specifically to the striking relationship between the physical body, the movements of the dural membrane and cerebrospinal fluid, and a person's traumatic history. I learned that shock, trauma, or stagnation anywhere in the body and energy bodies affect the rhythmic movements of the dural membrane, the sac containing the cerebrospinal fluid that surrounds and protects the brain and the spinal cord. The breath of life, I learned, expresses itself in this dural sac as a consistent tide—a calm ebbing-and-flowing motion upward to the sun and downward to the earth.

This sinuous tidal rhythm not only plays a significant role in expressing and distributing the potency and vital energy of the earth and the sun throughout the body but enhances the body's own self-healing and self-regulating capabilities. Time and time again, I witnessed physical tissues shift back into optimal alignment when the discerning fascia interpenetrating all tissues, the dural membrane, and the cerebrospinal fluid released its infrastructures of survival and all vibrations not congruent with the earth and the sun's fuel: love and compassion.

Like yoga, Qigong, Tai Chi, and other practices, craniosacral therapy, self-Reiki, and Reiki taught me that a human is first and foremost interconnected with the earth and the sun. To be fully alive and thrive is to be coupled with your indispensable grounding cord to the centre of the earth and your simultaneous impulse to grow upward to the sun. All living beings share this principal orientation, but trees, more than any other, palpably live these teachings and share them with us. Unfortunately, many of us suffer from estrangement from trees and our Sacred Tree-ness. Thankfully, I gradually learned to use visualizations in a meditative state to heal my fundamental and life-sustaining vertical axis and Sacred Tree—the aspect of me innately aligned with love and compassion.

UNDERSTANDING THE SACRED TREE'S CYCLICAL WISDOM

Several years later, while teaching a Reiki Level Two program focused on connecting the Reiki hand positions with the organs under the students' hands, I took notice each time a participant fumbled with a (by now) crumpled piece of paper to which she reacted with a conspiratorial nod. I finally went up to her on our last break on the third day and asked, "What is on that piece of paper that is so clearly in synch with this course?" She revealed a chart with lots of tiny markings seemingly produced by a mosquito. I reached for my reading glasses and gradually focused on the gold mine of concise information that would transform the container for my intuitive findings to this day.

My heart raced and I was instantly covered in sweat. It was the strangest experience to witness at a bespectacled glance what I had been discovering with my eyes closed for a decade. This chart not only contained information that jived with my findings but also organized it in such a way that I could recognize the building blocks of human experience at all levels—physical, emotional, mental, and spiritual—and observe the cycles of life and evolution in the making simultaneously. I encountered the cyclical wisdom of our Sacred Tree, the dynamic and regenerative cycle and counterpart to its interdependence with the earth and the sun.

Little did I know that for centuries Chinese shamans and healers had a predilection for writing, drawing, and creating charts in order to share the wealth of their wisdom and teachings with their students. At that point, I had no idea that any shaman anywhere had ever documented their philosophy, healing methods, and practice. Despite the fact that medical Qigong was pushed underground by the Chinese government during the Cultural Revolution forty years ago, this immense body of knowledge and practice is vibrant in many countries where practitioners in exile and their students continue to teach and document their tradition and discoveries.

However, on account of the political climate in China at the time, the emphasis of Qigong practices in China had shifted away from traditional philosophy and shamanism and increasingly focused on the martial arts applications and a more scientific perspective. Yet, medical Qigong is an extremely potent and involved energy medicine offered by a medical Qigong master who has studied Chinese medical theory and shamanic energy manipulation. The exercises and meditations we are more familiar with are the Qigong master's prescriptions for their patients to heighten the healing after the session. I absorbed some of this abundance in the context of a course in Toronto with Donna Oliver and continue to profit from this healing system in my intuitive explorations.

In a nutshell, the five foundational agents and energetic orbs in this system are the cyclical building blocks of your Sacred Tree and all living beings, including the earth and the sun. They are the five elements: wood, fire, earth, metal, and water. They are the five seasons: spring, summer, late summer, autumn, and winter. They are the five solid yin-organ groupings: liver, heart, spleen/pancreas, lungs, and kidneys/brain/reproductive organs. They are paired with the five hollow yang-organ groupings: gallbladder, duodenum/small intestine, stomach, colon, and bladder/sea of marrow. These energetic orbs are the vehicles of the harmonious, high-frequency emotions of compassion, inner peace, trust, integrity, and wisdom as well as the disharmonious, low-frequency emotions such as anger, shock, worry, grief, and fear. And on and on it goes. Please note that I break down disharmony into hot and cold expressions. This is my contribution to the Chinese system to facilitate diagnosis and healing. More on that later in Reiki Plus Plus: Level Two, and much more in the study tool and divination platform I created for self-Reiki and Reiki practitioners: *Sacred Tree for All Seasons: Reclaiming Your Capacity to Heal • The Guidebook and Oracle Cards.*

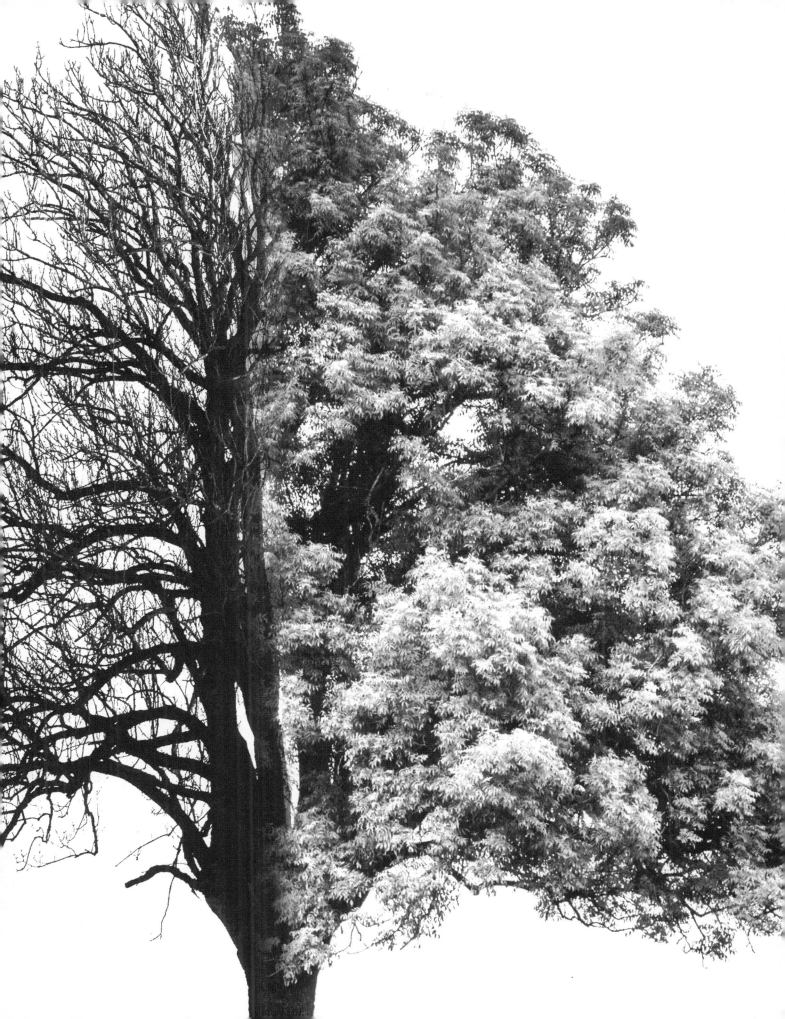

	WOOD 木	FIRE 火
ELEMENT		
SEASON	·Spring	·Summer
YIN ORGANS	·Liver	·Heart
YANG ORGANS	·Gallbladder	·Duodenum ·Small Intestine
EXTERNAL ORGANS	·Eyes and Third Eye	·Tongue
HARMONY	·Compassion	·Inner Peace
EXPLOSIVE DISHARMONY	·Anger	·Anxiety/Shock
IMPLOSIVE DISHARMONY	·Powerlessness	·Dissociation

EARTH 土	METAL 金	WATER 水
·Late Summer	·Autumn	·Winter
·Spleen ·Pancreas	·Lungs	·Kidneys ·Reproductive Organs ·Brain
·Stomach	·Colon	·Bladder ·Sea of Marrow
·Mouth	·Nose	·Ears
·Trust	·Integrity	·Wisdom
·Abandonment	·Excessive Grief	·Fear/Panic
·Worry	·Shame	·Overwhelm

PHYSICAL BODY	SACRED TREE
SUN	SUN
Head/Arms	Branches
	Base of Branches
Chest	Trunk
Abdomen/Legs	Roots
EARTH	EARTH

I AM A BEAUTIFUL SACRED TREE.

I have the power to draw the
life force through me.

I send my roots down
to the centre of the earth.

I pull the loving earth energy
into my heart until it is brimming
with enough unconditional love
to animate my branches.

When it does, I effortlessly
reach for the sky to receive
the nutrients of
the sun.

CHAPTER FOUR

THE JOURNEY BACK TO YOUR SACRED TREE

INVITING IN LOVE AND COMPASSION

As you may have read in my revised memoir, *ME TOO LOUD & CLEAR: How I Walked the Talk from Silence to Active Hope*, I was blackened to a crisp in the hell of my despair, loneliness, and unlove—not only because of my father's and maternal grandfather's extensive sexual abuse and my mother's betrayal but because I actively rejected and buried my truth and blocked the flow of my consciousness and memories for decades in order to survive.

I, unfortunately and quite unconsciously, pushed away my innate Sacred Tree wisdom and with it love and compassion for more decades than necessary to survive. I basically threw the baby out with the bathwater for my entire twenties and early thirties. It has to be the biggest irony ever. I now realize that to open to love once the epic crisis has subsided is to *sense, see, hear,* and *know* the not-so-warm-and-fuzzy aspects of my experience.

I had to concede, despite decades of conditioning, that when I invited and allowed traumatic experiences, mine and later those of others, to flow through me, I was essentially in service to the beautiful healing energy of love and compassion. To surrender to this powerful current and Sacred Tree wisdom is to accept the honour of becoming both a compassionate witness and caregiver in situ, *sensing, seeing, hearing,* and *knowing* the intricacies of an experience at whatever age the adversity, shock, trauma, and violence occurred. I ascertained experientially over and over again that intuitive perception is fundamentally the gift of love and compassion in action. It is an opportunity to be a loving presence and companion in a place and time when a younger self or fellow living being had no support. And this is the best thing ever!

It was nothing less than astounding to witness the mysterious ways in which everything in my life, including abuse and witnessing abuse through whatever lens I was studying or practising, all yielded happiness and abundance rather than sadness and depletion. It seemed to me that life was turned on its head! Everything I had perceived as a liability before became a potent asset. Rather than pain and suffering, the energy I opened to in self-Reiki or Reiki sessions was nothing less than Sacred Tree-ness in action.

Beyond being open to loving other people or welcoming other people's love, I opened up to loving everyone and the whole darn kettle of fish, even if it smells rotten and it sucks. In meditation or in private sessions and healing circles, I *sense, see, hear,* and *know* not only our true self and narratives but love and compassion—divine love, God, Durga, Buddha, Universe, life force, Nature, or whatever name you like—in action within myself and others at the best of times and the worst of times.

Unfortunately, I blamed "divine" energy for years for creating the mess and leaving me alone to deal with it. So of course I thought, "To hell with all of you 'Gods' or whoever and whatever you are. I'm going to sort this out on my own, thank you very much." It is a painfully distorted logic that made so much sense to me for so long. And yet this protective strategy inadvertently set into motion the high winds that fed the very flame I wished to extinguish: the cycle of violence and isolation. It's taken me years of watching and listening to love's horror show to trust and know that truth is not what bit me in the ass. Rather, it's my grandfather's, father's, and mother's abuse; their own abuse; or my own not-so-gracious actions, misdeeds, or violence. In other words, it's unlove, not truth, that bites us in the ass and tries to carry off chunks of our hide in its gnarly jaws.

Up until my introduction to self-Reiki and Reiki, all my interactions were coloured by love's perceived absence rather than informed by its magnificent unconditional presence. Given my upbringing and early adult years, this was a likely assumption. Yet, the more I practised self-Reiki and Reiki, I became increasingly aware that the compassionate earth and sun sing and sing generously all the time. Regardless of where I'm at or where my clients are at, they sing and patiently wait for our ears to hear them past the din of our day-to-day consciousness and drama. Furthermore, when we settle down enough, we can sense that their subtle and exquisite tones nourish, love, and support us, no matter what the hell is going on.

This teaching was a glorious and welcome shift in my perception: the nutrients in the earth and the sun sustain my well-being despite my past or present discomfort, wounds, and pain. In other words, to be ill, heartbroken, a victim, or a perpetrator does not cut you off from the vibrant energy of life and love. Although part of you is suffering and disoriented, you can nonetheless access the life force to soothe, recharge, nourish, reconfigure, heal, and release the imbalance and disharmony that has been plaguing you, whether for forty years or four hours.

When practising self-Reiki or Reiki, you are not suddenly a different person you can now love more, you are the whole blessed "mess" who deserves love and was love in action all along. The energy of life itself — love and compassion — is always present, no matter what.

ALIGNING WITH LOVE AND COMPASSION

As you well know from visceral experience, you're not getting anywhere without some adversity and trauma and you're not going anywhere you like without a lot of love and self-love along the way. Your Sacred Tree is the host for the entirety of human energetic experience on the earth plane: physical, emotional, mental, and spiritual. Therefore, you are in constant flux with incoming wholesome nourishment and unwholesome physical, emotional, mental, and spiritual mayhem in utero and after birth. Reiki and self-Reiki are imminently accessible tools to help you navigate through thorny growth to burgeoning and prospering. In other words, for thriving to really gain traction and well-being to blossom, you and your traumatized astronauts and architects of survival must settle back into harmonious, loving vibrations in your Sacred Tree—the aspect of you innately aligned with love and compassion.

And who are they? you might ask.

The traumatized astronauts are the aspects of your spirit, your soul fragments, who catapult out of your heart and Sacred Tree into a drifting trauma capsule when overwhelming adversity strikes. It stands to reason that when you are overcome by spiritual, mental, emotional, and/or physical pain, you lose sight of the pool of unconditional love in the world: your heart and Sacred Tree. The traumatized astronauts' counterparts, the architects of survival, are the valiant knights in shining or not-so-shining armour created by the traumatized astronauts to survive the adversity using whatever resources they can pull together under duress. In other literature, they are often referred to as "coping" or "survival" mechanisms—but that description, in my opinion, belies how incredibly brilliant, beautiful, and lovable they really are.

It's never too late to throw a party and wholeheartedly invite your entire menagerie!

MEETING YOUR TRAUMATIZED ASTRONAUTS

As mentioned, we can describe the wounded aspects or your spirit as traumatized astronauts who float outside your Sacred Tree and heart of hearts. As life would have it, adversity strikes us all sooner or later, so it's a given that you have traumatized astronauts floating outside your heart consciousness. For instance, let's say at age four or so you experienced a jolting charge of adversity, overwhelmingness, and/or pain, and in response an aspect of your spirit or soul hurtled out yet remains attached by a lifeline, much like an astronaut to a spaceship. Although the traumatized astronaut remains attached to you and your innate source of Universal Love in your spiritual heart, it is nonetheless trapped in its own capsule of unlove and pain until it is acknowledged and guided back to the love in your heart of hearts and Sacred Tree.

Although you can lose track of experiences or outright forget them, your spirit or soul never loses consciousness or relies on verbal categorization and understanding. It traces your every move, experience, thought, and emotion and is always guiding and protecting your astronauts, including the more far-gone ones. Thus, it is absolutely feasible to heal all traumatized astronauts, including the ones on very long lifelines. The healing process simply requires a proportional amount of time, practice, and patience in relation to the distance. For instance, it may require a deeper meditative practice and state to attune to the murky blur of whatever drug or substance, unconscious state, or pre-verbal experience you are encountering.

Regardless of the distance, your Sacred Tree invites you to go fishing and lovingly connect with the little or not-so-little floating astronauts stuck in the experience of adversity or abuse. These traumatized astronauts have literally been fixed within the intensity of the experience, right smack in the middle of it, without any sense of it having ended. They do not know the love, safety, creation, service, or whatever joys and personal power you have experienced since that moment. They are completely and utterly cut off from the resources you have. They are still bundles of terror, horror, fear, helplessness, shame, and all the other intense emotions or sensations that the traumatic experience generated.

The pain contained in these disembodied time capsules is the unbeneficial energy often referred to as energy cysts, which you can release and heal with Reiki-infused energy. When you compassionately reach, touch, embrace, and love without judgment or conditions the wounded spirit fragments with the support of Reiki energy, you can break the isolating seal of trauma. The traumatized astronaut is no longer alone or trapped in its time capsule of unlove and confusion because Reiki energy helps you be there in heart, mind, and spirit.

Hence, Reiki energy can guide the spirit fragment back into your Sacred Tree, where it is treated to an exquisitely delightful bubblebath or a fabulously cozy bed or whatever else is loving, safe, and comforting. Subsequently, the Reiki-infused atmosphere facilitates the release of the anguish, physical pain, sorrow, shame, self-hatred, judgment, fear, rage, terror, or whatever from the forsaken capsule. It follows that the embraced spirit fragment gradually harmonizes and recalibrates all aspects of its physical, mental, emotional, and spiritual energy fields to the vibration of love.

This journey back to your Sacred Tree is a key juncture in the healing process where I believe a lot of confusion arises. While you release the painful gack in the capsule (every client including myself is all over that part), you also must welcome that hurt aspect of the self into your heart. In other words, you do not throw the baby out with the bathwater or cut the astronaut's lifeline and send them hurtling into space. In fact, it's only when you reel the traumatized astronaut back into the heart that you can truly release the trauma and unbeneficial energy causing dis-ease. You must efficiently release the bathwater while hanging on to the baby and loving them to bits!

It's fair to say that most of us can visualize the process of embracing a child aspect who is clearly hurt, and you can imagine that young child fragment softening into your compassionate acknowledgement of their pain and embracing with relief your comforting and soothing presence. I've witnessed this process daily in my practice. However, it's not always such an immediate or welcoming reunion. For instance, it can be less predictable when you encounter a wounded teenager astronaut. They might express their pain with rage rather than tears or look at you like you just stepped off a spaceship: "Like, what the fuck, *now* you come to me with all that love shit." Or you meet astronauts who really think they have their shit together and their ducks in a row: "I'm fine. Really, I'm fine" or "I've got it under control, thank you very much." It might take some time before they trust you enough to consistently show up, hang out, and eventually open up to change and healing.

Or it might be you who has a hard time showing up with compassion and generosity. You might still perceive that wounded child, teenager, young adult, or adult self as actually guilty of doing something bad. For instance, you might still believe that you deserved the harsh discipline, physical abuse, neglect, and/or rejection. Or you might still be hiding behind a thick veil of secrecy so that no one knows what horrible thing you did. You might still think that you asked to be touched by your father, uncle, or whomever—that *you* were doing the big, bad, and disgusting thing. There is nothing quite as potent as shame to stall the process of compassionate witnessing. As Brené Brown describes in her book *I Thought It Was Just Me (but it isn't)*, if shame is "the intensely painful feeling or experience of believing we are flawed and therefore unworthy of acceptance and belonging," then it makes sense that you can expect nothing more than a tenuous, half-hearted, and labyrinthine process of integration at first. Fear and self-blame might bare their fangs for quite a while before you open to the compassionate and generous acknowledgement and witnessing of your suffering.

To heal is to love those astronauts and welcome them back into your heart of hearts and Sacred Tree — the aspect of you innately aligned with love and compassion.

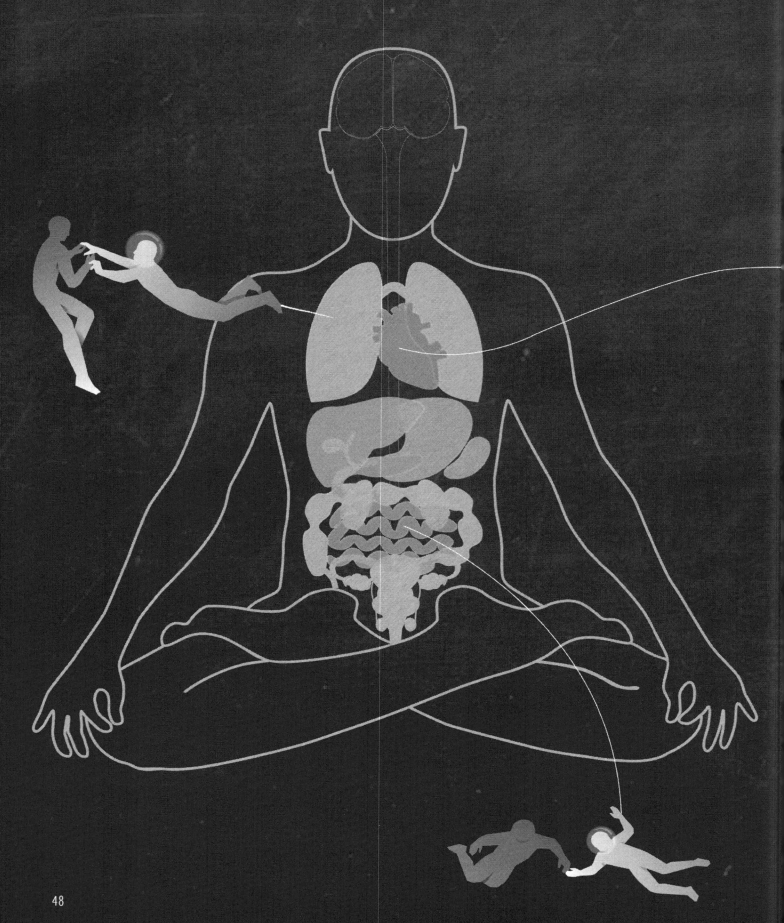

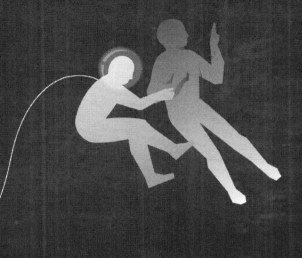

The potency of the adversity, and your reaction to it, determines the traumatized astronaut's distance from your Sacred Tree and the length of the lifeline.

    a. The more intense the charge, the farther away the astronaut/soul fragment is.

    b. The distance is even greater if you experienced any of the adversity in an altered state of consciousness created by anaesthetics, drugs, and/or alcohol or if the event itself produced a concussion, loss of consciousness, or other altered states.

    c. Furthermore, the lifeline is particularly long if the adversity occurred before verbal skills were developed.

    d. The lifeline is extremely long if the adversity occurred during your very different experience of corporality as an infant in your birth mother's womb.

    e. The lifeline is exponentially extended when the trauma was experienced by a caregiver or ancestor; in other words, if the trauma is intergenerational.

    f. The lifeline is comparatively extended when the trauma occurred in a past lifetime.

MEETING YOUR ARCHITECTS OF SURVIVAL

I am loath to say it, but there's a whole other layer to deal with. While your plethora of traumatized astronauts float in space, an army of determined, and often angry and despairing, architects of survival are doing whatever they need to do to survive the adversity. For every astronaut, there is an architect of survival in high gear. For years I collided with the contentious, addicted, judged, and hated architects of survival (my own and that of clients) without recognizing them as the resourceful counterparts of the traumatized astronauts.

It became painfully clear that without acknowledging their determination and creativity, transformation and liberation was a slow and arduous process yielding precarious harmony at best. Quite the reverse occurred when Reiki-infused love and compassion flowed to them too. Once I witnessed the power and beauty of these brave knights in shining armour, they, too, gradually softened into the love bath, thereby harmonizing their mandate with love rather than with whatever pain instigated their genesis. It comes as no surprise, really, that judging, fighting, and/or hating those aspects of the self spun the wheels deeper in the mud. I launched a reframing campaign years ago. This book is a continuation of my impassioned plea for all of us to shift away from violence within and without.

All that said, their process of integration can be more exigent. The clever architects of survival are just as stuck and, if anything, even more desperate than the traumatized astronauts. For one thing, they're all exhausted. They're hyper-vigilant and have been 24/7 since the threatening and hurtful events occurred. They've been using whatever resources—and I really mean whatever they had available to them—to orchestrate survival: disembody now, forget everything, play dead, pass out, lash out, get really stoned, become a sex kitten even if it is your father, yell, fight back, do art, don't do art, run faster, jump higher, skate faster, keep busy, get better grades, strive for a promotion, get tenure, get thinner, make more money, get a bigger house, get a new cottage, keep improving yourself, fuck as much as possible, party hardy, be brave and courageous, run for the hills … Whatever it is, do it without fail because your life depends on it. These architects are trapped in a tornado of life-or-death necessity and survival.

And did I mention that they are stubborn? These architects mean business; not only are they single-mindedly focused on their life-or-death mission, but they are also trapped in a time capsule similar to the astronauts. They use whatever resources they had available to them at the time they came into being in that threatening and hurtful moment. For example, remember the trauma that occurred at age four and sent one of your astronauts hurtling? Since then, your very powerful four-year-old architect is doing whatever it can with whatever tools are available, all at the service of preserving your integrity—or your life. If all it can do is cry, then so be it. If that gets the attention you need, then so be it. If you are seven and the only way you can be tenderly cared for is to be sick, then so be it. You get sick. If you are thirteen years old and discover the mind-numbing bliss of liquor to get away from the crazy shit going on at home, then so be it. You get drunk. If you are fourteen and the only way not to be beaten up by your brothers and father is to become a "man," then so be it. You suck it up and get tough. If you are fifteen and the only way to be in with the cool crowd or any crowd is to have sex, then you have sex, whether you really want to or not.

The point is that whatever the resource or strategy, it "worked" at the time and has many times since. And it's going to "work" ad infinitum if survival is your only goal, though I doubt it. Survival is a bare minimum baseline at best. Besides, there is no point judging these architects of survival for not helping you thrive over long periods of time. That isn't their job. Survival, per force, is a more immediate kind of business. For instance, you know all too well that there is nothing like a crisis to thwart the prioritization of your genius. These forsaken heroes are hooked into the adversity that created them, so it follows that for as long as you implement their strategies and directives, you remain powerless on one level or other, and disconnected from love and compassion and your Sacred Tree-ness in one way or another.

Moreover, healing the architects of survival can be tricky because many are relegated to the doghouse and are totally soused in shame when, in fact, they deserve quite the opposite; they, too, have succeeded in helping you survive. These guys often double up as your "dirty" little secrets. Whether you compulsively shop online, take ketamine at night and then stick cocaine up your nose in the morning, stay hooked to strained sex work despite having a more fulfilling job, only have sex with your spouse to keep the marriage going, watch porn a lot, or binge eat, you need to compassionately acknowledge, love, and celebrate these strategies and the architects' achievements without judgment. The new clothes helped you feel better at an event, the ketamine numbed you out good, and the cocaine got you to work in the morning, the sex work clients are familiar and easy somehow, the kids are happy in the private school your spouse pays for, your numbing orgasms give you a break from despair, or the excess food helps you forget your powerlessness for a while, even if it's only for a short while.

Conversely, the strategies used by the architects don't always seem like they actually thwart your life and health. It's one thing to look at an addiction to a prescription or over-the-counter pharmaceutical and think, "Hmm, not so good in the long run" or to acknowledge that you get sick to receive love: "Hmm, not so good in the long run." But to think that being brave or very productive is "not so good in the long run" is often an unexpected stretch. The key is to understand that bravery generally hinges on adversity to overcome; it presupposes the presence of threat or fear; and super-productivity often implies that you are worthless without your achievements. In other words, these seemingly positive qualities and impulses are often hooked into an underbelly of fear, shame, and unlove.

Unfortunately, until you love many of your architects of survival back to health with self-Reiki or compassion-infused healing energy, you tend to host quite the dedicated crew who create havoc, pain, disorientation, dissociation, addiction, and illness. It's only when you release these architects of survival from their duties that you can really be true to your essence, genius, and service, thereby transcending the limitations of your abusers, abuse, overwhelmingness, and confusion. The key is to honour the architects of survival by:

    a. compassionately witnessing the agony that engulfed you when you created them,

    b. honouring the service they performed at the time and since,

    c. recognizing their limitations without judgment,

    d. releasing hatred, frustration, and impatience,

    e. welcoming change and the transformational energy of love and compassion, and

    f. letting compassion and love win.

Generally, we more readily offer love to the parched and traumatized astronauts who, in turn, gulp it down gladly. The architects of survival, on the other hand, often respond with resistance and fear. Their very nature was formed by adversity and unlove and their duty is to fight deadly danger. If love penetrates their field, the unlove and their *raison d'être* will dissolve. As one of my students very aptly said, "My architects are so scared! They feel like they're dying!" In light of this, these valiant fighters have a greater distance to cover to unreservedly veer away from unlove and eventually trust transformation and freedom. Their healing and integration journey is markedly different and requires even more tenderness, compassion, patience, and generosity. Eventually, along with the victimized astronauts, they also rest and heal in the five-star love vibes in your heart of hearts.

Activating your built-in alchemical bells and whistles consciously shifts your experience from a tentative and fearful crawl to a turbo-infused joy ride.

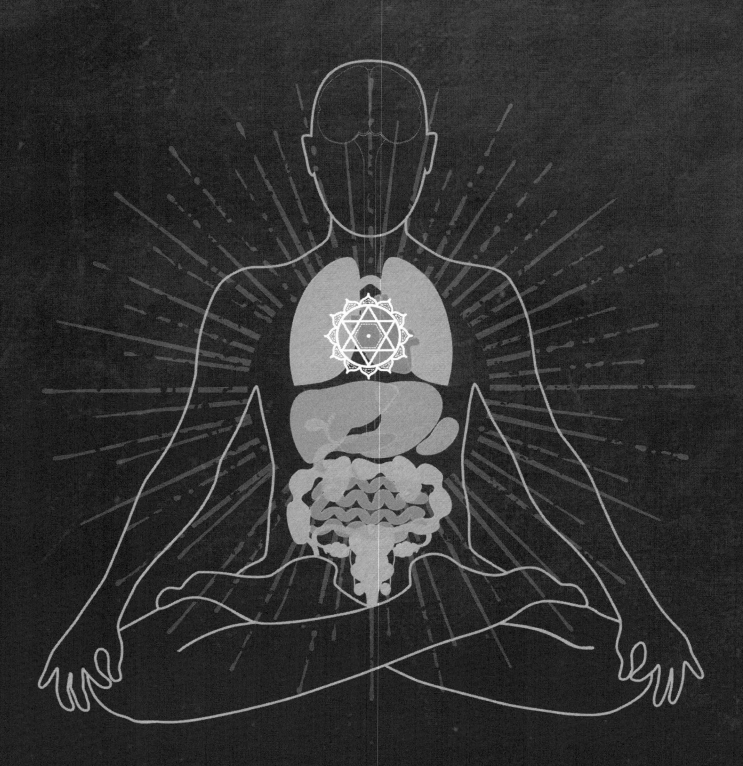

TRUSTING YOUR SELF

Let's just say that, generally, none of this is instantaneous or immediately accessible. First, you tend to host a vast number of acknowledged but not yet integrated traumatized astronauts and architects of survival. Second, you often host just as many whom you don't remember, whom you deny, and/or who are still obscured by shame. Third, you generally host many more surreptitious astronauts and architects created and fuelled by conscious and unconscious religious, cultural, and social biases; dogma; and expectations. And last, you have absorbed, virtually by osmosis, your caregivers' tragic astronauts and nefarious, if potent, architects. These vibrations are so tempestuous and brawny that they imprint your energy bodies with their signatures along with the imprints of your ancestors' astronauts and architects. Needless to say, it can be a life's work to untangle the threads of your fragmented essence.

As daunting as this may seem, your physical and energetic bodies are designed to accomplish this task. Although it may feel like it sometimes, you are not forced to stagger up the rocky and tortuous mountain path while shackled and barefoot. You actually inhabit a powerful vehicle designed to propel you forward to your destination. Like a bird, you have been given wings to fly. Each organ, energetic orb, and current in your wondrous energy bodies is a specialized transformer with the capacity to transmute alchemical trauma back into love. In other words, you are specifically designed to alchemically transform the astronauts' and architects' intensity. Although alchemical trauma is love in action anyway, you are nonetheless built to learn, grow, and evolve closer to and back to love, whether you know it or not.

It's love for the whole crew that's needed 24/7! Although this can be a rather daunting task, it is a powerful "YES!" to the process of life, living, and thriving.

DEDICATING YOUR SELF TO SERVICE

It is obvious to me now that my long struggle was not so much about getting out from under the thumb of my perpetrators; rather, it was to drag myself out of the state of unlove and all its toxic manifestations. That was the heart of the problem (pardon the pun), and it lived inside me like a pernicious poison. In the end, unlove and uncompassion, more than terror and horror, were the source of my pain and suffering.

You, too, have the potential to flow with the energy of love and compassion every day, no matter what others have put you through in the past or are still inflicting upon you today. The magic that fuels love and compassion is the same life force that nourishes a beautiful rose. And all roses have a thorny stem that later produces a bud, which then blossoms, shares its beauty—and later withers and dies. This journey is embedded in the logic of the plant's being-ness.

You have this perfect logic of growth and Nature in you. You, too, follow the laws of birth, thorny adversity, growth, beauty, generosity, and death. All living beings are in it together, the earth and the sun included. We all bear the universal gifts of love, compassion, and generosity. For instance, I am constantly reminded that I am not a healer or an artist or whatever; I am simply called to share the gifts of love, compassion, self-healing, and transformation with others. It is my way of being part of the solution and in synch with the energy of life and love. Your life purpose is coextensive with your reawakened innate ability to love and self-heal, and your life path involves sharing this medicine with others in your particular and unique way.

To be in service is to actively self-heal, recognize your innate genius and path, and share your loved, strong, happy, connected, and vibrant voice in whatever way most efficiently supports you and all living beings.

What is your unique expression of love?

In *The Tibetan Book of Living and Dying*, Sogyal Rinpoche succinctly defines the healing force of love and compassion in action:

> I know and I firmly believe that there is no need for anyone on Earth to die in resentment and bitterness. No suffering, however dreadful, is or can be meaningless if it is dedicated to the alleviation of the suffering of others. We have before us the noble and exalting examples of the supreme masters of compassion, who it is said, live and die, in the practice of Tonglen, taking on the pain of all sentient beings while they breathe in, and pouring out healing to the whole world when they breathe out, all their lives long, and right up until their very last breath. So boundless and powerful is their compassion, the teachings say, that at the moment of their death, it carries them immediately to rebirth in a Buddha realm.
>
> How transformed the world and our experience of it would be if each of us, while we live and as we die, could say this prayer, along with Shantideva and all the masters of compassion:

May I be a protector to those without protection,
A leader for those who journey,
And a boat, a bridge, a passage
For those desiring the further shore.

May the pain of every living creature
Be completely cleared away.
May I be the doctor and the medicine
And may I be the nurse
For all sick beings in the world
Until everyone is healed.

Just like space
And the great elements such as earth,
May I always support the life
Of all the boundless creatures.

And until they pass away from pain
May I also be the source of life
For all the realms of varied beings
That reach unto the ends of space.

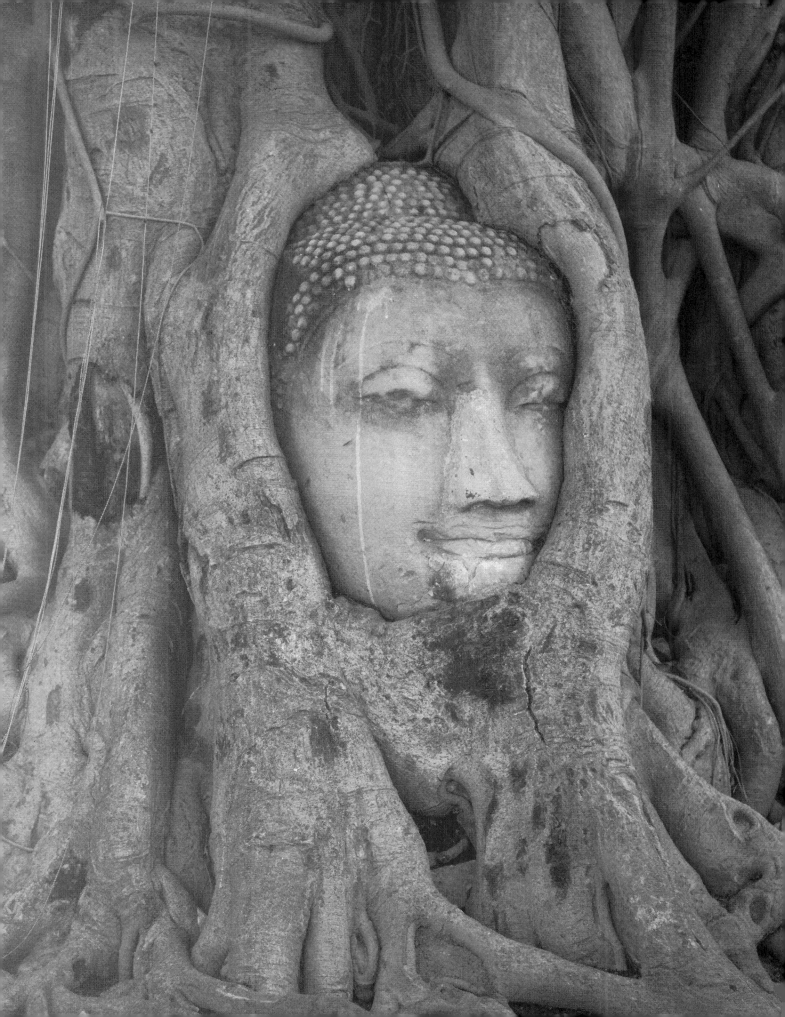

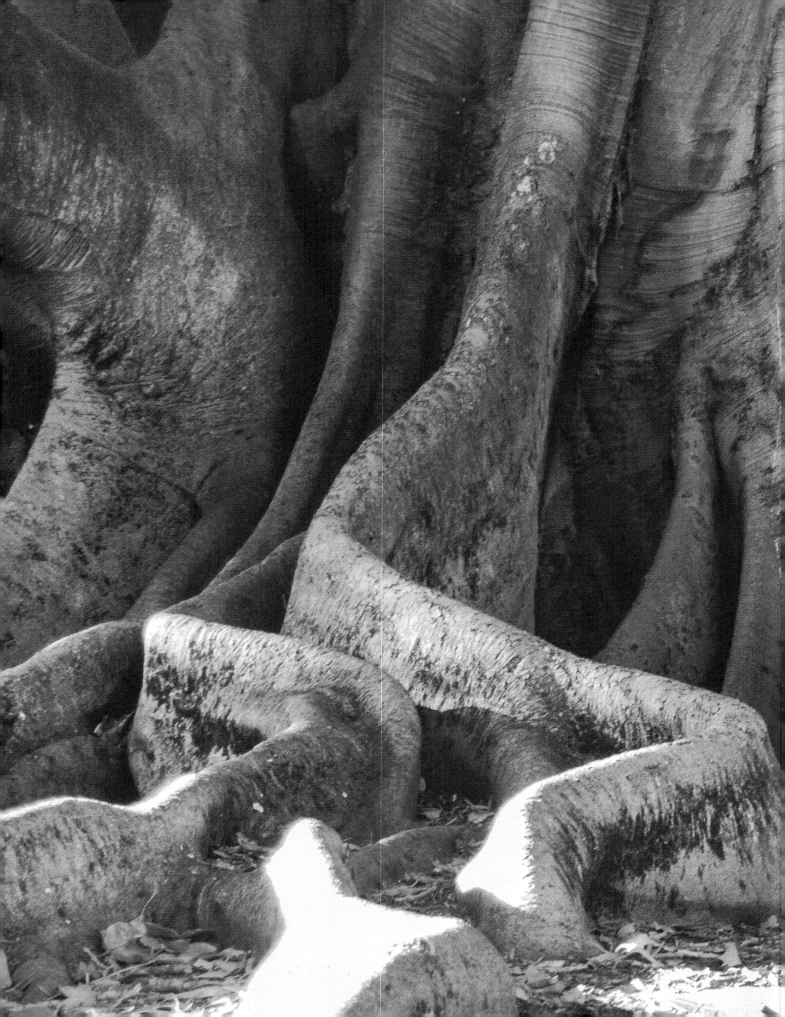

PART TWO
REIKI PLUS PLUS
LEVELS ONE, TWO, AND THREE

REIKI PLUS PLUS
LEVEL ONE

CHAPTER FIVE
LEARNING THE REIKI BASICS

WHAT IS REIKI?

The word *Reiki* derives from two Japanese characters: *Rei*, meaning "universal or spiritual," and *ki,* meaning "energy or life force." Reiki refers to the energy that animates everything and is harnessed by many different therapeutic practices, including meditation, yoga, various martial arts, and the healing touch: a relaxing, nurturing therapy that uses gentle touch to assist in balancing physical, emotional, mental, and spiritual health and well-being. The Chinese posited the existence of a vital energy, which they called qi or chi. An ancient Indian yogi tradition speaks of prana, the breath of life, and kundalini, the divine Shakti energy. Kabbalah, the Jewish mystical practice, refers to these same energies as the astral light. Many esoteric teachings—such as those of Rudolf Steiner, the Austrian scientist, philosopher, and founder of Waldorf education, and those of Native American medicine people—describe the human energy fields in great detail. According to all these conceptions, this universal energy is the basic constituent and source of all life.

The human organism, then, is not just a physical composition of molecules. You comprise dynamic energy fields that surround and penetrate your material body. The fundamental energy fields are as follows: the physical, emotional, mental, and spiritual. Your material tissues are shaped and anchored by these vital energy fields, which are perceived by trained practitioners as pulsing and flowing webs of light. Most dis-eases, for instance, are initiated in one of these energy fields and then transmitted to your material body, sometimes becoming far more than the mere absence of ease or disharmony; they can become serious illnesses. The aim of self-Reiki and Reiki therapy is to allow the energy life force to flow without restriction through your physical, mental, emotional, and spiritual energy fields by eliminating the blocks and hindrances created by trauma, adversity, negative mental patterns, and/or spiritual despair.

Reiki is a channel for the energy that is in everything through a specific lens, one that facilitates your conscious interaction with ancient principles of life, living, and healing. In so many religions and spiritual practices, the energy of life in all its splendour and mystery is presented to you through various faces, whether it be Kali, Krishna, and Ganesh; or God, Jesus, Mary, and the Holy Spirit; or Buddha, white, or green Tara. Reiki is just that—an energy signature, a phone number if you will, that represents an aspect of the whole. It contains the whole while allowing you to grasp and interface with a more manageable aspect of the vastness and to focus it on you or others to activate self-healing.

Reiki is essentially a "laying on of hands" healing system. The practitioner's gentle and light touch replenishes the body's energy fields, rebalancing the currents and chakras (spinning spheres of energetic activity) and facilitating the release of blocked energy. Reiki practitioners not only build on their ability to contain and transmit heightened amounts of ki, but they also develop an inner perception that allows them to sense things beyond the normal range of the five senses. It is this type of sensing that allows the practitioner to recognize the blockages that are lodged in the subtle bodies.

THE ENERGY BODIES AT A GLANCE

PHYSICAL BODY	ENERGY BODIES	SACRED TREE
SUN	SUN	SUN
Head/Arms	SPIRITUAL	Branches
Neck	MENTAL	Base of Branches
Chest	EMOTIONAL	Trunk
Abdomen/Legs	PHYSICAL	Roots
EARTH	EARTH	EARTH

土

WHEN CAN REIKI HELP?

SUPPORTING THE PHYSICAL ENERGY BODY

Self-Reiki and Reiki therapy supports and informs the healing of physical dis-ease and chronic illnesses of all kinds, including headaches, migraines, chronic fatigue, endometriosis, thyroid conditions, chronic yeast infections, ovarian cysts, eczema, digestive disorders, irritable bowel syndrome, colitis, and cancer, as well as those arising from accident or surgery. It's particularly helpful when health issues have not responded well to traditional Western medical treatment because self-Reiki and Reiki reawaken intuitive perception. Reiki energy thereby activates your ability to perceive the contraction and trauma that is creating the physical unease or dis-ease to begin with. When you access, recognize, and soothe the root of the disharmony, the life force and love can flow without restriction again. This potent energetic release and emotional resolution activates a transformational healing process in the physical body.

"Our culture habitually denies the insidious and pervasiveness of sex-related issues. I first learned in my medical practice that abuse against women is epidemic, whether subtle or overt. I saw how abuse sets the stage for illness in our female bodies."

— Christiane Northrup, M.D. and author of
Women's Bodies, Women's Wisdom: Creating Physical and Emotional Health and Healing

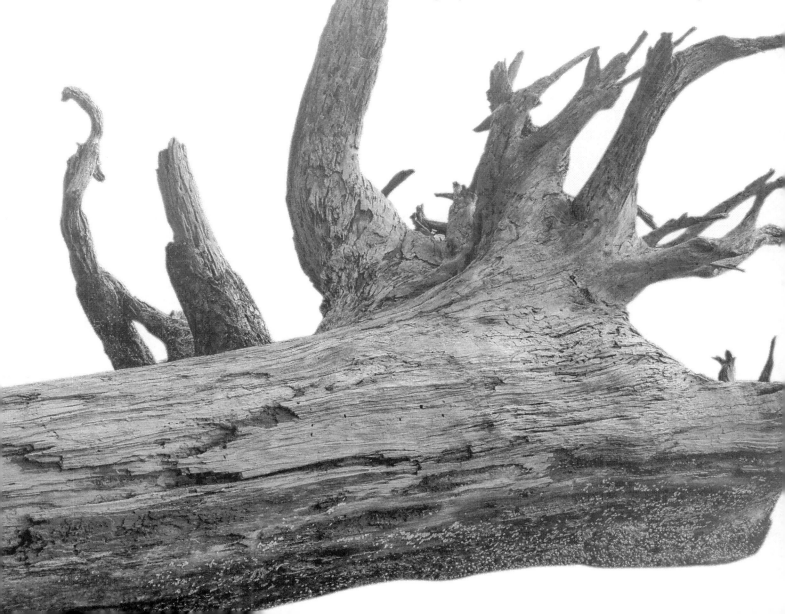

"Repression — dissociating emotions from awareness and relegating them to the unconscious — disorganizes and confuses our physiological defences so that in some people these defences go awry, becoming destroyers of health rather than protectors."

— Gabor Maté, M.D. and author of *When the Body Says No*

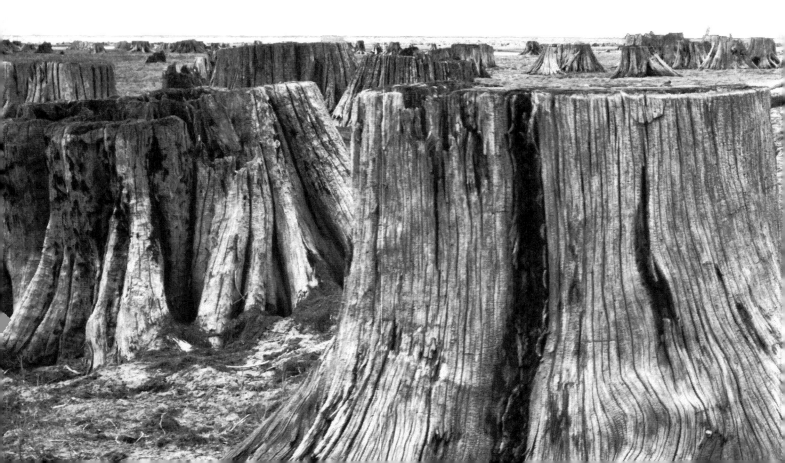

SUPPORTING THE EMOTIONAL ENERGY BODY

Self-Reiki and Reiki therapy supports and informs the healing of emotional/
psychological strain and distress such as anxiety, insomnia, panic attacks,
chronic fatigue, depression, overwhelm, dissociation, and other stress-related
dis-eases, including those arising from sexual, physical, and emotional abuse
and traumas. All too often, traumatic narratives are warehoused in your
emotional energy body rather than being healed. Repressing and storing
these negative experiences works in the short-term, as it helps you survive an
event you don't have the resources to process, but in the long-term
it creates unease and/or dis-ease. Self-Reiki and Reiki are excellent tools
to locate and access the various stockpiles of low-frequency emotions you
are now strong enough to acknowledge, heal, and release. They bring
a soothing and loving energy to the contractions and blockages due to
trauma and adversity, thereby restoring trust and emotional well-being
and flow.

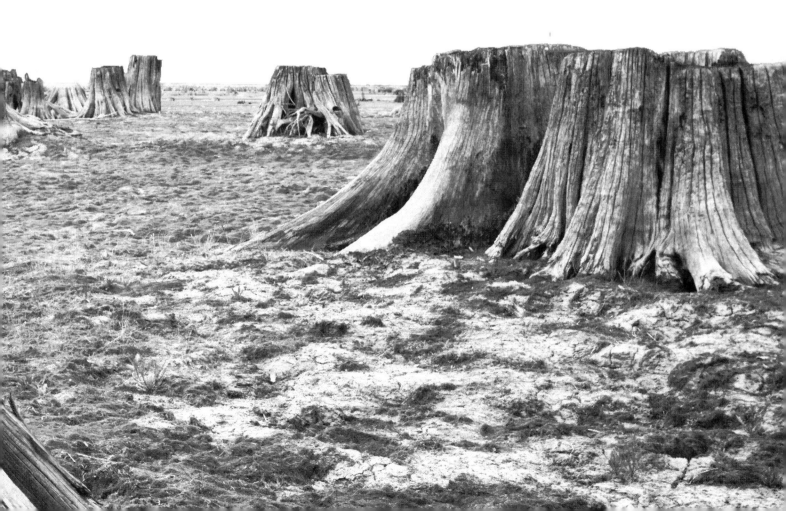

SUPPORTING THE MENTAL ENERGY BODY

Self-Reiki and Reiki invigorate your third eye, the foremost portal for intuitive perception. In doing so, your capacity to tap into your innate wisdom and guidance is strengthened. As such, it unifies your day-to-day consciousness, including your limiting belief systems and other blind spots, with your innate spiritual baseline, genius, and life purpose. Therefore, self-Reiki and Reiki proficiently reveal any intrusive, harmful, and denigrating interference due to social and cultural programming, constructed familial mythologies reinforcing hierarchy, systemic discrimination, colonization, misinformation, and indoctrination. For instance, if you believe you are a second-class citizen because you are a woman, black, or queer, you can count on self-Reiki and Reiki energy to root out these limiting belief systems and unconscious biases and to restore your innate dignity, purposefulness, and magnificence.

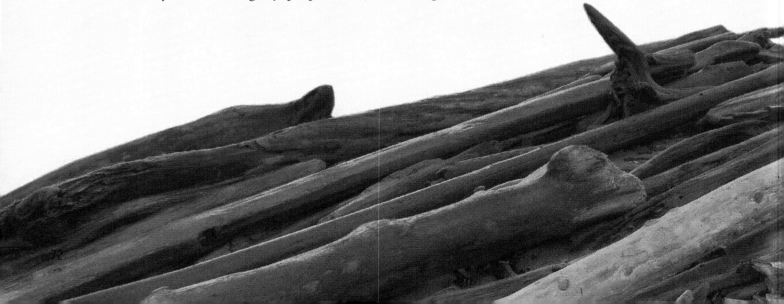

"Feminism involves so much more than gender equality and it involves so much more than gender. Feminism must involve consciousness of capitalism (I mean the feminism that I relate to, and there are multiple feminisms, right). So it has to involve a consciousness of capitalism and racism and colonialism and post-colonialities, and ability and more genders than we can even imagine and more sexualities than we ever thought we could name."

— Angela Davis, political activist, academic, and author, in her 2013 speech "Feminism & Abolition: Theories & Practices for the Twenty-First Century"

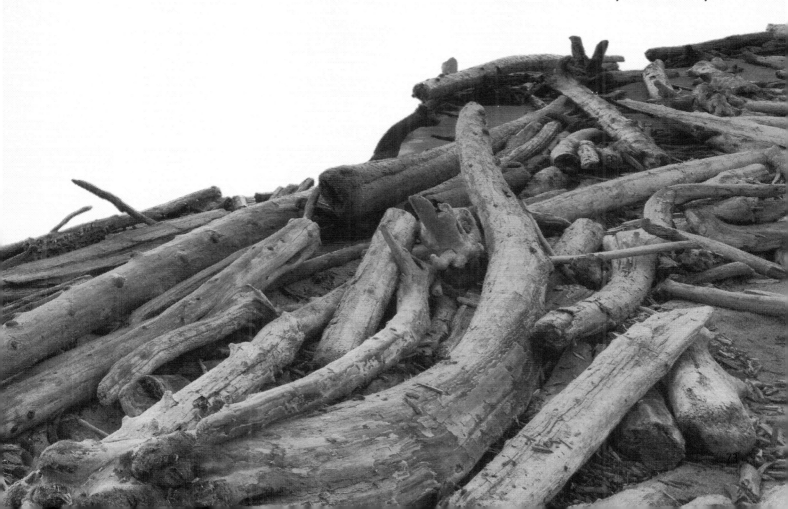

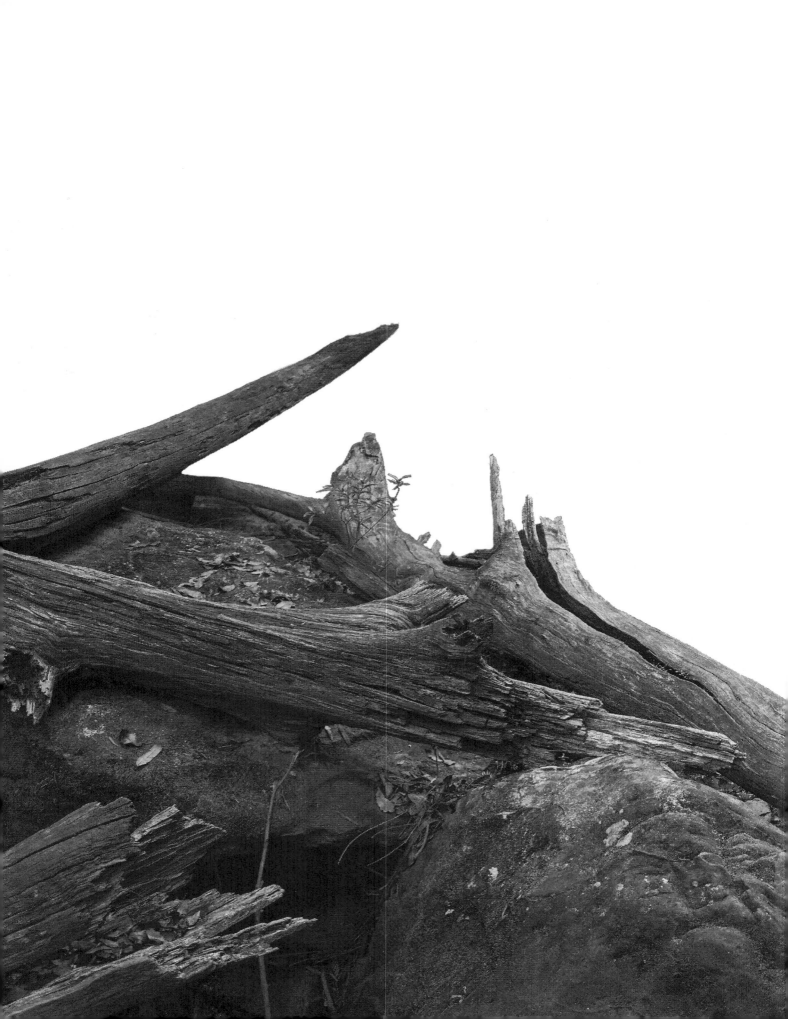

SUPPORTING THE SPIRITUAL ENERGY BODY

Self-Reiki and Reiki therapy supports and informs the healing of spiritual malaises, including religious indoctrination, oppression, domination, overmanagement, colonization, self-sacrifice, depression, and/or creative blocks. For instance, if your family's or faith's political and organizational infrastructure, beliefs, conventions, rules, rituals, and/or practices do not honour and celebrate your personal power, authority, and freedom, then self-Reiki and Reiki reawaken your heart's wisdom and with it your self-worth, discernment, and confidence. Reiki energy untangles and extracts the authoritarian opinions and judgments, thereby creating space for your innate wisdom, personal authority and power, and purposefulness to emerge. This kind of trauma can lay waste to your sense of life having meaning and can decimate your ability to listen to yourself. By leading you home to your core self, Reiki energy fosters your birthright to self-trust, self-determination, and inner peace.

"If you think of the universe as a vast electrical sea in which you are immersed and from which you are formed, opening your creativity changes you from something bobbing in that sea to a more fully functioning, more conscious, more cooperative part of that ecosystem."

— Julia Cameron, *The Artist's Way: A Spiritual Path to Higher Creativity*

THE PATH TO SELF-HEALING

Self-Reiki is a powerful tool to activate the energy channels and centres in your Sacred Tree, its roots, core, and branches. Through its application, you learn how to channel the life force through your energy bodies. You actively draw in the energy of life itself and focus it on particular aspects of your being, much like shining a flashlight on your congested liver, nervous stomach, or the sadness in your chest. Let's face it, without self-inquiry and conscious engagement with your malleable physical, emotional, mental, and spiritual energy fields, you generally face more of the same kinds of problems, conflicts, tensions, pain, and dis-eases. Energetic imbalances can resonate throughout your entire being, thereby creating a vicious cycle affecting your physical, emotional, mental, and spiritual bodies. A disharmony in any one of your four realms can trigger the cycle. Conversely, shifting your energetic flow to an optimal vibrational level in one realm can reverse the cycle and eventually fuel a metamorphosis on all levels. You can literally start changing your life from the inside out!

Your transformational journey gains traction when:

a. You register that a return to health and harmony requires personal energetic work such as self-Reiki to create changes in all four energy fields (spiritual, mental, emotional, and physical), something that surgery, legal/illegal drugs, and many forms of talk therapy won't accomplish.

b. You acknowledge that your illnesses, dis-eases, and manifestations of disharmony are nothing other than messages your spirit is attempting to transmit: "Something is wrong. You are ignoring something very important. You are not listening to your whole self." You honour, listen, comprehend, and heed your body's sacred messages and messaging system. You thereby aim to uncover and eventually heal the root of the energetic dysfunction, illness, and disharmony rather than turn in circles and manage only the symptoms.

c. You learn to connect with your innate self-healing capacity and fount of love no matter what is going on. Self-Reiki inspires you to access the nutrients in the earth and the sun despite illness, disorientation, or despair. In other words, to be ill, heartbroken, or a victim does not cut you off from the vibrant energy of life and love. Although an aspect of yourself is suffering, you nonetheless have the power to soothe, recharge, nourish, reconfigure, and release the imbalance and disharmony.

CAN ANYONE PRACTISE SELF-REIKI AND REIKI?

It is essential to receive a Reiki attunement, an initiatory process offered in Reiki workshops worldwide. Reiki attunements (Levels One, Two, and Three) open and expand the ki-holding capacity in your energy channels that run through the centre of your body, arms, and legs. They clear your channels of energy obstructions, balance your chakras, and replenish all your energy bodies. Heavenly ki energy, carrying the four sacred Reiki symbols, enters your crown chakra, heart, third eye, and hands. Earthly ki is drawn through your legs and lower energy centres to the heart. In a mere ten minutes, the attunement turns the light on, reconnecting you with your capability to self-heal.

The best way to strengthen your innate self-healing capacity and learn Reiki is to practise often and let the energy teach you. I recommend doing a self-Reiki session daily after receiving the first attunement. The more self-Reiki sessions you do, the more effectively you cultivate your channel and capacity to draw higher and more potent Reiki vibrations. It's also a good idea to be attuned more than once to intensify your self-practise, even if you repeat a Level One attunement again. The attunements meet you where you are. If you worked through a big piece and experienced a significant release, the next attunement will revitalize and stimulate your energy flow and connection that much more. It's also beneficial to be attuned by different Reiki masters. Some practitioners have cultivated a more potent connection than others.

Additionally, it is most important to support your self-healing path by receiving Reiki treatments from a Reiki master or energy healer at least a few times a year. Periodically checking in with an experienced practitioner who can substantiate your discoveries and process can reveal some of your blind spots, complete some of the work you don't know how to take further, and boost your vibrational level, creating a robust framework for your self-practice. It is a prerequisite to expand your knowledge, update your baseline, and coax you to go further. It's especially useful to reach out when your self-practice is sagging. The insights and surge of energy can inspire you to get back on it and audaciously explore further or go deeper.

If your outer world needs to be transformed, the process must begin within. Self-healing is nothing less than self-transformation!

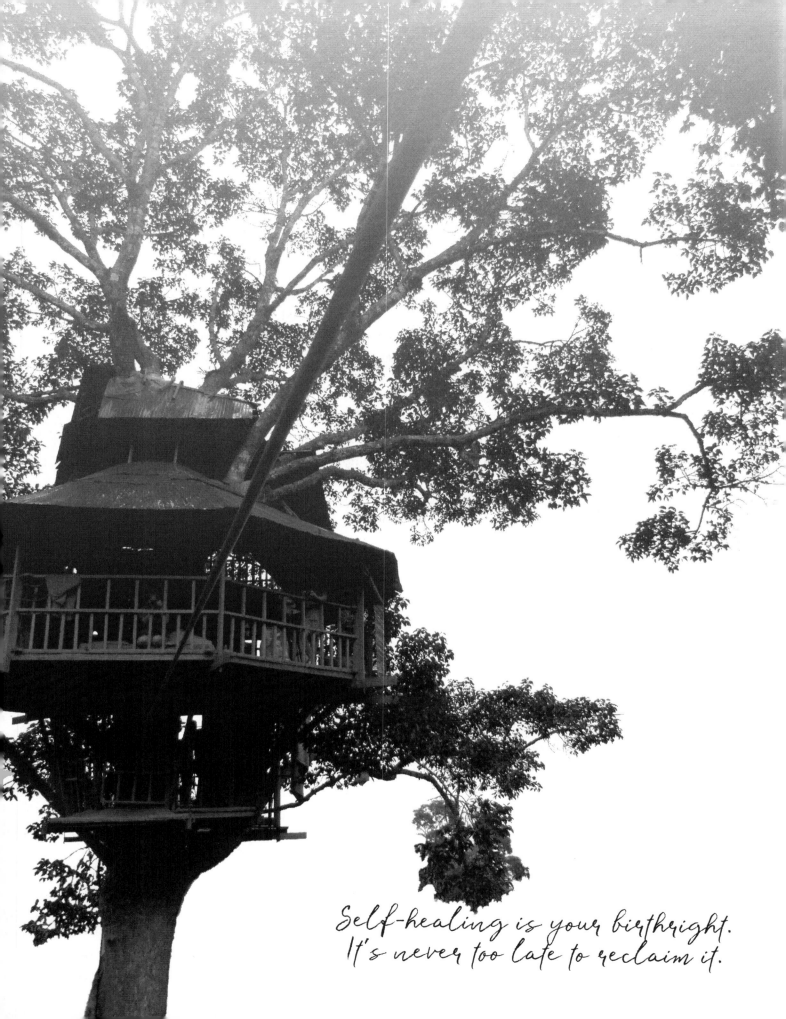

Self-healing is your birthright.
It's never too late to reclaim it.

Furthermore, bear in mind that Reiki is a sacred practice and healing process—yours and that of others—that requires a private, calm, and safe environment. Do not practise Reiki if you, your friend, or your client has consumed alcohol or recreational drugs. In other words, it's not a party trick. If you are drawn to practising on others, it is essential to take into consideration the Canadian Reiki Association Code of Ethics, whether you are a member of this association or not. Their guidelines are sound and should be honoured in all circumstances. Basically, when it comes to ethics, there are no exceptions.

THE HISTORY OF REIKI

Reiki was discovered and developed by Dr. Mikao Usui, who was born August 15, 1865, in Japan. At a young age, Usui studied Kiko, the Japanese version of Qigong, a Chinese discipline designed to improve health through meditation, breathing practices, and slow-moving exercises. Kiko focuses on the development of ki and includes methods of healing through the laying on of hands. It requires that one build up a supply of healing energy through the use of certain exercises before employing it. When using the Kiko method, one is prone to depletion, a key issue that took root in Usui's mind. He travelled all over Japan, China, and Europe in pursuit of knowledge and understanding of medicine, psychology, religion, and spirituality. Due to his enhanced psychic abilities, he joined the metaphysical group Rei Jyutu Ka, where his spiritual education continued.

In 1914, Usui decided to become a Buddhist monk. In March 1922, he travelled to Mt. Kurama on a twenty-one-day retreat. There he fasted, chanted, prayed, and meditated. Toward the end of the retreat, a great and powerful spiritual light entered the top of his head; this light was the Reiki energy coming to him in the form of an attunement. It was an enlightening experience: he now knew he could heal others without his energy becoming depleted. Usui used Reiki on himself at first and then on family members. He moved to Tokyo in April 1922 and started a healing society named Usui Reiki Healing Society. He also opened a clinic in central Tokyo and began teaching and giving Reiki attunements. When a huge earthquake disrupted the life of the city in 1923, more than 140,000 people were killed and thousands of people were left homeless, while many others were injured or became physically ill. Almost everyone was emotionally traumatized. Usui and his students worked day and night to help as many as they could.

In 1925, Usui opened a much larger clinic and began travelling all over Japan, driven by the desire to make the technique available to everyone. He taught two thousand students and trained sixteen teachers. The Japanese government recognized him with the KunSan To award for meritorious service to others. He suffered a fatal stroke while teaching a class on March 9, 1926.

Hawayo Takata was responsible for bringing Reiki to the West. Thanks to her, Reiki has spread all over the world. Born in Hawaii on December 24, 1900, Takata worked on sugar plantations from a very young age. When her husband died, she again worked on plantations to support her family. She developed a lung condition, abdominal pains, and eventually had a nervous breakdown. She journeyed to Japan to visit her parents and to seek help for her health, eventually going to Dr. Hayashi, a former student of Usui who had left to start his own Reiki clinic. After four months of treatments, Takata healed completely. Her recovery inspired her to study Reiki so she could maintain her health when back in Hawaii; she earned her second degree and worked in the clinic for one year. In 1937, she returned to Hawaii. Hayashi followed her and together they taught Reiki and gave treatments. Takata established her own clinics in Hilo and Honolulu. She became a well-known healer and travelled to the U.S. mainland and to other parts of the world, teaching and giving treatments. She initiated twenty-two Reiki masters before her death on December 11, 1980.

After Takata's death, one of the twenty-two masters she had trained decided to disregard some of Takata's restrictive rules and high fees. Iris Ishikura began charging a very moderate fee and in some cases taught for free. By the mid-1980s, several hundred Reiki masters charged lower fees and began supplying written material and class workbooks. Reiki is now a practice readily accessible in many parts of the world.

"In times like these, the happiness of humanity is based on working together and the desire for social progress. This is why I would never allow anyone to possess it (Reiki) just for himself!
Each of us has the potential of being given a gift by the divine, which results in the body and soul becoming unified. In this way (with Reiki), a great many people will experience the blessing of the divine.
First of all, our Reiki Ryoho is an original therapy, which is built upon the spiritual power of the universe. Through it, the human being will first be made healthy, and then peace of mind and joy in life — will be increased."

— Dr. Mikao Usui, founder of the Reiki healing system and author of
Reiki Ryoho Hikkei (Reiki Healing Art Handbook)

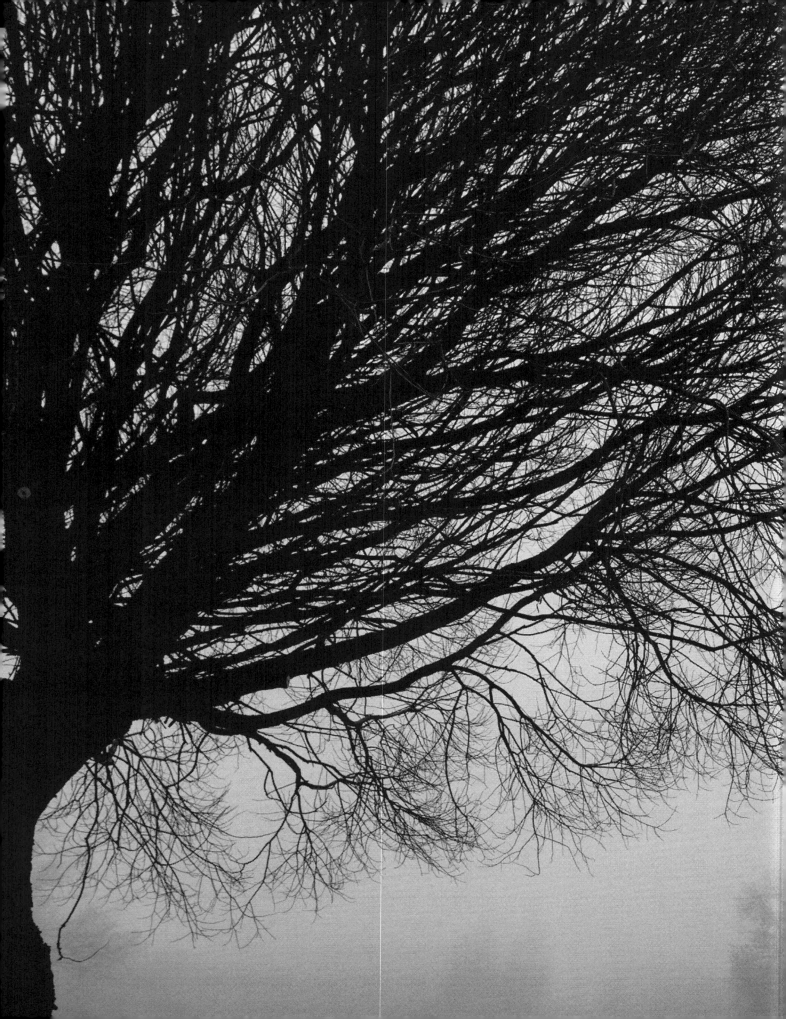

REIKI PRINCIPLES

The Reiki principles provided by Dr. Mikao Usui are spiritual guidelines. They are the foundation of Reiki as a spiritual path and self-healing method. They were studied, used in meditation, and chanted by Usui and his students. Consider their meaning and application in your life. Combined with practice, daily effort to observe the principles is what makes Reiki a way of life. The principles encourage you to awaken to who you are.

Just for today do not anger.
Just for today do not worry.
Just for today be grateful.
Just for today work diligently.
Just for today be kind to all living beings.

JUST FOR TODAY ...

The fundamental teaching that anchors each principle is a reminder to be present in the here and now. HUGE! The bad news is that you most likely battle with varying levels of subtle or pervasive dissociation. You probably have learned to survive by numbing yourself with addictions, medication, distractions, entertainment, media, intellectual knowledge, overachieving, underachieving, and a whole host of other options. As far as I'm concerned, numbness is a pandemic. It's not a matter of if but rather a matter of degree.

a. Some of you acknowledge its impact on your ability to self-heal and be in service to others and make wholesome choices consistently enough;

b. Some of you acknowledge its impact yet strain and sweat to moderate numbing activities and choices;

c. Some of you acknowledge its impact and work persistently to gradually shift out of a mammoth combination of addictions consistently enough;

d. Some of you acknowledge the impact yet embrace change only in fits and starts;

e. Some of you acknowledge its impact yet resist change;

f. Some of you are still foggy and do not perceive the extent to which you are checked out of your Sacred Tree.

"Just for today" reminds you to be present and to recognize the seemingly endless and often very creative ways in which you seek to feel less and engage less with your inner life. For many of you, this is a colossal journey in and of itself. It is a path that suggests embracing your inner experience without trying to control it, bury it, or neglect it. To live in the now is to embrace compassionate self-awareness and mindfulness day by day, moment by moment.

JUST FOR TODAY DO NOT ANGER

Right off the bat, this first principle reminds you that anger is a trustworthy indicator that you are experiencing a significant disturbance and disharmony. As painful and disruptive as anger is, it usually covers up an even more painful emotion such as grief, abandonment, fear, terror, shame, humiliation, powerlessness, hopelessness, despair, shock, and/or trauma. If you recognize anger stirring within you and interrupt its destructive outward expression, you have an opportunity to recognize the source of the fire rather than impulsively hurt others and/or yourself. *Just for today do not anger* is a call to feel, know, and engage in radical self-awareness, mindfulness, and self-healing. To anger less is to awaken your innate kindness by exploring, examining, naming, and compassionately voicing your truth within and without.

JUST FOR TODAY DO NOT WORRY

This teaching is a pertinent reminder to use your emotional energy for life-sustaining action, love, and healing. When you routinely worry about something or someone, it perpetuates the impact of unhealed trauma and the flight–fight–freeze response. In general, worry is nothing other than fear camouflaged as a more or less tolerable daily discomfort and habit. Yet fear is the polar opposite of love. To be in its grip is to be cut off from the life-giving and healing energy of love. Like anger, worry obscures the source of the turbulence and interferes with your self-knowledge, awareness, and healing. To face your fear head on is to embrace the process of uncovering and healing the wounds, adversity, shock, and/or trauma that distanced you from love in the past and continues to do so in the present.

In addition, worry is often fear disguised as love. It is my observation that the significant presence of worry in parent–child relationships is all too often justified as an expression of love. It's a cultural distortion and recipe for disaster to say that if parents worry they are loving their children. Parents will worry, that is par for the course. But in and of itself, it is not the expression, manifestation, or gift of the essential energy of love. Worry is not love in action; it is a subtle or overt, destructive, and detrimental perpetuation of fear and the cycle of violence.

JUST FOR TODAY BE GRATEFUL

Yes, generally you are grateful for the flowers and trees, the mountains and valleys, the rivers and oceans, and for what we culturally agree is beautiful, nourishing, and comforting. But are you able to be grateful and honour your parents, elders, teachers, and life story no matter what? In other words, do you honour the support and unconditional love you have experienced and conversely the judgment, disrespect, violence, and conditional love you have suffered? Gratefulness is a call to recognize your blessings, loving Nature and truth in all its facets, as well as the adversity and trauma. It presents an opportunity and invitation to sit with the truth of your experience with honesty, clarity, presence, and grace.

Your unreserved and active engagement with the wild and often painful twists and turns of your life and the characters who inhabit it sets a powerful healing energy into motion. Climbing into your Sacred Tree with your eyes wide open does nothing less than prompt a nascent trust in your innate alchemical power to transform trauma into wisdom and inner peace. At first you may cautiously discover and ascertain your inherent interconnectivity with love in all circumstances. Eventually, you may recognize and celebrate love, including alchemical trauma, as the trustworthy organizing principle of evolution on the earth plane.

JUST FOR TODAY WORK DILIGENTLY

The key here is to work hard at what matters, NOT the work you are imposing on yourself to make money to gain material possessions and status, NOT the work you push through to receive external validation so you feel better about yourself, NOT the work you think you should do because your father/mother or whomever approves of you more, NOT the work that keeps you so busy you have no time to feel, and NOT the work that you perform competitively to win and beat others to the top. In other words, NOT the work that serves to quell the fear of being a pauper or unsupported, that dulls the ache of self-loathing, that creates the illusion that you are more lovable because of certain accomplishments or commitments, that numbs you and blocks access to your inner self, or that perpetuates the contaminated yang and patriarchal power dynamic (that of power over others) rather than the cultivation of personal power and authority.

This teaching is a call to initiate the effort and discipline to learn and practise mindful presence in your Sacred Tree. The work that matters is the journey of healing that provokes the shift out of fear and into love. It's the quintessential trek that reveals your genius and service and energizes their manifestation.

JUST FOR TODAY BE KIND TO ALL LIVING BEINGS

Sure, easy-peasy! But wait a second, this is not just about small dogs and super-sweet babies, it's about consistently showing up for yourself with kindness, respect, and love. This teaching builds on all the previous principles: be mindfully present; delve below the choppy waters of anger to know and heal the pain that dwells on the ocean floor; face your fears and dismantle the cycle of violence so you can embrace the life-sustaining energy of love; honour and embrace the good, the bad, and the ugly so you can flow with grace; keep your nose on the track and align your effort with your genius and service; and discover the power of love within and without to mobilize your yearning and healing.

When you learn to tap into the magnanimous unconditionality of self-love, you experience a deep knowing that your spirit is anchored in a most wondrous Sacred Tree with roots firmly attached to the centre of the earth and branches stretching up to the sun, no matter what is going on. You see, sense, and celebrate not only your true self but Universal Love—divine love, God, Durga, Buddha, Universe, Nature, or whatever name you like—in action within you at the best of times and the worst of times. You also know and trust that your channels are capable of receiving a booster shot of love and Reiki healing energy in a self-healing meditation or in a session with a client no matter what adversity and turmoil is unfolding.

"Only when we can devote ourselves without being prejudiced by our thoughts and feelings will we become an instrument for the universal life energy."

— Dr. Mikao Usui, founder of the Reiki healing system

CHAPTER SIX

EXPLORING SACRED TREE ANATOMY: THE VERTICAL AXIS

FROM EARTH TO SUN AND SUN TO EARTH

Whether you are in a state of harmony or disharmony, your entire being expresses its relationship to the earth and the sun in an energetic dimension including the physical, emotional, mental, and spiritual realms. Your Sacred Tree is blessed with major energy vortexes and pools rooted within your central and vertical energetic channel, which flows between the earth and the sun. In this chapter, we will focus on seven internal portals (the chakras), two of the external chakras (the Earth Star and the Sun Star), and three internal energetic reservoirs, the dantians.

The chakras and dantians (among a myriad of other energetic gateways beyond the scope of this book) oversee, regulate, and shape your Sacred Tree's transformational and alchemical potency. These energy vortexes are some of your spirit's most trustworthy teachers and guides in its quest to evolve and grow. These innate allies are with you every blissful or traumatized step of the way. In other words, Universal Love in action in all its flavours of harmony is literally right there in you, whether tuned up and imminently accessible or temporarily tuned out and submerged under the gack of trauma and confusion.

While I will describe these systems briefly without elaborating on the vast body of knowledge already available, I offer you a framework to tap into the power and wonder of your Sacred Tree anatomy and its fertile interdependence with the earth and the sun. For further study, I highly recommend *Eastern Body, Western Mind: Psychology and the Chakra System as Path to the Self*, the must-read book about chakras by Anodea Judith, *and Anatomy of the Spirit: The Seven Stages of Power and Healing*, a seminal book by Caroline Myss.

CHAKRAS AND DANTIANS AT A GLANCE

SUN	SUN	SUN	SUN
SACRED TREE	BODY	CHAKRAS	DANTIANS
Branches	Above Head	Sun Star Chakra	Upper Dantian
Branches	Head/Arms	Seventh Chakra	Upper Dantian
Branches	Head/Arms	Sixth Chakra	Upper Dantian
Base of Branches	Throat	Fifth Chakra	Upper Dantian
Trunk	Chest	Fourth Chakra	Middle Dantian
Trunk	Chest	Third Chakra	Middle Dantian
Roots	Abdomen/Legs	Second Chakra	Lower Dantian
Roots	Abdomen/Legs	First Chakra	Lower Dantian
Roots	Below Feet	Earth Star Chakra	Lower Dantian
EARTH	EARTH	EARTH	EARTH

土

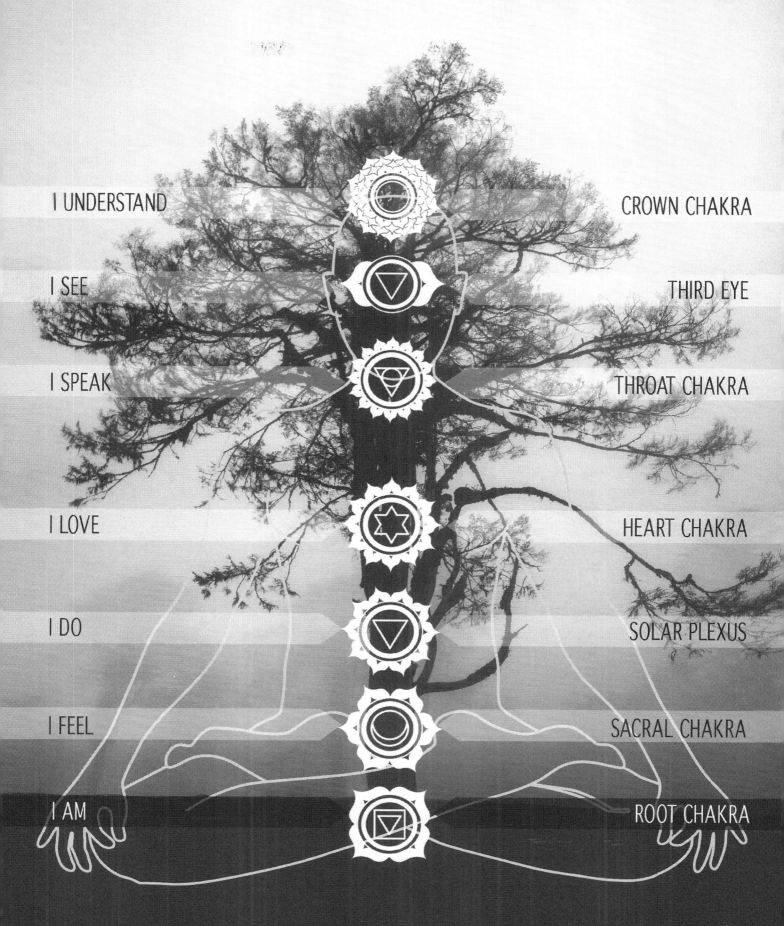

I UNDERSTAND   CROWN CHAKRA

I SEE   THIRD EYE

I SPEAK   THROAT CHAKRA

I LOVE   HEART CHAKRA

I DO   SOLAR PLEXUS

I FEEL   SACRAL CHAKRA

I AM   ROOT CHAKRA

91

CHAKRAS

The chakra system has exploded into popular culture via the widespread study and practice of yoga asanas. Therefore, it is the most common language and system used to describe the architecture of your energy bodies when teaching energy medicine modalities. Reiki practitioners, in particular, often focus on the chakra system as a tool for diagnosis and healing. Although it says a lot about a super beautiful and exciting shift in the dominant culture, this flood of chakra information has eclipsed the power and brightness of your less glittery and more slithery organs; hence, the emphasis on the organs and the cyclical wisdom of their energetic orbs in Reiki Plus Plus: Level Two.

That said, the more celebrated chakras of the four-thousand-year-old Indian yogic tradition are an integral part of your energetic vehicle to support and facilitate your evolutionary quest to reclaim and calibrate your Sacred Tree. The word *chakra* literally means "disk" or "wheel" and describes the spinning pools of bio-energetic activity emanating from within your central energy channel. Each chakra is a colourful funnel extending outward from the central energy channel. There are seven of these major pools stacked from your feet to your head. The seventh chakra (crown) and first chakra (root) have one funnel extending up and down respectively; and the second chakra through to the sixth have two funnels, front and back, extending from your central energy channel past your skin and into your aura.

While many students and practitioners focus on these seven portals, I highly recommend working with two of the external chakras as well: namely, the Earth Star Chakra below your feet and the Sun Star Chakra above your head. Engaging with these two additional external chakras not only enlivens your energetic awareness by virtue of connecting you consciously with energy outside your physical periphery, but it greatly amplifies your Sacred Tree's fortitude and flow between the earth and the sun.

CHAKRA HARMONY

Each chakra is a reservoir for a distinctive flavour of harmony. These high-vibration attributes of the life force are programmed deep in the core of your mind–body interface. When flowing, these innate teachers instigate, guide, and nurture your physical, emotional, mental, and spiritual functioning and well-being.

THE EARTH STAR CHAKRA

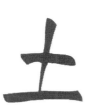

is a high-performance first or root chakra. It is your spiritual gateway to the living multidimensional spirit of Mother Earth, along with her mineral, animal, and plant realms. It is the premier tool to replenish your earth/yin/Shakti energy, to increase your communion with the sacred energy of Mother Earth, and to develop your affinity with magic. As we yogis love to say: the more connected to the earth you are, the higher you fly! Hence, this chakra is not second to the Sun Star Chakra. Both these portals are essential conduits to the primordial energies of life and love. You thrive when your earth/yin/Shakti star and sun/yang/Shiva star are efficient conduits for the harmonious and simultaneous flow of your downward manifestation current and upward liberation current (more on this at the end of this chapter). Therefore, it expands your trust in the healing power of change, transformation, and evolution as well as in balanced and harmonious daily living.

THE FIRST CHAKRA (Muladhara or Root Chakra)

anchors the central energetic channel to Mother Earth and the earth realm. Hence, it strengthens your umbilical cord to Mother Earth and establishes your primary vertical orientation between the earth and the sun. Keep in mind, the seed must first be planted in the earth and then it grows and evolves. It stands to reason that a tree needs strong roots to thrive and be resilient to seasonal conditions as well as challenging periodic conditions. Without strong roots, the tree topples.

THE SECOND CHAKRA (Svadhisthana, Sacral, or Moon chakra)

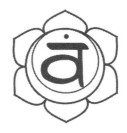

is the storehouse of unconscious karmic imprints and mental impressions, including those accumulated from past lives. You evolve and transcend unwholesome karma and imprints by consciously and mindfully engaging in relationships with empathy, nurturance, enjoyment, creativity, sexual health, and the willingness to change and grow. It's no wonder your small intestines and colons so often shriek their discontent and demand much attention! You are not going anywhere lovely without untangling these knots.

THE THIRD CHAKRA (Manipura or Solar Plexus Chakra)

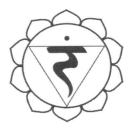

radiates its light throughout the entire cellular structure of the physical body and supplies power to the vast network of energy channels and meridians in the energy body, much like the sun shining on all the planets. When this fire burns like a steady Olympic flame, low-frequency emotions are less likely to stagnate or destabilize your energy fields. Hence, you are empowered, dynamic, reliable, self-disciplined, and confident and thus relaxed enough to be light, spontaneous, and playful.

THE FOURTH CHAKRA (Anahata or Heart Chakra)

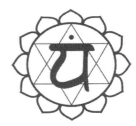

is the wish-fulfilling tree. When you awaken this chakra, you are inspired and manifest desires in alignment with your highest and greatest good. Compassion and unconditional love flow through you into the world. As a result, you experience contentment and inner peace. This luminous lucidity and productivity fosters order, serenity, and healthy boundaries.

THE FIFTH CHAKRA (Vishuddha or Throat Chakra)

is the distinguished bridge between the earthly realm and the spirit realm. When awakened, it helps you discern between pure and impure energy. You thereby align your personal will with the earth/sun will. In other words, your spirit's purpose manifests on the earth plane and your choices on the earth plane support your spirit's purpose.

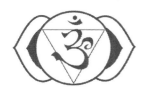

THE SIXTH CHAKRA (Ajna or Third Eye Chakra)

is an intuitive gateway to wisdom. When awakened, it has the capacity to purify impure energies and burn away the fog of ignorance and illusion. You see beyond the duality of egocentric contraction (desire/aversion, pleasure/pain, life/death, etc.) and access deeper realms of wisdom beyond sensory perception.

THE SEVENTH CHAKRA (Sahasrara or Crown Chakra)

is your primary gateway to the sun and infinite time, space, and wisdom. While it funnels the flow of sun/yang/Shiva energy into your central channel, the other chakras transform this life-affirming energy. It is an intuitive gateway to immortal planes of consciousness and celestial communication.

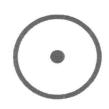

THE SUN STAR CHAKRA

is often referred to as the "seat of the soul." Located above the head, it is not the soul per se, but it contains your spirit's energetic templates—all the reasons why you chose to incarnate at this particular juncture and in this specific context. When awakened, this high-performance seventh chakra fuels nothing less than spiritual bliss, awakening, and enlightenment.

THE HARMONY IMPRINTS OF THE UPPER CHAKRAS

CHAKRA	COLOUR	LOCATION	PHYSICAL AFFILIATION	HARMONY IMPRINTS
Sun Star	White or Gold	Twelve Inches Above the Head	Whole Body	·Celestial Yang Union ·Spiritual Consciousness ·Bliss ·Ecstasy ·Self-Knowledge ·Grace
Seventh	Violet	Top of Head	·Brain ·Pineal Gland	·Open-Mindedness ·Mindfulness ·Devotion ·Thoughtfulness ·Comprehension ·Serenity
Sixth	Deep Blue	Brow and Base of Occiput	·Brain ·Hypothalamus ·Pituitary Gland ·Endocrine System	·Archetypal Awareness ·Self-Reflection ·Clear Perception ·Intellectual Discrimination ·Imagination ·Intuition
Fifth	Light Blue	Throat and Neck	·Neck ·Throat ·Esophagus ·Lungs ·Small Intestine ·Colon/Rectum	·Self-Expression ·Creativity ·Clear Communication ·Good Listener ·Discernment ·Enthusiasm
Fourth	Green	Centre of Breast Bone	·Heart ·Lungs ·Diaphragm ·Thymus Gland ·Vagus Nerve	·Compasssion ·Unconditional Love ·Self-Love ·Imagination ·Contentment ·Healthy Boundaries

THE HARMONY IMPRINTS OF THE LOWER CHAKRAS

CHAKRA	COLOUR	LOCATION	PHYSICAL AFFILIATION	HARMONY IMPRINTS
Third	Yellow	Navel or Solar Plexus	·Liver ·Gallbladder ·Spleen ·Pancreas ·Stomach ·Duodenum	·Dynamism ·Empowerment ·Reliability ·Self-Discipline ·Confidence ·Spontaneity/Playfulness
Second	Orange	Navel or Above Pubic Bone	·Kidneys ·Bladder ·Colon ·Small Intestine ·Reproductive Organs	·Healthy Bonds ·Nurturance/Empathy ·Enjoyment/Self-Control ·Sexual Health ·Creativity ·Willingness to Change
First	Red	Perineum	·Kidneys ·Bladder ·Adrenals ·Colon ·Small Intestine ·Reproductive Organs ·Spine	·Survival ·Group Acceptance ·Vitality ·Presence ·Right Livelihood ·Safety ·Stability
Earth Star	Brown or Black	Twelve Inches Below Feet	Whole Body	·Anchor in Mother Earth ·Earth Energy Purveyor ·Respect for the Earth ·Interdependence with All Living Beings ·Mystical Solidity ·Yin Footing

CHAKRA DISHARMONY: EXPLOSIVE VERSUS IMPLOSIVE

Each chakra lives your life with you. These specialized organizational centres receive and assimilate your experiences. Therefore, when you experience high-vibration emotions, the chakras absorb the benefits. When you experience adversity, each chakra operates like a hospital or healing ward charged to help you process the disharmonious vibrations analogous to its specialty and vocation. If you nourish and fortify your innate "medical staff" and teachers physically, emotionally, mentally, and spiritually with self-Reiki, Reiki, meditation, physical movement joining mind–body–spirit, and cleansing, you raise the vibration of your chakras and thus benefit from their resources, resilience, and wisdom.

Conversely, the chakras' efficiency can weaken over time if suppressed low-frequency emotions and vibrations, adversity, and/or trauma are extreme or persist. In other words, if the "medical staff" and teachers are inundated with trauma or low vibrations due to unwholesome activities, they become destabilized and less efficient. Often it is said that the chakras become blocked. This is a confusing descriptor because when a chakra's function is compromised, it becomes either explosive or implosive. The word *blocked* only speaks of implosive disharmony, not explosive disharmony. If a chakra's disharmony is explosive, it needs to be purged. If a chakra's disharmony is implosive, it needs to be nourished. With training and practice, Reiki practitioners sense this imbalance reliably and purge or nourish the chakra accordingly.

    a. When a chakra's disharmony is explosive, its energy is zingy and agitated with the flavour of disharmony opposite to its honourable vocation and specialty. Low-frequency emotions such as scornfulness, pomposity, aggression, overintellectualization, excessive talking, jealousy, arrogance, sexual addiction, or greed spew outward. The chakra needs to be quieted, soothed, and purged.

    b. Conversely, when a chakra is burdened by heavy, low-frequency emotions such as alienation, apathy, lack of imagination, shyness, self-doubt, powerlessness, or rigidity, it is said to be implosive. The chakra sinks inward and needs to receive energy—the chakra needs to be tonified and nourished.

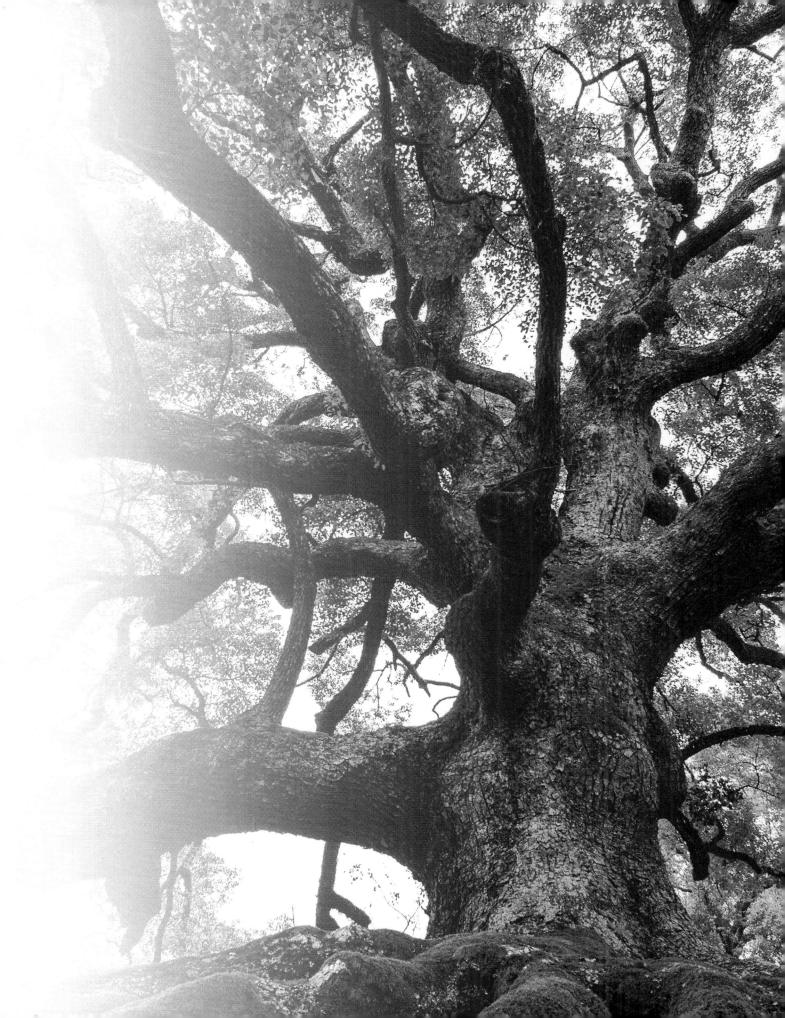

HARMONY IMPRINTS	EXPLOSIVE DISHARMONY	IMPLOSIVE DISHARMONY
·Celestial Yang Union	·Contempt	·Disorientation
·Spiritual Consciousness	·Distrust	·Meaninglessness
·Bliss	·Doubt	·Purposelessness
·Ecstasy	·Scornfulness	·Obedience/Submission
·Self-Knowledge	·Mockery	·Conservatism
·Grace	·Foregone Conclusions	·Sycophancy
·Open-Mindedness	·Influential Control	·Spiritual Bypassing
·Mindfulness	·Superiority	·Dissociation
·Devotion	·Spiritual Addiction	·Boredom
·Thoughtfulness	·Pomposity	·Cynicism
·Comprehension	·Overintellectualization	·Skepticism
·Serenity	·Illusion	·Incomprehension
·Archetypal Awareness	·Overintellectualization	·Insensitivity
·Self-Reflection	·Overrationalization	·Stubbornness
·Clear Perception	·Overauthorization	·Rigidness
·Intellectual Discrimination	·Inaccurate Perception	·Lack of Imagination
·Imagination	·Obsessions	·Indifference
·Intuition	·Delusions	·Denial
·Self-Expression	·Excessive Talking	·Fear of Speaking
·Creativity	·Gossip	·Shyness
·Clear Communication	·Loudmouthed	·Unclear Communication
·Good Listener	·Inability to Listen	·Lack of Creativity
·Discernment	·Refusal to Communicate	·Bafflement
·Enthusiasm	·Use of Silence to Control	·Disappointment
·Compassion	·Codependence	·Remoteness
·Unconditional Love	·Neediness	·Criticism
·Self-Love	·Demanding	·Intolerance
·Imagination	·Jealousy	·Selfishness
·Contentment	·Self-Sacrificing	·Insecurity
·Healthy Boundaries	·Poor Boundaries	·Lack of Sincerity

THE DISHARMONY IMPRINTS OF THE LOWER CHAKRAS

CHAKRA	HARMONY IMPRINTS	EXPLOSIVE DISHARMONY	IMPLOSIVE DISHARMONY
Third	·Dynamism ·Empowerment ·Reliability ·Self-Discipline ·Confidence ·Spontaneity/Playfulness	·Aggression ·Competition ·Confrontation ·Belligerence ·Arrogance ·Deceit/Manipulation	·Low Self-Esteem ·Shameful ·Victim Mentality ·Weak Will ·Unreliability ·Poor Self-Discipline
Second	·Healthy Bonds ·Nurturance/Empathy ·Enjoyment/Self-Control ·Sexual Health ·Creativity ·Willingness to Change	·Sexual Addiction ·Seductive Manipulation ·Obsessive Attachments ·Emotional Dependancy ·Martyrdom ·Poor Boundaries	·Lack of Desire ·Denial of Pleasure ·Fear of Sex ·Sexual Repression ·Inner Emptiness ·Excessive Boundaries
First	·Survival ·Group Acceptance ·Vitality ·Presence ·Right Livelihood ·Safety ·Stability	·Greed ·Hoarding ·Fatigue/Laziness ·Inertia ·Fear of Change ·Rigid Boundaries	·Fear or Chronic Fear ·Fear of Death ·Restlessness ·Poor Focus ·Chronic Disorganization ·Financial Difficulties
Earth Star	·Anchor in Mother Earth ·Earth Energy Purveyor ·Respect for the Earth ·Interdependence with All Living Beings ·Mystical Solidity ·Yin Footing	·Conventionality ·Predictability ·Routine/Habits ·Banality ·Imitation ·Forgery	·Avoidance ·Disinterest ·Alienation/Dejection ·Scarcity ·Passivity ·Freeloading

SIMULTANEOUS UPWARD AND DOWNWARD FLOW

Your Sacred Tree's central energy channel runs vertically in front of your spinal cord. Its life-affirming current connects to the earth via your Earth Star Chakra and to the sun via your Sun Star Chakra. The animation and collaboration of all nine primary chakras generate a brilliant crystalline column of white light flowing simultaneously to and from the sun, and to and from the earth. This meaningful, efficient, and simultaneous flow between all these teachers and allies encourages your spirit to flow upward from the earth to the sun to transcend the earth plane and soar toward universal oneness and, conversely, to flow downward from the sun to the earth to support your spirit's genius and manifestation on the earth plane.

a. When the upward flow (aptly named the "current of liberation" by Anodea Judith) doesn't get off the ground, you can be unconsciously or consciously stuck in routines and patterns, or constantly thrown back to survival issues, or feel trapped, powerless, victimized, or paralyzed. Hence, your growth and evolution toward compassionate and loving consciousness is hindered.

b. By contrast, when the downward flow (aptly named the "current of manifestation" by Anodea Judith) is impeded, you may become confused and aimless—without a sense of purpose or direction. Or you may fly high, dream big, and brim with ideas but are unable to make commitments or get the traction you need to carry seed ideas and inspiration to fruition and completion.

The union and harmonization of both currents is the foundation for your well-being and freedom. Therefore, the health, strength, or value of your Sacred Tree or chakra energy system is not contingent on climbing hierarchical echelons or a singular upward attainment of success. Your upper chakras are NOT more powerful or more important than your lower chakras. In other words, the sun/yang energy is NOT more important than the earth/yin energy, and your branches are NOT more important than your roots. Your life force must flow up and down through all the chakras simultaneously for you to experience both quintessential expressions of harmony: transcendence and fulfillment.

All your chakras are an integral part of your spirit-expanding and life-sustaining ecology. Each flavour of harmony built in to each chakra is a building block of life and love in action. If one chakra is excessive or deficient, hence blocked, your flow of liberation and manifestation is diminished. If many chakras are blocked, then the flow is thwarted. Thriving harmony and growth are the result of yang and yin in respectful, dynamic, and loving collaboration. A healthy chakra system exemplifies teamwork, universal respect, and harmony par excellence!

SELF-INQUIRY AND SELF-HEALING IN ACTION

I suggest that you use the chakra and dantian charts in this chapter to identify which harmonies and disharmonies describe your typical experience and state of being at this time. Create your own lists or charts to map out your current harmony and disharmony patterns.

If most of the harmonious vibrations you identified are in the same chakra, these innate healers are the most accessible guides on your journey right now. Inviting these specific high-frequency emotions into your self-Reiki and meditation practices stokes your evolutionary journey. Accordingly, the disharmonies you identified within these chakras or dantians are the most fluid and readily healable.

If most of the disharmonious vibrations you identified are excessive, then this chakra or dantian needs to be purged—you must release the excess energy. If most of the disharmonious vibrations you identified are deficient, then this chakra or dantian needs to be nourished—you must tonify this depleted chakra or dantian. Either way, purging your excessive chakra or dantian and/or nourishing your depleted chakra or dantian supports your besieged innate healers, thereby reactivating your powerful transformational and evolutionary matrix and self-healing capacity.

	SUN	SUN
CHAKRAS	**UPWARD LIBERATION FLOW:** From Earth to Sun	**DOWNWARD MANIFESTATION FLOW:** From Sun to Earth
Sun Star	·You transcend the ego and awaken to spiritual consciousness.	·You activate a contemplative state of mind in meditation, Nature, or other mindfulness practices to connect and invite inspiration.
Seventh	·You actively cultivate the spiritual dimension of your being. ·Your innate spiritual compass and other sagacious teachers inform and guide you.	·An inspiration stirs your spirit. ·You open-mindedly yet discerningly discover its relevance and alignment with your life purpose.
Sixth	·You acknowledge the power of your intuitive perception and innate spiritual guidance. ·You receive this wisdom and act upon it.	·The inspiration provokes your genius. ·The seed idea ferments while you discover and explore its relevance to your evolution.
Fifth	·You are discerning and your choices on the earth plane align with your spiritual curriculum.	·Your seed idea evolves into a project in a specific medium or form.
Fourth	·You tune in to the loving and compassionate teacher in your spiritual heart. ·You align with your true nature, which is hardwired for love and compassion.	·You fall in love with your project.
	EARTH	EARTH

	SUN	SUN
CHAKRAS	UPWARD LIBERATION FLOW: From Earth to Sun	DOWNWARD MANIFESTATION FLOW: From Sun to Earth
Third	·You shift your focus from how and why you relate to people around you to how you relate to and understand yourself.	·You kick into gear and do whatever is necessary to get ready for production.
Second	·You develop healthy bonds, relationships, and partnerships beyond or within the tribe (one on one) to satisfy personal and physical needs.	·You love what you do, and you do what you love.
First	·You situate yourself within your biological tribe, culture, and nation as well as with the traditional beliefs that come with this package. ·You develop a sense of belonging or not belonging, depending on what this context represents for you.	·Your work is presented and/or distributed.
Earth Star	·You are made of the earth, are nourished by the earth, and will return to the earth. ·You acknowledge the interdependence of all living beings and act accordingly.	·Your project serves as a catalyst for a new community and broader-reaching conservation and healing.
	EARTH	EARTH

DANTIANS

Ancient Daoist teachings describe three important energetic centres, the dantians, in the central energy channel located in your abdomen, heart, and head. They are important points of reference in Qigong, Tai Chi, martial arts, traditional Chinese medicine, and Daoist meditation. The Chinese word *dantian* is often translated as "elixir field" or "field of energy." While the life force energy enters your body through the first and seven chakras and circulates in the central energy channel, these powerful reservoirs collect energy, store it, and transform it before distributing it to all your organs, tissues, auras, and energetic bodies (physical, emotional, mental, and spiritual).

The **lower dantian** is the first and foundational cauldron for the liquid-like earthly ki. As such, it is the root of your Sacred Tree and invigorates your physical body and umbilical cord to the centre of the earth. It is also the epicentre of your gut feelings—the conduit for your physical body's intuition and messaging system. The formidable network of neurons in your gut–brain dantian are mercifully capable of sending and receiving impulses, recording experiences, and responding to emotions before the mind.

The **middle dantian** is your cauldron and reservoir for emotional and mental vibrations. As such, it is the trunk of your Sacred Tree and the epicentre of your heart consciousness and compass. It transforms the liquid-like earth energy of the lower dantian and the radiant light from the upper dantian into a steam-like energy. Hence, it regulates your mind–heart–earth connection and instigates and inspires mindful presence, empathy, order, and emotional and mental clarity.

The **upper dantian** is the funnel and reservoir for the radiant light from the sun. As such, it is the branches of your Sacred Tree and the epicentre of your spiritual awareness and interdependence with all living beings. The heavenly ki has a luminous, ethereal, vapour-like quality that balances and orients the energy of the three dantians.

DANTIANS AT A GLANCE

DANTIANS	LOWER DANTIAN	MIDDLE DANTIAN	UPPER DANTIAN
LOCATION	Abdomen	Chest	Head
ELEMENT	Earth	Fire	Light
CHAKRAS	First and Second	Third and Fourth	Fifth, Sixth, and Seventh
PHYSICAL AFFILIATION	·Vagina and Penis ·Uterus and Prostate ·Kidneys and Bladder ·Colon ·Small Intestine ·Spleen	·Heart ·Lungs ·Thymus Gland	·Brain ·Dural Membrane ·Cerebrospinal Fluid ·Bone Marrow
RESPONSIBILITY	·Reservoir for Earthly Ki and Reproductive Essence	·Reservoir for Mental/Emotional Vibrations	·Reservoir for Heavenly Ki
HARMONY	·Health ·Vitality ·Physical Stamina ·Personal Power ·Anchor in Earth ·Stability ·Gut Feelings	·Clarity ·Order ·Tranquility ·Inner Peace ·Serenity ·Empathy ·Emotional Awareness	·Compassion ·Unconditional Love ·Spiritual Orientation ·Devotion ·Psychic Perception ·Visions ·Intuition
DISHARMONY	·Feebleness ·Lethargy ·Powerlessness ·Purposelessness ·Instability ·Insecurity ·Fear	·Anxiety ·Shock ·Heartache ·Excessive Grief ·Suppression ·Numbness ·Dissociation	·Contempt ·Skepticism ·Cynicism ·Disorientation ·Misperception ·Pessimism ·Doubt

SPIRITUAL — UPPER DANTIAN

EMOTIONAL AND MENTAL — MIDDLE DANTIAN

PHYSICAL — LOWER DANTIAN

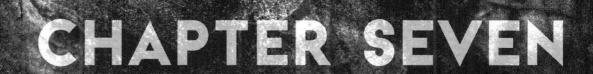

CHAPTER SEVEN

APPLYING REIKI PRACTICE FUNDAMENTALS

JOSHIN KOKYUU-HO BREATHING

The Japanese phrase *Joshin Kokyuu-Ho* means "breathing exercise to purify the spirit." Dr. Usui invites you to use this breathing exercise at the beginning of a treatment to ground yourself before entering the treatment room or during a session to magnify the strength of your connection to the earth when you encounter a block. You can also use it any time of the day to ground your energy on Reiki healing energy.

The Joshin Kokyuu-Ho breathing technique:

a. magnifies your connection to Reiki healing energy,

b. clears your central channel so you can be a more efficient conduit for ki energy,

c. teaches you to consciously draw in the energy from the cosmos and collect it in your lower dantian, and

d. reminds you that the energy does not belong to you but is simply the all-pervading life force coming through you.

The lower dantian is important for Reiki practice because it is the Sea of Qi, the reservoir of earth energy. It also activates your centre of gravity— the perfect place of balance. When open and charged, the lower dantian contributes immensely to feeling grounded and connected to the centre of the earth. To breathe into it activates the here-and-now orientation of the conscious mind, thereby helping you feel more calm, strong, and intuitive.

JOSHIN KOKYUU-HO BREATHING

STEP 1	Inhale through your nose and imagine drawing Reiki energy into your body through the crown chakra. Pull the energy down to your lower dantian, located two fingers below your navel.
STEP 2	When the breath reaches your lower dantian, keep it there for a few seconds without straining yourself. Find your own rhythm. Visualize this breath expanding and permeating your entire body.
STEP 3	Exhale through your mouth and imagine the energy flowing out through your fingerstips, the palm of your hands, the tip of your toes, and the soles of your feet.

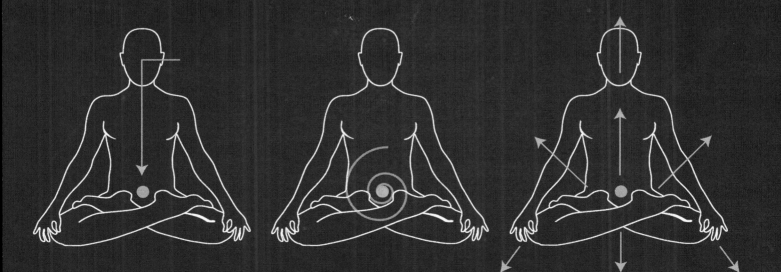

KENYOKU CLEANSING RITUAL

The Japanese word *Kenyoku* means "dry bathing." Dr. Usui invites you to use this cleansing technique before entering the treatment room and after sessions when the client has left.

The Kenyoku cleansing ritual:

a. brings you to the present moment,

b. strengthens your energy bodies,

c. purifies your physical, emotional, mental, and spiritual energy bodies, and

d. detaches the energy of clients, situations, thoughts, and emotions that do not serve the session.

KENYOKU CLEANSING RITUAL

STEP 1	Stand in a comfortable position, feet shoulder-width apart.
STEP 2	Place your right hand on the left side of your chest, over the collarbone. Now stroke down gently across the chest to the right hipbone. Do the same with your left hand, starting on the right side of your chest, over the collarbone. Stroke gently down toward your left hipbone. Repeat the motion with your right hand.
STEP 3	Place your right hand on your left shoulder and stroke down gently the outside of your left arm and the top of your left hand, past the fingertips. Do the same stroke with your left hand from your right shoulder over the outside of your right arm and the top of your right hand, past the fingertips. Repeat this motion once more with your right hand.
STEP 4	Do the same stroke with your left hand from the right shoulder over the inside of your right arm and palm, past the fingertips. Repeat the same motion with your right hand.

REIJI-HO OPENING PRAYER

The Japanese word *Reiji* means "indication of the spirit" or "indication of the Reiki energy." Dr. Usui invites you to do this prayer just before starting the session.

The Reiji-ho opening prayer:

a. opens your central channel like a hollow bamboo for the sacred energy to flow through,

b. activates your intuition,

c. helps you pay attention to intuitive messages, and

d. guides your hands and attention to where they are needed in the session.

REIJI-HO PRAYER

STEP 1	Sit or stand in a comfortable position and close your eyes.
STEP 2	Fold your hands in front of your heart and ask for the energy to flow through you freely.
STEP 3	Ask for the healing and well-being of your client on every level.
STEP 4	Bring your folded hands up to your third eye and ask Reiki to guide your hands to wherever they are needed.
STEP 5	Follow your hands and begin the treatment.

BYOSEN BODY SCAN

The Japanese word *byo* means "sick" and the word *sen* means "line." Dr. Usui invites you to begin the session with a full body scan. Take note of the areas you are called to and work on them in sequence during the session or keep information in mind while practising the introductory positions. While scanning the body, you may feel heat, magnetism, pressure, or just a deep knowing that you have found an ailing body part. You may also experience an uncomfortable feeling in your hand, which may move up your arm and sometimes even your shoulder. This sensation is called *hibiki*. Stay with it. Let the sensation trace back down your arm and out of your hand. This unpleasant register is caused by the dissonance of positive Reiki energy directed to a negatively charged body part.

BYOSEN BODY SCAN

STEP 1	Scan the front of the body in a slow downward movement along the centre line, holding your dominant hand an inch or two above the client's body, palm facing down. Keep your other hand on your own lower dantian.
STEP 2	Be sure to keep your hand at least six inches outside the client's energy as you draw it back to the head.

INTRODUCTORY HAND POSITIONS AND SEQUENCE

This formal sequence is traditionally taught in Reiki Level One. It involves a series of hand positions in a specific sequence embracing the entire body. When all parts of the body are covered evenly, by default you receive a harmonizing treatment. This specific sequence of hand positions acts like "training wheels" for practitioners who are beginning the practice of self-Reiki and Reiki. As you gain more experience, you can feel free to follow the intuitive information retrieved during the Reiji-ho prayer or Byosen body scan. I describe this more intuitive approach and treatment protocol in Level Two.

In general, hold all the fingers of each hand together, including your thumbs. This allows you to read energy more intensely and creates a clear and condensed signal for the body. The energy not only gets dissipated when your fingers are spread apart, but it may also increase the client's unease. For instance, it's far less likely to feel invasive if you explore the body with the heel of the hand with all fingers joined before you settle into a hand position than if you approach the body with your fingertips or with spread fingers.

☞ If you only have time for an abbreviated session, please include the following hand positions:

> 1 Biological Eyes, Sixth and Seventh Chakras
>
> 4 Rear aspect of Sixth Chakra, Seventh Chakra, Medulla Oblongata
>
> 9 Third Chakra
>
> 10 Biological Heart, Fourth Chakra, Lungs
>
> 12 Reproductive Organs, Small Intestine, Colon, Bladder, First and Second Chakras
>
> 13 Knees
>
> 14 Ankles
>
> 15 Feet, Earth Star Chakra

☞ If you only have ten minutes or if you feel really tired or upset, simply rest in Position 10: Biological Heart, Fourth Chakra, and Lungs.

INTRODUCTORY HAND POSITIONS AT A GLANCE

#	HAND POSITION	BODY
☞ 1	HANDS OVER EYES	Biological Eyes, Sixth and Seventh Chakras
2	HANDS OVER TEMPLES	Right and Left, Brain Hemispheres
3	HANDS OVER EARS	Ears
☞ 4	HANDS UNDER HEAD	Rear Aspect of Sixth Chakra (Third Eye), Seventh Chakra, Medulla Oblongata
5	HANDS OVER THROAT	Throat, Fifth Chakra
6	HANDS OVER LOW RIGHT RIB CAGE	Liver, Gallbladder
7	HANDS OVER LOW LEFT RIB CAGE	Spleen, Pancreas, Stomach
8	HANDS BELOW RIGHT RIB CAGE	Duodenum
☞ 9	HANDS OVER STERNUM	Third Chakra
☞ 10	HANDS OVER WHOLE CHEST	Biological Heart, Fourth Chakra, Lungs
11	HANDS BELOW LEFT AND RIGHT RIBS	Kidneys
☞ 12	HANDS IN A V OVER ABDOMEN	Reproductive Organs, Small Intestine, Colon, Bladder, First and Second Chakras
☞ 13	HANDS OVER AND UNDER KNEES	Knees
☞ 14	HANDS OVER ANKLES	Ankles
☞ 15	HANDS ON SOLES OF FEET	Feet, Earth Star Chakra
16	SMOOTH AURA	Whole Body

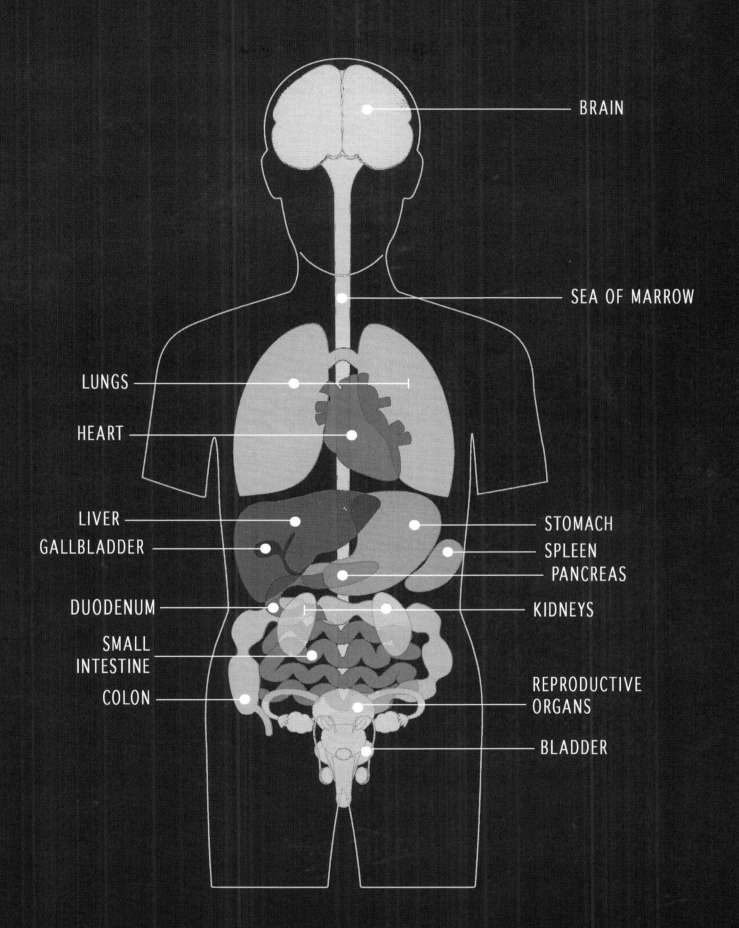

BRAIN

SEA OF MARROW

LUNGS

HEART

LIVER

GALLBLADDER

DUODENUM

SMALL
INTESTINE

COLON

STOMACH

SPLEEN

PANCREAS

KIDNEYS

REPRODUCTIVE
ORGANS

BLADDER

117

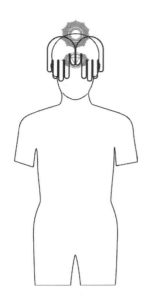

INTRODUCTORY HAND POSITIONS

☞ 1. BIOLOGICAL EYES, SIXTH CHAKRA, SEVENTH CHAKRA

Place the hands over the eyes to the right and left of the nose, from the forehead to above the mouth.
It strengthens the optimal functioning of the seventh chakra and sixth chakra—the third eye—which is an absolute precondition for intensive holistic healing.

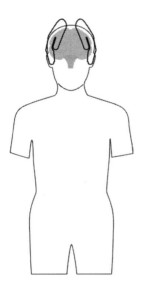

2. BRAIN HEMISPHERES

Cover the temples with the fingertips reaching to at least the cheekbones.
Balances the two brain hemispheres. Increases self-healing and healing capacity. Rekindles our vivid connection to our core self and spirituality.

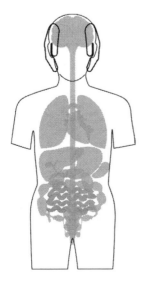

3. EARS

Cover the ears.
The outer ear has reflex zones and acupuncture points for practically every area of the body. Therefore, Reiki here awakens all organ systems and increases the body's ability to absorb Reiki energy.

☞ 4. REAR ASPECT OF SIXTH CHAKRA, SEVENTH CHAKRA, MEDULLA OBLONGATA

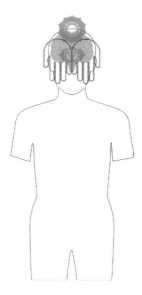

Slide the hands under the back of the head, and be sure to cover the centre of the back of the head.
Calibrates the rear aspect of the sixth and seventh chakras and the medulla oblongata located directly between the brain stem and the rest of the brain. This "reptile brain" is responsible for regulating survival bodily functions such as breathing, heart rate, and the flight–fight–freeze mechanism. Lacking language, its impulses are instinctual. Reiki here has a very relaxing effect. Many people "doze off" into a meditative state. Do not interrupt. Profound integration of suppressed emotions, narratives, and traumas can occur in the liminal state.

5. THROAT, FIFTH CHAKRA

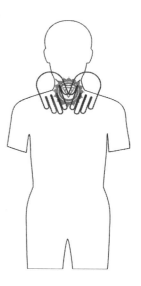

Hover hands approximately two inches above the throat.
Be sensitive and especially gentle here because it can easily feel uncomfortable or threatening when hands encircle the throat. At most, only allow the edge of your hands to rest on the jaw. Better yet, float an inch or so above the throat.

The throat chakra is the bridge between our spirit and this earth plane existence. Calibrating this centre increases our discernment and ability to align our choices with our spirit's goals.

6. LIVER, GALLBLADDER

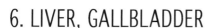

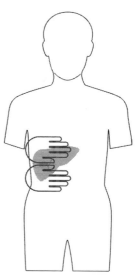

One hand covers the lower ribs on the right side above the navel, up to the centre of the body. The other hand is placed directly below the navel.
In traditional Chinese medicine (TCM), the liver is the mother of the heart; hence, it is the energy centre for the highest spiritual vibration: compassion. TCM doctors say that although the heart stores the spirit, it is the liver that can unbalance the spirit. In light of this, don't be shy about hanging out a long time with the liver and gallbladder.

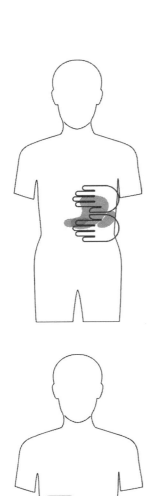

7. SPLEEN, PANCREAS, STOMACH

One hand covers the lower ribs on the left side above the navel, up to the centre of the body. The other hand is placed directly below the navel.

The spleen, pancreas, and stomach are the yin and yang organs of the earth orb. Considering the pandemic disconnection from yin and earth energy, it is most beneficial to recalibrate this triad.

Also, the spleen is the largest lymph node. Considering the prevalence of cancer at this time, it is especially relevant to increase the flow of the lymphatic system. The pancreas regulates blood sugar levels. Considering the scale of sugar addiction in most individuals, it is sound advice to assist this organ triad.

8. DUODENUM

Place hands below the rib cage on the right side.

The duodenum is the vital organ between the stomach and small intestine. Very few people even know they have one! Yet it distinguishes nutrients from waste and emotionally distinguishes truths from untruths. It is therefore the most efficient bullshit detector in our bodies. In my books, irritable bowel syndrome should be called "irritable duodenum syndrome."

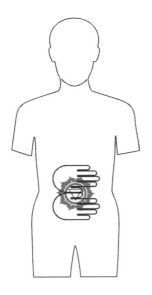

☞ 9. THIRD CHAKRA

The hands are placed above and below the navel on the centre line of the body.

Most of us are locked into a very excessive or very deficient imbalance here. It is essential to unwind the persistent patterns of overachieving or underachieving. With foes such as aggression and competition, or shame and a weak will, we are virtually sure to have some serious work to do here.

10. BIOLOGICAL HEART, FOURTH CHAKRA, LUNGS

One hand is placed on the upper chest horizontally and the other vertically on the heart area between the breasts. Include this hand position in all sessions. The biological heart on the left of the chest, the spiritual heart and fourth chakra in the centre of the chest, and the lungs are often accessed by only one hand position because we frequently work around clients' breasts and their choice of bra. Place your hands, with all fingers joined wherever you can, to respect the client's comfort and safety.

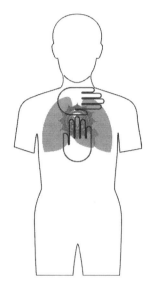

Take your time! This is Grand Central Station. Reiki on both hearts nurtures our healthy "yes" and healthy "no." It promotes self-love as well as our capacity to become devoted to tasks and other people. Reiki on the lungs releases suppressed and stored grief. We are perennially isolated when it comes to processing our grief in modern society. It is my sense that we suffer the most from the absence of communal grieving rituals more than any other rituals built in to indigenous cultures and harmonious communal living.

11. KIDNEYS

Place hands horizontally on the lower right and left ribs (at the height of the kidneys) so that two fingers rest beneath the ribs. Include this hand position in all sessions. The kidneys habitually store unacknowledged memories of fearful experiences and adversity. The charge of these emotions and toxins is like icy water congealed in these organs. Dr. Usui recommends that you treat the kidneys for at least fifteen minutes if there has been any kind of poisoning or shock.

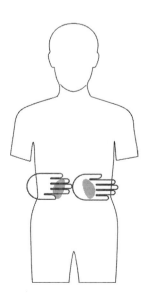

Also, in light of systemic caffeine and sugar addiction, these overstimulated and fatigued glands (due to adversity and excessive chemical stimulation) often hit a wall sooner rather than later. Reiki here can deactivate the flight–fight–freeze response. Although withdrawal from stress hormones can cause sensations of bone-deep fatigue, it is an opportunity for a new, healthier hormonal equilibrium to emerge.

It takes time for the whole being to shift into a sustainable hormonal ecology focused on evolution and thriving rather than survival.

☞ 12. REPRODUCTIVE ORGANS, SMALL INTESTINE, COLON, BLADDER, FIRST CHAKRA, SECOND CHAKRA

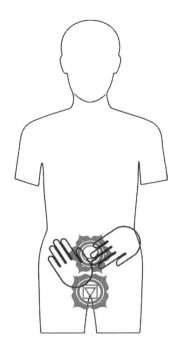

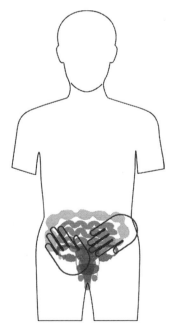

Hands are placed in a V, reaching the top of the pubic bone.

Do not approach the pubic bone with the tips of your fingers. This touch can feel threatening. Establish your position with the heel of your hands.

Reiki here is like having an area code access rather than a specific phone number. Once you make a connection, decipher which organs are signalling for attention, then shift your hand position accordingly. For instance, if called to work on the small intestine, shift your hands to the upper centre of the abdomen; if called to work on the uterus or bladder, shift your hands to the centre just above the pubic bone; or if called to the ovaries or colon, shift your hands to either side of the centre.

The intestines and colon can easily become congested with yeast, bacteria, parasites, and rotting fecal matter. Dr. Usui recommends placing your hands on the two upper corners of the colon to facilitate elimination and detoxification, and placing a hand on the centre of the abdomen to stimulate the small intestine.

Be extra respectful, gentle, and mindful of this minefield of suffering in light of the patriarchal and sexist biases that women have endured for centuries. Take into account the likelihood of stirring sexual trauma and other intensity such as birthing, infertility, miscarriages, and abortions, to name a few.

Virtually every low-vibration emotion and most news media and entertainment pull us away from our earth mother's abundant gifts and life-sustaining rhythm. We are distracted and unplugged at best and careless and self-centred at worse. Reiki here rebuilds our foundation and roots, hence increasing our receptivity to healing, transformation, and wholesome interdependence.

☞ ## 13. KNEES

Place both hands on the front and back of one knee and then on the other.

Energy easily becomes congested in large joints. It is very important to clear the knees to augment receptivity to earth energy.

☞ ## 14. ANKLES

Wrap both hands around one ankle and then the other.

The next largest joints on the way to the feet also need to be cleared to ensure grounding. Moreover, the ankles house secondary chakras responsible for our ability to create the conditions of personal survival, means of support, security, and well-being under unusual or quickly changing circumstances—literally, the capacity to think on our feet.

☞ ## 15. FEET, EARTH STAR CHAKRA

Place each hand on the sole of each foot from the toes to the middle area. Be sure to cover the big toes.

It is essential for grounding and concluding the session. It is necessary to strengthen the connection to the centre of the earth. Grounding not only balances the energy flow within the body but also harmonizes and strengthens the aura and the Earth Star and first chakra.

16. SMOOTHING AURA

Smooth the aura at least three times by sweeping hands along the entire body from head to feet.

Ask if the client feels well and has a clear head. If this is not the case, treat the knees, ankles, and feet one more time to ensure that the client is grounded. Then smooth the aura again.

REIKI PLUS PLUS
LEVEL TWO

CHAPTER EIGHT

UNDERSTANDING THE
REIKI SYMBOLS AND MANTRAS

INVOKING THE ENERGY WITH THE REIKI SYMBOLS

In general, one of the key features of Reiki Level Two training is the introduction of three of the five sacred Reiki symbols. While the master symbol is studied in Level Three, you implement the attunement symbol in Level Four Teacher Training. In light of this, you can skip this chapter if you are attuned to Level One only. Traditionally, you wait until you have received a Level Two attunement to work with and activate the various symbols and mantras consciously and specifically.

The traditional symbols and mantras used in Reiki are sacred representations and mantras embodying the Reiki healing energy. When invoked during a meditation or a session, they intensify the potency and specificity of the transmission. Although the practitioner's hands focus the energy on specific areas of the body, client, animal, plant, or crystal, invoking the symbols heightens the flow of the universal life force and directs the energy to specifically clear physical, emotional, mental, and/or spiritual blocks.

The symbols are also training aids to increase your vibration, learn how to direct the energy to the various levels, strengthen your capacity to transmit, and improve your intuition. They are powerful tools to help you integrate the Reiki healing and spiritual vibration into your being. It is essential to develop a personal practice with the symbols and/or mantras to increasingly perceive, experience, and embody their qualities. Knowledge of their technical function alone is not sufficient. The goal is to learn the right quality of attention and to experience the frequency that the symbols and mantras activate. Once these vibrations and energy signatures are integrated, they are activated whether you actively use the symbols and mantras or not.

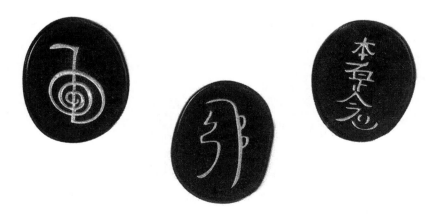

Conventionally, Reiki students and practitioners focus on the visual symbols in their meditation, personal practice, and sessions. To become familiar with each symbol, I recommend that you mindfully draw each shape over and over again, as many times as is necessary to absorb each pattern. If a symbol is drawn incorrectly, do not cross it out or improve it; instead, simply start over. Once you are familiar with each symbol, I recommend that you use your index finger to draw the symbols on your palms before or after your daily meditation practice. During a session, you can visualize the symbol in your mind's eye or draw the symbol with your hand in the air over the client's body.

Although it is less common, it is also possible to chant the Reiki mantras to activate the symbol's power. This is the method I tend to choose in sessions and attunements. Many authors deduce that Dr. Usui chanted the Reiki mantras in the same way he used mantras for achieving spiritual harmony and inner peace as a practising Buddhist. The word *mantra* divides into two parts: *man*, which means "mind," and *tra*, which means "transport or vehicle." Reiki mantras, like Buddhist mantras, are powerful sounds or vibrations. When spoken or chanted often, they focus your mind and open your channel to the specific vibrational field of the mantra.

In several spiritual disciplines, it is recommended that you chant mantras 108 times a day for 40 consecutive days to embody and imprint their vibration. After receiving Level Two attunement, I recommend that you start with chanting the first symbol, Cho-Ku-Rei, for 40 consecutive days, then move on to the second symbol, Sei-He-Ki, and complete the sequence with the third, Hon-Sha-Ze-Sho-Nen. After receiving Level Three attunement, you can chant the master symbol, Dy-Kyo-Myo. You can keep count by using a mala (Buddhist prayer beads), a circular string of 108 beads with the 109th bead (called the "Guru Bead") hanging perpendicular to the counting beads. Traditionally, the mala is held resting over the third finger of the right hand, and the beads are brought toward you, one by one, using the thumb. Each bead counts one repetition of the mantra. If you want to chant a second cycle, do not cross over the Guru Bead. Turn around and count the beads all the way back. Then you turn around again if you want to chant a third cycle. It is said that if you never cross the Guru Bead and never count it as a normal bead, it symbolizes the infinity of the spiritual practice.

CHO-KU-REI (CR)

FIRE SYMBOL & MANTRA

"Increase power of Reiki energy now!"
"Focus Reiki energy more intensely in this place!"

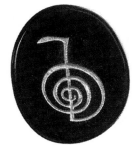

Concentrating on Cho-Ku-Rei:

- Intensifies the flow of Reiki energy. Known as the "light switch," this symbol can be used several times in a treatment to increase the power of the transmission.

- Awakens the spiritual essence of every being or object.

- Focuses the healing energy on issues related to physical reality, the element of yin, and earth ki such as physical health, physical health regimens, and financial issues.

- Concentrates the energy. The counterclockwise direction in which the symbol is drawn focuses the Reiki energy in a specific place. It can be used several times in a treatment to direct the energy to specific locations on the body.

- Increases the power of the other symbols and mantras.

SEI-HE-KI (SHK)

WATER SYMBOL & MANTRA

"Focus the Reiki energy on the emotional and mental bodies now!"

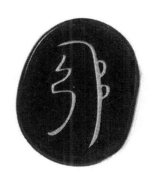

Concentrating on Sei-He-Ki:

- Focuses the healing energy on issues related to the mind, the element of yang, and heavenly ki such as emotions, feelings, beliefs, habits, and attachments.

- Facilitates the release of old, stored emotions, thereby releasing the emotional sources of physical illness. You may use SHK repeatedly in sessions. For instance, draw this symbol on the crown chakra at the start of the healing if you know that emotional issues are front and centre, use it to promote calm if the recipient is upset and distraught or, conversely, if the recipient is attempting to release emotions but can't seem to speak or cry.

- Dissolves disharmonious, unwelcome, and unsupportive thought patterns as well as out-of-date belief systems in the subconscious. It simultaneously supports the process of updating perceptions, strategies, and belief systems.

- Aligns the upper chakras. It escalates your spiritual development, thereby increasing the flexibility and vitality with which you approach situations and adversity. It also protects you from the loss of heart consciousness through attachment to the material world.

- Supports the growth and flow of love and compassion. SHK helps you develop a deeper understanding of the spiritual heart. You learn how to be with yourself in the here and now as well as experience yourself and others with a more open heart.

HON-SHA-ZE-SHO-NEN (HS)

ETHER SYMBOL & MANTRA

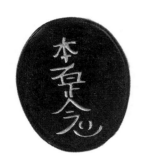

"The Buddha within me connects with the Buddha within you now!"

Concentrating on Hon-Sha-Ze-Sho-Nen:

- Awakens you to the spiritual interconnection between the seemingly disparate material and immaterial realms of experience.

- Connects you to light energy and heart consciousness, that is, your ability to extend your mind beyond the boundaries of time and space. It charts the pathway for energy and information to travel through space, allowing you to connect with spirit guides in other dimensions and human beings in other locations. As such, it is the primary symbol used for distance or absentee healing.

- Encourages a progressive expansion of consciousness, thereby broadening possibilities. The HS symbol is the next step in the journey after working with the SHK symbol to clear emotions and belief systems on the subconscious level that thwart growth.

- Bolsters your fortitude to embrace the spiritual goal of producing wholesome karma despite adversity. It boosts your resolve and resilience when faced with the daunting option to succumb to or transcend the cycle of violence. All perpetrators were victims, yet not all victims need be perpetrators. HS helps us focus your energy to transcend the cycle of adversity by not hurting others no matter what was/is done to you.

- Focuses the conscious mind and energy on new choices and actions. It increases mindfulness, commitment, and effectiveness.

CHO-KU-REI

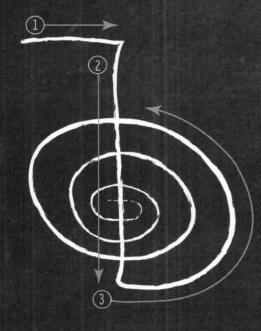

HON-SHA-ZE-SHO-NEN

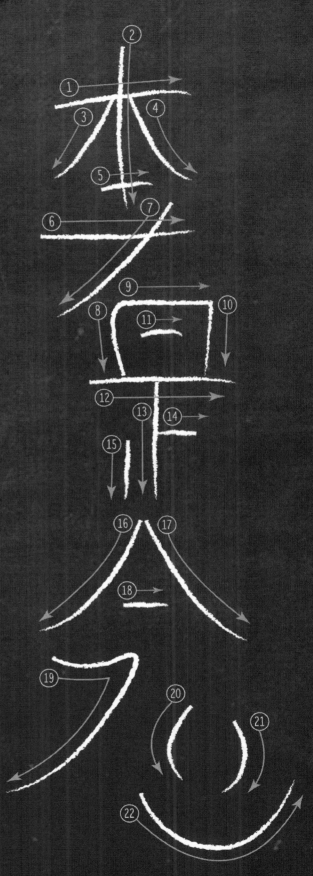

SEI-HE-KI

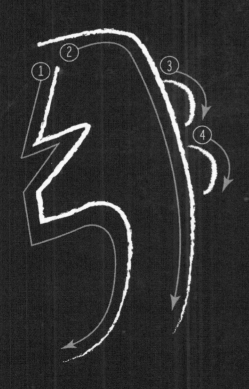

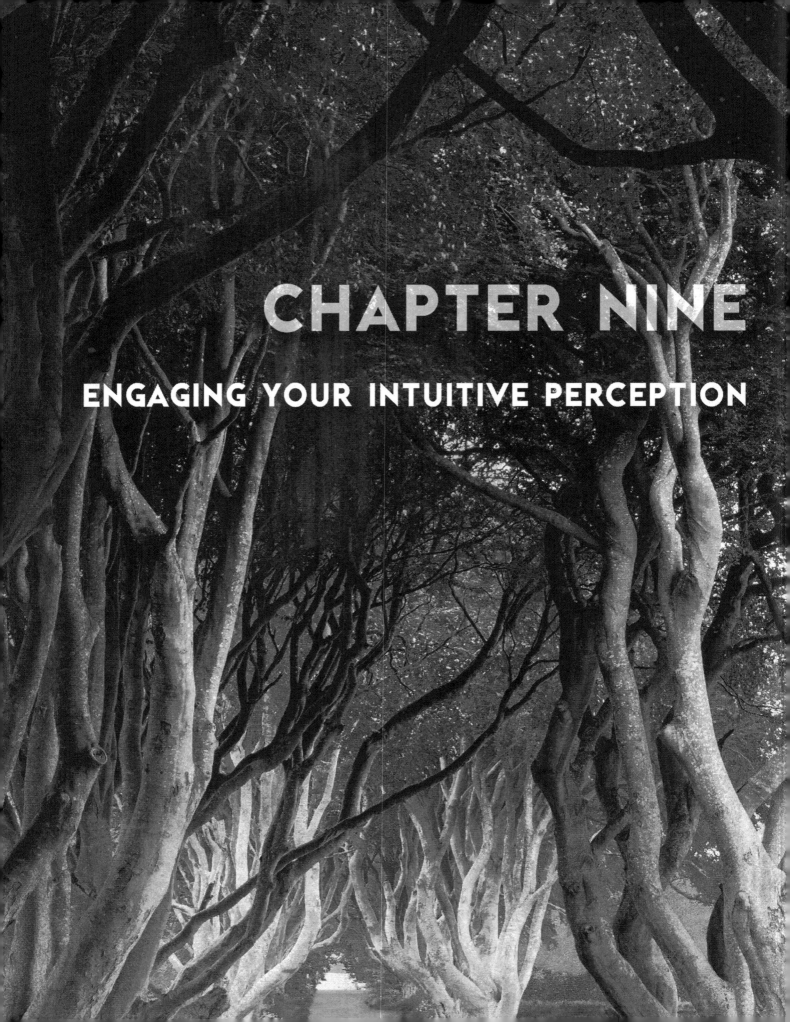

CHAPTER NINE
ENGAGING YOUR INTUITIVE PERCEPTION

CONVERSING ON A SPIRIT LEVEL

Intuitive perception—whether it's clairsentience, clairvoyance, clairaudience, or claircognizance—is not a unique gift. Each of these is an innate ability that I and many others have reawakened. You can intuitively and compassionately *sense* (clairsentience), *see* (clairvoyance), *hear* (clairaudience), and *know* (claircognizance), sometimes all at once or in various increments depending on the day or situation. Hence, you have the innate ability to lovingly and compassionately witness the ravages of violence, unlove, and isolation in yourself and in others.

So many friends, students, and clients have asked me, "How does it work?" "What is it like?" or "What the hell are you doing?" that you would think I have a pat answer by now, but I don't. Let me try to express in words the formless experience behind my closed eyelids and in my heart. After placing my hands on a client's shins, I help settle their energetic patterns into an interdependent flow with the earth's field as well as with the sun's. In other words, I remind the client's fields of their Sacred Tree-ness and capacity to be in harmony with the earth and the sun, love and compassion. Once the client has softened into this fundamental flow, their innate Sacred Tree wisdom comes to the foreground rather than the usual, everyday brain, intellectual brain, monkey brain, worry-bunny brain, or totally traumatized brain—or whatever part of themselves that runs the show rather than their core self. They essentially soften into a meditative state: their breathing deepens and their anxiety and distractions quieten.

Once the client has softened into the field of love and compassion, and I with them, their self-healing wisdom can reach me and mine can reach them. In other words, we engage in a blessed form of communication: we enter into a conversation on a "spirit level." Although the client makes the effort to come in for the session through snow, rain, or strained bank accounts, their spirit floats in knowing exactly why they are here and what the next item is on their self-healing agenda. With love and compassion working much like a crystal in a radio, the client's wisdom speaks up and out past the usual static, and my third eye then begins to receive and interpret the data expressed by the client's core self and inner wisdom.

Most of the time, I experience a mix of *sensing, seeing, hearing,* and *knowing,* more or less all at once. For example, when working with a client processing a traumatic experience, I may *see* only a face and *sense* a motherly presence or role, whether caregiving or not, whether biological mother or not. Then I might *see* the space where the given event is occurring. I might *see* a fridge and the corner of a kitchen counter or an expanse of mangled grass with a fence in the distance. I then *sense* whether we are in the client's childhood home or at school or wherever. The third download might be of the figure in movement. By the quality of the movement, I *sense* violence, rage, impatience, or simply a gesture communicating unlove. I may *hear* a voice sounding like the teacher in the Charlie Brown animation. Sometimes I *hear* words and sentences, but mostly I simply *know* the meaning of what is being said. The tone comes through loud and clear. This is most helpful when the scenes are unfolding in a language foreign to me. Then I might *sense* a wrenching pain in my right shoulder. I recognize that this sensation is not my own, that this is the client's experience. I learn and receive what it feels like to be yanked by one arm and dragged by their mother in the kitchen or by a bully in the schoolyard. I might also sense sadness, dejection, numbness, and fear. I learn and receive the emotions the client felt in these circumstances. I witness what it feels like to be them in that specific moment.

The gift is not in my senses, eyes, ears, or brain, nor is it in yours; love and compassion is simply our innate potential and true self in alignment with the life force and our life purpose. Hence, compassionate witnessing is our natural and fundamental state of being. This is the biggest irony of all: the thing we are most often frightened of is love in action and the compassionate witnessing of love in action. It is love itself that we *sense, see, hear,* and *know.* But we don't always like—in fact, we mostly don't like—what love has to show, say, or share.

For a long time, the love running through my life was the voice that expressed the truth about my childhood experiences with my abusive grandfather, father, and mother. In that sense, love made me scream, cry, and tremble with horror. Often, we silence the voice of love because we decide that love is happiness and should be, well, "happy." We distort and reduce happiness to a happy pill akin to a shot of cocaine (or whatever your fave is) that makes everything go away, while happiness is quite the opposite: it is a shot of everything that is, in all its wondrous mystery, without censorship or an overriding judgment deciding what is good or bad, "happy" or sad.

CLAIRSENTIENCE: SENSING

In the past ten years of teaching, I have found that all students access clairsentience, the kinesthetic intuitive language, within a few days of training. It's a little sneaky though because the information comes to you in the form of sensations in your own body. For example, your upper back suddenly feels tight or tingly or you suddenly feel nauseous and headachy. The key word is *suddenly*. You felt fine a minute ago but suddenly you are not so comfortable, or grounded, or clear-headed. The key is to realize quickly that these are not your feelings or sensations but those belonging to the client. If you do not attach to these sensations and remain clear that your body is now expressing your client's stuckness and dis-ease, pain and discomfort do not develop or take hold in your body. The sensations remain in the realm of perceptions. They are the kinesthetic language in action.

It is crucial to cultivate a clear distinction between empathy and compassionate witnessing. If you latch on to the sensations and carry them for the client, you are responding empathically; you literally feel what the client is feeling. Your vibration therefore lowers to match theirs; for example, you, too, sink into despair. When you compassionately witness, you sense what the other is feeling while still vibrating at the high frequencies of love; you don't literally feel or carry the other's sensations and thereby join them on their lower frequency. It is vital to maintain a healthy, vibrant, and clear channel for the higher vibrations (I will elaborate more on the daily practices that support this later) to be assured that you are compassionately witnessing rather than empathically taking on the burden of another's suffering.

It works like magic if the encounter is fully embraced by the practitioner and the client alike. You must both fully engage in your soul's purpose to heal, and when you do, the sensations are imprinted with your clear intention. On the other hand, if the client is not truly embracing the opportunity to take in the full extent of the experiences that surface during the session, then you can become burdened with their trauma. If they are not pulling their weight, so to speak, it requires more vigilance. In my experience, this situation most often comes up when the client is offered the session for free by a family member, friend, or me. The financial commitment mostly symbolizes a conscious decision to engage in transformative action. It's an effort to pay, and with it

INUITIVE PERCEPTION AT A GLANCE

CLAIRSENTIENCE	CLAIRVOYANCE	CLAIRAUDIENCE	CLAIRCOGNIZANCE
Sensing	Seeing	Hearing	Knowing

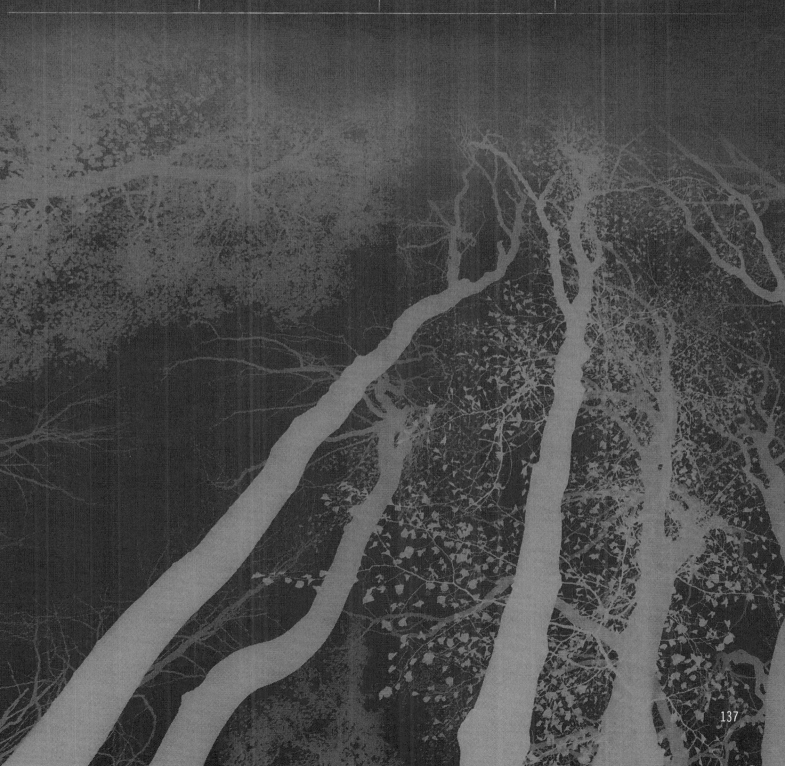

comes a willingness to make the effort required to open up to self-healing. With a freebie, there is often the erroneous notion that you, the practitioner, are doing the healing when in fact you are simply a guide to the client's own source of self-healing, wellness, and wisdom. It is essential that you both commit to the contract. If you don't, the session is a simple fluff-and-buff, feel-good temporary relaxation experience for them and an energy drain on you.

When you develop kinesthetic compassionate witnessing, your body sensations and emotions become progressively more suspended during sessions. Eventually, your body even shuts down symptoms like a runny nose or unsettled bowels when the first client enters your office in the morning. I've had to literally run for the Kleenex box or the washroom the minute the last client is out the door. To your detriment, you are "magically" exactly where you left off before sessions. This is most useful on days when you are experiencing personal or professional challenges. Emotions are put on hold, your service takes the front seat, and your potentially distracting turmoil takes the back seat.

This works well especially if you are "on your game," meaning if you have rested, meditated and practised yoga, eaten well, and have avoided caffeine, chocolate, and sugar. By contrast, if you do not adequately prepare for sessions and the ocean is murky and agitated, it will remain so in the session. It's paramount to acknowledge that unlike a dissociative state, being in "kinesthetic service mode" is about being very present, grounded, and in your body. Clairsentience, after all, manifests in your body. You have to be in it to receive the messages. It's only by supporting your well-being that your whole body can serve as sensitive, perceptive, and precise antennae that will guide your healing sessions despite surface turbulence.

A felt-sense is more than enough. Work with it! Waiting for the big visuals is a trap you can easily fall into. Gold mines of information thus remain untapped.

CLAIRVOYANCE: SEEING

Although the three other intuitive languages—whether it be images, language, or thoughts—are less easily accessed and developed, they are somewhat simpler to focus on and decode. Basically, once these three innate channels of communication are reopened, it's more straightforward: you "see" or you "hear" and/or you "suddenly understand." The information comes barrelling through a funnel—you don't have to look through your whole body. And it's easier to recognize an image, message, or download as external and not yours.

Truth, however, can present itself in vague visual images or no image at all. For example, if the victim's eyes were closed or the abuse took place in a dark room, there is literally no movie for anyone to see, even if you consider yourself clairvoyant. There is no third-person point of view or special lighting conditions that amplify your ability to *see* in the dark. You both, client and practitioner, drop into the situation as it was, *seeing* what was literally seen or looked at.

How baffling visual clues can sometimes be is best exemplified by one particular client's sessions. Every time I dropped into her experience of being violated the first time she was penetrated, I saw blue. I asked my client if the walls were blue in the room where she first had intercourse. "It was in my bedroom. It wasn't painted blue." To make things more complex, my client perceived her first experience as perhaps not ideal but nonetheless a loving encounter with her much older boyfriend. My *sense* that a violation occurred the first time she "made love" failed to diminish even if the mysterious blueness I perceived seemingly did not fit. We looked at other relationships to find violation and could not.

Months later and many sessions later, we dropped into the same scene. This time, my client was open to *sensing* that her first experience at fourteen years old was indeed far from ideal when suddenly she exclaimed: "Oh my God, I was staring at the world map pinned on my bedroom wall. I was obsessed with the Caribbean Sea. I dreamt of escaping to that sunny paradise one day." That small papery expanse of blue and its promise of happiness in paradise pervaded her vision and helped her distort her perception of her first sexual encounter. All she and I could *see* was that tiny blue portal of hope out of her stark reality. First, she had dissociated, and, second, she had created a fantasy, holding on to this perception to protect herself from the sordid truth that she was not ready or willing that afternoon to go "all the way." "My boyfriend made the decision for me! Oh my God, I was a cruise ship director for ten years! I was numb with 'happiness' on the blue seas. It was my job to be 'happy' and make sure everyone else was 'happy.' I ran away from myself and worked around the clock to forget my truth and make my dreams a reality. You have no idea! It's 24/7 on cruise ships."

Be patient. A fleeting image, colour, or shape is enough. Don't wait for the big production movie with great shots and lighting. Soften into the poetic and emotional dimension of the visual presenting itself. Let the plot unfold!

*Fear can be a huge hurdle.
Meditate, dance, practise yoga, or do
whatever you know will reunite you with
love and compassion.*

CLAIRAUDIENCE: HEARING

Aside from learning to settle into a meditative state, you need to cultivate trust before your intuitive perception flows. You may crash into the many walls erected by overbearing parents and caregivers, dogma, popular culture, language, left-brain dominance, and whatever else before *sensing, seeing,* and *hearing* clearly. There is lots of gunk out there, and it has been dumped again and again on your precious intuitive antennae. For example, a student who mostly *hears* just like I mostly *see* had to learn how to hear, listen, and trust his high self and guides first. It is only when he could embrace the guidance and teachings within himself that he could harness his skill to *hear, listen,* and share when practising Reiki Plus Plus on someone else.

This student had to learn that the most trustworthy guidance comes from within, not from authority figures, family, friends, colleagues, teachers, doctors, or whomever. For instance, he remembered that he used to hear and talk to ghost-like angels in his childhood bedroom without fear. It was only after his family and church referred to these entities as evil-doers that he became afraid of these whispering visitations and did everything he could to shut them down. He had to unlearn his family's Christian dogma. His panic was amplified when he watched a few scary movies about ghosts. He also had to reframe popular culture's chronic distortion—through the lens of fear rather than love—of life's mysteries and the hereafter.

To make matters worse, he also often asked his siblings if they could hear them too, and when he repeatedly received "You're crazy!" as a response, it only escalated his efforts to ban the devil from his bedroom so he wouldn't be crazy as well as evil. Poor little guy, he prayed fervently to be normal, pure, and sane—in other words, deaf to all wise whisperings. His core self and inner wisdom were of course patient enough to stick around until he could soften into their embrace and love. He now knows, most of the time, that he has reopened his channels to his intuitive wisdom, not some crazy-ass scary and perhaps evil energy.

CLAIRCOGNIZANCE: KNOWING

I often refer to this experience of *instant knowing* as a thought blog or download. A huge amount of complex information involving all levels of the human experience (physical, emotional, mental, and spiritual) suddenly appears fully formed, organized, and accessible in your consciousness. Claircognizance basically entails a swift access and knowing in an instant or a few minutes. A clear example of a massive download stands out for me. Late one drizzly night in Toronto, my partner and I head out to a music event at Lee's Palace on Bloor Street West. Even though it's not my thing to be out late anymore, I am pumped because this ten-piece band, unknown to me until then, combines contemporary beats with Mexican mariachi instrumentation and phrasing. I'm crazy about multiple trumpets passionately shrieking, especially mariachi-style. Well, it sure was worth the wet late-night trek. By 1 a.m., the four trumpets blast the first six notes of their grand finale "solo" and a portal opens. My great-aunt's voice soars in above the notes and delivers a passionate and particularly involved message.

In the space of—What? Four minutes? How long can a trumpet quartet solo be?—*ma tante* Blanche did nothing less than download a most prescient plot on a very touchy topic: she quite unexpectedly instructed me how to come out to my mother the very next day. Like, what? Within a few minutes she essentially laid out the why and the how of this entire operation. She was loud, louder than four trumpets remember, and clear that I had to call my mother tomorrow and reveal the depth of my relationship with my partner, its history, my history, and my joy. My partner and I glide to a Kinko's copy centre a few blocks east on Bloor, she on a wave of ecstatic rhythms and I on the sheer intensity of my aunt's blaring announcement. Despite the store's harsh fluorescent lighting and the usual mayhem of getting blueprints printed out, I hold on to the new scenario and succinctly let my partner in on what just happened and what's happening tomorrow. I then adhere to silence in order to hold on to the emotional experience and the subtleties of my aunt's message.

Let's face it: I have a mere twelve hours to integrate the wisdom of my aunt's memo and trust the plot enough to go ahead with something I have delayed and avoided for close to twelve years. Yet not a bone in my body puts on the brakes. I change my schedule, barely sleep, and devote my heart and mind to the task. At 3 p.m. a huge dragonfly hovers above my slumped body in my deck chair. "It's time," she signals! I dial my mother's number, she answers, and it takes me more than one and a half hours to speak the truth in my heart in the form my aunt laid out. I wish I had a recording. My aunt had definitely created one of the best monologues of all time. My mother laughed, she cried, and most importantly she listened and heard, not usually one of her strong points. Who knows what all was going on for her at this juncture, but my aunt cleverly perceived our mutual openness to truth, respect, and love on that specific day.

Be open at all times!
You need not be in meditation, the temple, or in a Reiki Plus Plus or self-Reiki session. Intuitive perception is active and heightened awareness moment to moment. It's nothing less and nothing more than love and compassion on all levels: physical, emotional, mental, and spiritual.

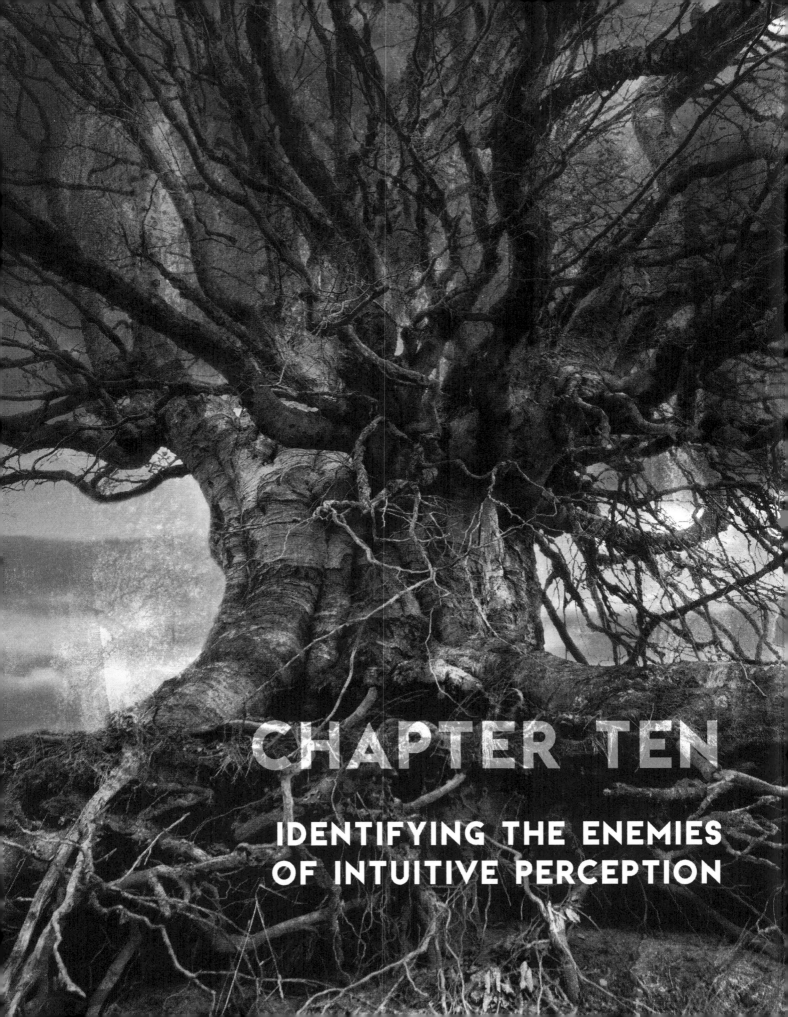

CHAPTER TEN

IDENTIFYING THE ENEMIES OF INTUITIVE PERCEPTION

DENIAL AND SELF-LOATHING

Long before *ma tante* Blanche tapped me on the shoulder, I was shaking off the crusty remains of my victimization and messy survival—and with them denial and self-loathing. I had to start by remembering, in other words *sense, see, hear,* and *know,* enough of my abusive past to dismantle my denial—enemy number one of my third eye and intuitive perception. I fumbled and fell yet moved closer to unconditional love and compassion every time I focused and cleared another layer of lies and confusion. Although forgetting and denial is sometimes absolutely essential for your survival, in time, when you recover enough of your truth, you also unearth your most essential and valuable innate intuition and wisdom. It is with consistent practice and focus that you incrementally stop rejecting and judging yourself and start loving yourself, no matter what the hell you were doing or no matter what was being done to you. You thus gain clearer and clearer intuitive perception.

Compassion in action starts with compassionately witnessing yourself without restraint, fear, judgment, criticism, or the itty bitty shitty committee.

LOOKING OUTWARD RATHER THAN INWARD

Another block to developing heightened perception that I perceive in almost all my students is their anxious preoccupation with learning how to intuitively perceive in others, as though they are trying to learn to see through skin and bones. The key to amplified compassionate perception is to recognize that there is nothing out there to *sense, see, hear,* and *know.* Everything you really need to intuitively perceive is within yourself. By opening up to the act of witnessing yourself in all your horror and so-called fuck-ups, you tap into your innate ability to intuitively *sense, see, hear,* and *know.* And we are back at enemy number one: denial and self-loathing.

I, too, used to believe that to *sense, see, hear,* and *know* was to intuitively perceive something outside, implying that I could see through skin and brain cells or what have you. Yet the wall you learn to see through is still within yourself; it is the wall of day-to-day consciousness, denial, and lack of compassion. When clients exclaim, "How do you know that?" and then under their breath claim that I am psychic or just plain weird but they respect me anyway, they are missing one crucial piece of the puzzle: I am still looking in the same place, whether with a client or in a self-healing session. I am not *sensing, seeing, hearing,* and *knowing* them; I am perceiving their experience and witnessing it within my third eye. I am doing the same thing I did in the bath for years and now practise on my meditation cushion.

First, you learn to do it within yourself and for yourself. Then, you practise compassionate witnessing on command. Eventually, you're simply plugged in whether alone or with a client.

LOOKING FOR PROOF

The third most significant block to intuitive perception I witness in my clients and students is their focus on getting big visuals. Most expect wisdom and traumatic pasts to present themselves as nothing short of a film with full production values that rolls before both biological eyes and the third eye. But memories and wisdom are not attended to by a film crew who captured the event from the outside. "Proof" and truth are not found in big visuals only. Awareness blossoms when you compassionately witness the emotions and whatever sensory information is presenting itself without stubbornly waiting for the proof and truth to present themselves as footage you could conveniently show in a courtroom. Relying only on big visuals is a waste of valuable information, healing energy, and time!

When you settle into inner truth rather than proof, you can cultivate a more responsive and fluid relationship with the wisdom that intuitive perception brings to the surface.

ACCULTURATION

The fourth interference most students and clients crash into is the many walls and fabrications erected by overbearing caregivers, teachers, clerics, and politicians. Most of us have been force-fed a suffocating meta-narrative that chokes the great mystery of life. For instance, you may have been subjected to dogma and doctrines created to control their devotees. Or beliefs set in place by organized religions to tragically undermine personal power and authority as well as innate wisdom. Or you became engrossed with patriarchal intellectual and scientific authorities who continue to weave a tiny grid within which the whole world and human experience apparently transpires. Or all of the above in sequence or at once! This noxious combination feeds an immensely myopic and human-centric superiority complex. Unfortunately, this blinkered attitude continues to flourish in "modern" or "civilized" or apparently "rational" individuals.

Popular culture and dominant narratives can also prevail over your imaginations, uniqueness, and dignity. Profit-driven television, movies, and media can fabricate a web of external expectations that entangle your spirit with confusion and skewed values and priorities. The same applies when you are bombarded with the tidings and personae that people chose to present on Facebook and other forms of social media. When your inner world is crowded with an array of fictionalized characters and fabricated personal mythologies, it potentially distorts your perception of the world and your place in it. The generated emotions such as shame, self-loathing, sadness, discontent, despair, and alienation create an invasive network of noisy low vibrations in your physical, emotional, mental, and spiritual being.

Also, fear-inducing spins on world events can create enough anxiety to tip you over into a flight–fight–freeze ecosystem. Knowing everything that is going on does not necessarily make you more compassionate or loving. Therefore, it is important to select news sources produced by writers, academics, artists, and activists who are not affiliated with corporate entertainment providers. And even then, it is best if you consume it judiciously. Unfortunately, the rampant proliferation of propaganda and misinformation clouds and often damages your intuitive antennae. The onslaught can create enough confusion, doubt, and skepticism to interfere with your capacity to tune in to the many levels of subtle energies and your self-healing potential.

Lack of trust in your innate wisdom prevents you from acting on your intuitive hunches and insights. The less you act on your wisdom, the less accessible it becomes. It's a horrible catch-22!

UNFAMILIARITY WITH SACRED TREE ANATOMY

Often, clients and students overestimate the role that intuitive perception plays when I compassionately witness their suffering. Although *seeing* through skin and bones and studying anatomy or medical Qigong are not prerequisites for most Reiki certifications, I would not be the practitioner I am today if I navigated the surface of the body not knowing and understanding what organs and energy bodies are under my hands. Although you do not manipulate the body physically when practising Reiki or Reiki Plus Plus, and are not educated enough or certified to do so, you are interacting with the energetic ecosystems of the physical body, including its organs, energetic orbs (presented later in this section), dantians, and chakras. When you recognize the organ or energy body, and know its energy matrix and its physical, emotional, mental, and spiritual dynamics, you can orient yourself more rapidly and work more efficiently. In other words, your intuitive perception knows which radio channel to tune in to. You're not vaguely searching high and low in the great mystery. You specifically check in to the particular ethos and aspect of the human experience this organ orb, dantian, or chakra specializes in.

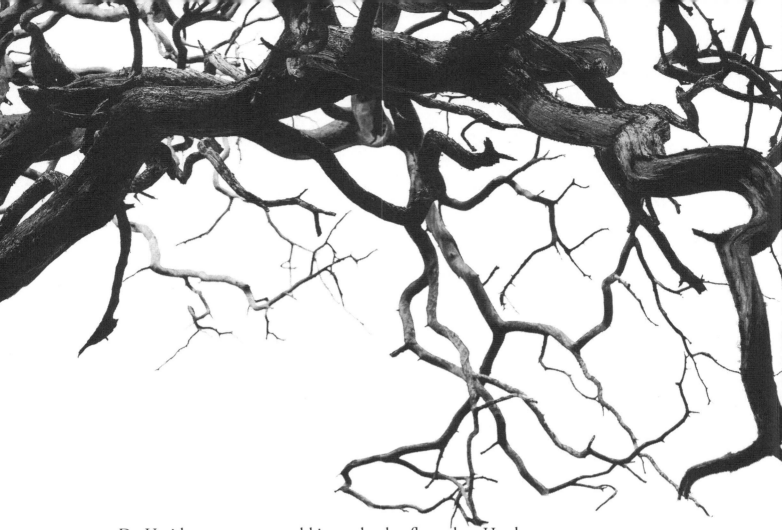

Dr. Usui knew anatomy and his notebook reflects that. He also wrote about the physical, emotional, mental, and spiritual forces at work in any given site in the body. I highly recommend *Surface Anatomy: The Anatomical Basis of Clinical Examination* by John S. P. Lumley and *Netter's Anatomy Flash Cards* by John T. Hansen to get a clear and solid introduction to the noteworthy headliners of the physical body. As a visual person, I found it most helpful to study the diagrams by propping the book or cards on the table where I was most likely to eat alone. Daydreaming on the images while eating actually burned them in my mind's eye with relative ease. I then supported this passive approach by actively reading about health in general and medical Qigong and traditional Chinese medicine in particular.

It's a crying shame that Reiki practitioners are not encouraged to know and interact with the energy bodies and the organs more consciously and precisely.

TOXICITY AND DISSOCIATION

Toxicity and dissociation tend to feed off each other. As you can imagine, being clogged up or "out of body" does nothing for your intuitive perception. If you ever completed a cleanse, you might have noticed how much you learned about engaging with your organs and body from this process alone. First, you had to educate yourself enough to cleanse safely and productively, or if you had a more complex health issue, you were educated by your naturopath, nutritionist, or other expert to navigate an intricate cleansing sequence. Usually, a detoxifying cleanse and a shift in your approach to eating is an eye-opening process of self-discovery and heightened physical and intuitive awareness. It is experiential anatomy and "in-your-body" training worth its weight in gold.

The food you put in your mouth, and whatever else you put in your body, speaks volumes of where you are at physically, emotionally, mentally, and spiritually. When you lift the dense veil of accumulated toxicity and shed toxicity-inducing eating habits, you not only experience more optimal functioning in your physical organs, but you gain fluidity and clarity in your Sacred Tree and intuitive perception as well.

Besides, understanding what you eat, why you eat it, when you eat it, and how you feel about what you eat is the most efficient way to nurture conscious in-your-body living and intuitive flow. The very tangible and physical experience of eating nutritious foods and cleansing quickly turns into a journey into the anatomy of your Sacred Tree. If you stick with the program long enough, you experience the gradual unveiling of your spiritual heart and the love and compassion within. Perhaps to your surprise, you will find this part of you intact, loving, and powerful no matter what has been done to you or what you have done to yourself or others. Eventually, you experience the essential energy of the sun and the earth, Shiva and Shakti, yang and yin, or whatever *you* call it, living with you and through you 24/7. Consequently, you discover the most energizing and nourishing energies of all: unconditional love and compassion.

When you're plugged in, healthy, and vibrant, your intuitive perception is thankfully included in the package.

STRESS HORMONES

Last but certainly not least is the seventh enemy of intuitive *sensing, seeing, hearing,* and *knowing,* the powerful ecology of fear: your stress hormones. A calm and meditative state is essential to maintain clear access to intuitive perception and instant insights. The messages are muddled, static-y, and intermittent if your mind and heart are not clear and you are not fully present in your body and connected to the earth and the sun. If worries and fear are getting the better of you, the flight–fight–freeze hormonal imbalance will hinder your channel. There's nothing quite as potent as adrenaline to get in the way of intuitive perception. Once the alert signals in your medulla oblongata (reptile brain) are hopping like ants in a hot skillet, the third eye (sixth chakra) immediately above it has no chance in hell to be a clear and calm enough surface on which to register insights.

Your intuitive perception can therefore remain buried or suffer if you do not rectify systemic disharmony in your life. This can range from being enmeshed in a codependent relationship all the way to being disempowered in a violent relationship, from eating too much sugar to snorting too much cocaine, from habitually working late nights to being a driven workaholic, or from unhealthy boundaries to compulsive self-sacrifice. Whatever the dissonance, if it is chronic or addictive, then among the long list of hindrances and suffering, you will also end up with a veiled third eye.

Yet, beyond life's infinite cocktail of situations that induce fear, you all too often unconsciously encourage and produce more stress hormones by consuming certain foods or substances and by engaging in disruptive activities. The message is clear: it is not only essential to heal your traumas and shift your emotional, mental, and spiritual ecosystems away from fear but also to learn to interact consciously with the physical manifestation of fear in your body. Many habits and avoidable imbalances trigger fear in your physical ecosystem and pull you away from accessible and infinitely available love, compassion, and heightened perception. In other words, the fear-soup you simmer in daily is not all linked to the traumas in your past or the stressors you are invariably exposed to every day; you actually have control over part of it in the here and now.

For instance, refined sugar, agave syrup, too much natural sugar or glucose, caffeine, wheat, all GMOs, MSG, alcohol, starchy foods, and rich fatty foods catapult your body into overdrive. You are then indelibly trapped in the old flight–fight–freeze response, thereby promoting the production of stress hormones, the reviled drugs of fear that steer your physical ecosystem away from the vibrations of love and compassion. Nicotine, prescription drugs, and recreational drugs are of course huge contenders, creating imbalances that reinforce survival rather than thriving, thereby driving you further away from your Sacred Tree. The trick is to cultivate emotional, mental, spiritual, and physical wellness in order to be a clear vessel for the very high vibrations of love and compassion. It's not just a list of don'ts; more importantly, it presents a luxuriant menu of activities and practices that support rather than detract from your Sacred Tree.

To ensure that you lower your production of stress hormones and achieve a workable level of compassionate presence, prepare in whatever way is necessary every day: go to bed early, especially if you have sessions the next day, to ensure that you are well rested and refreshed. First thing in the morning, practise chanting, meditation, yoga, or other formal spiritual practices, including writing, to support your inner peace and stillness. Integrate these practices into your scheduling. For instance, you can set aside the first hour and often more of your workday for meditative preparation. Only after that do you schedule in clients. Avoid a flurry of email communication (especially those dealing with contentious issues in your personal or professional life), business transactions, and vigorous cleaning or activity before treatments or self-Reiki. Create a clear home, workspace, and practice room, free of clutter, paperwork, storage, and dust. Support the energy in your home and workspace with clear and clean crystals, daily smudging, and energy clearing.

You can also block off one to two hours after sessions to practise meditation or body–spirit movement to clear your energy field and to maintain cardiovascular fitness, as well as to cultivate strength, alignment, and flexibility. Spend time in Nature. Schedule several retreats a year, where you can do many more hours of practice. Every few weeks, you can book craniosacral therapy, Reiki, Thai yoga massage, rolfing, or whatever else supports your well-being. Continue to read and learn from teachers such as Sally Kempton, Adyashanti, Sogyal Rinpoche, Vishnu Devenanda, Sivananda, Gabor Maté, Mandaza (Augustine) Kandemwa, Nelson Mandela, and so many others.

Basically, if you do not adhere to these logistics—and especially if your body is dragged down into the ecology of fear by any of the noxious effects of foods and substances such as caffeine and turbulent and ungrounded activity—then clairsentience, clairvoyance, clairaudience, and claircognizance are less available to you, and by extension to your clients.

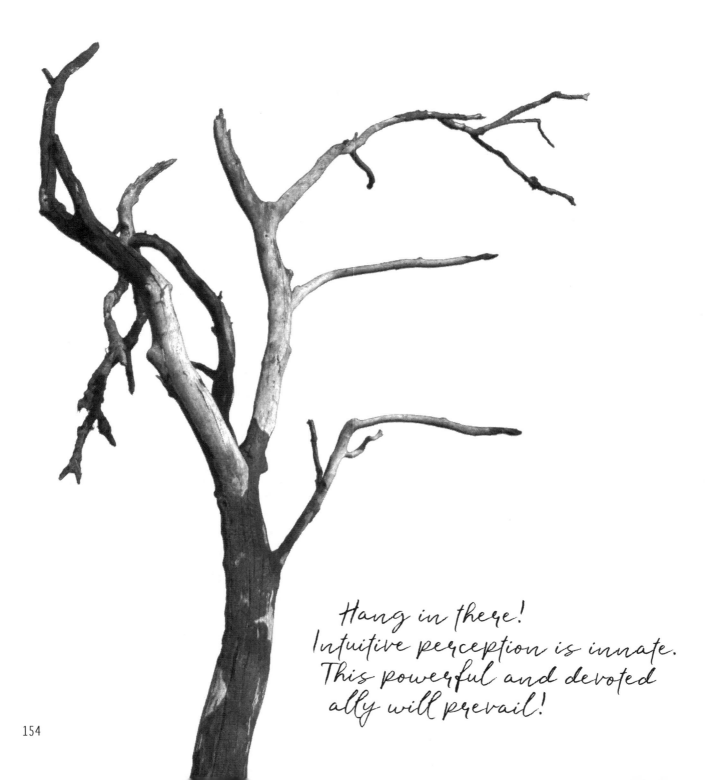

Hang in there!
Intuitive perception is innate.
This powerful and devoted
ally will prevail!

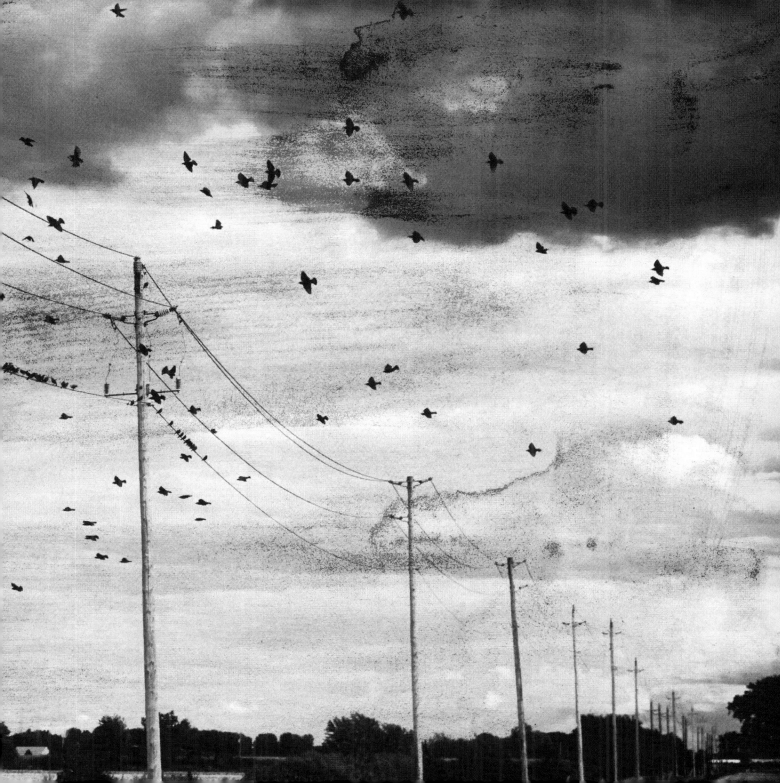

CHAPTER ELEVEN
PERFORMING DISTANCE REIKI

WHAT IS DISTANCE REIKI?

Distance Reiki or distance healing is the pearl of Reiki Level Two training. It is extremely effective and is a great way for clients to continue their work with practitioners when one of them is out of town and for practitioners to treat clients or family who live in other cities. For most students (and clients, for that matter), this is the most woo-woo aspect of the Reiki practice because practitioners can send therapeutic healing vibrations and energy patterns to a person who is physically distant from them.

Yogis and energy healers have recognized for centuries what modern astrophysicists and quantum scientists have only recently become aware of: concrete reality is a mere illusion of solidity. We are actually made of energy vibrating at different pitches that coagulate in various forms, objects, and beings we see with our biological eyes. For Reiki practitioners who intuitively work with energy, healing is therefore a matter of balancing and transmitting higher vibrations and manifestations of the life force—they can sense and alter that incorporeal energy and thus access it outside of the conventional limitations of time and space.

When I studied Reiki, it took me months to actually try doing distance Reiki. A friend of mine essentially had to be in enough distress while I was away in Montreal for me to schedule a phone session with her. Although I had experienced distance sessions and had no doubt of their validity and effectiveness, my trepidation was rooted in my fear of failure: "How am I going to actually activate the energy and reach her in her home, in her body, and in her spirit in Toronto?" For others, it's a total dominant culture clash: "Like, right, the energy will travel through the phone and thin air and actually heal someone in another city?!?"

Whatever the source of the resistance, whether it's self-doubt or skepticism, it's totally worth facing because this practice is extremely powerful and it's a fantastic way to learn how to transcend time and space. I mean, WOW! In every moment of the experience you are reminded that your materiality is nothing more than an agreed-upon reality system with lots of rules and limitations created and reinforced by conscious or unconscious religious, social, cultural, familial, ancestral, political, scientific, and intellectual biases.

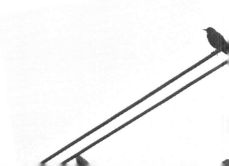

As far as I'm concerned, the best part of this radical experience is that you don't need to take a powerful drug or cultivate your spiritual awakening for decades with various ascetic practices to shake the foundation of your conscious and unconscious beliefs and biases enough to taste the wonders of love and compassion in action. You just need to pick up your smartphone :) and go for it! And if it seems low-key and odd the first time, try again. Distance healing can instigate a paradigm shift that altars your self-perception and your default biases and interactions with the "known" world.

Distance Reiki can be the beginning or continuation of an easeful rather than fearful relationship with the mystery.

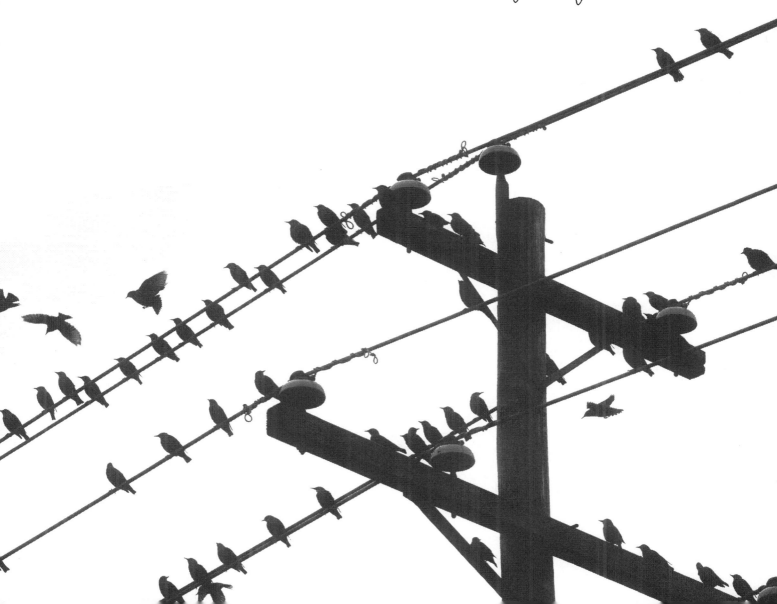

THE DISTANCE REIKI METHOD

Despite the fact that the concept and inner workings of distance Reiki are rather puzzling and mysterious, the method is simple:

- The client and the practitioner (separately, in their own spaces) settle in a quiet room where they will not be disturbed. Both close the door, dim the light, light a candle, or burn white sage.

- The practitioner can sit quietly in a chair with legs and arms relaxed or on the floor in lotus position. The client can sit as well; however, they are most often more comfortable lying down.

- Once settled in, the client calls at the appointed time. After a brief check-in, the practitioner begins the session.

- The practitioner invokes the Hon-Sha-Ze-Sho-Nen (HS) symbol and mantra.

- If the practitioner normally remains in verbal contact with the client, they can remain online together. If the practitioner usually reports findings at the end of the session, then the practitioner may go offline after the check-in and call the client back when they are done.

- The practitioner can use a pillow or cushion as a surrogate body to apply their hands on and focus their concentration.

- The client receiving distance healing often feels what is happening. As their energy shifts, they sense the movement and release of energy; see colours and images; and experience emotions, memories, and sensations such as numbness or tingling.

- If they worked offline, the practitioner calls the client back and both report on their experience.

In general, the Hon-Sha-Ze-Sho-Nen symbol and mantra is underused and underexplored. In addition to the distance healing method described above, it can be used to ignite your spiritual focus, transcend distance, or create a calm process even when you are working with clients in your office.

- You can invoke the HS symbol whenever you feel entangled in day-to day consciousness. The HS symbol can kindle your spiritual fire and awareness.

- You can sense and send energy to the client's head even when you are working on their feet, or you can access the kidneys, for instance, from the front of the body. This, too, is distance healing.

- You can sense and send energy to a child playing on the floor of your office with their favourite toy or reading a picture book rather than creating stress for both the child and the caregiver by insisting that the child lie still on your treatment table. That said, please advise the caregiver before the session not to bring energetically disruptive electronic devices such as iPads.

- You can sense and send energy to an infant who is nursing or sleeping on the caregiver's body rather than potentially stressing them with demands that interfere with their sense of safety and comfort. It's usually enough that they are not at home and perhaps meeting you for the first time.

- You can sense and send energy to a mother while she is nursing or attending to her infant's needs. She does not need to arrange for a babysitter or disrupt the infant's routines more than necessary.

- The clients who usually opt for distance healing are caregivers inviting the practitioner to work with their children as it's often the least disruptive choice for both of them. Caregivers who opt to work on the phone can nonetheless talk to their child about Reiki, introduce them to you and your work, and let them know when it is happening.

DISTANCE REIKI STUDENT EXERCISE

Here's a simple way to learn and practise distance Reiki:

- Sit in chairs about six to twelve feet apart and facing away from you Reiki practice-buddy.

- The practitioner practises distance Reiki in silence for ten minutes.

- The recipient first reports to the practitioner what they experienced.

- Then the practitioner describes their perceptions, focus, information, and images to the recipient.

- Both talk and elaborate on their shared experience.

- Switch back and forth and repeat the exercise at least four times.

This simple and quick exercise yields amazing results. My students are generally amazed by how often their sensations as either the recipient or the practitioner and vice versa match and complement each other in unexpected ways. Also, it's often in doing this simple exercise that students open up to a more metaphoric and imagistic language. My sense is that this context drives the left brain out of dominance and allows for more right-brain hemisphere activity. It's a safe, easy, and fun way to move away from conscious reasoning and left-brain linearity and to explore and develop intuitive perception.

THE ETHICS OF DISTANCE REIKI

It's important to bear in mind to only practise distance Reiki if the energy is welcome. The rules of engagement are not different for distance Reiki. The receiver or a child's caregiver (valid up to about age twelve) must give you informed and wholehearted permission to do the session. If you are concerned for someone and for whatever reason you don't have their consent, then pray for the person rather than do a Reiki session. It is crucial to understand the absolute necessity of honouring this guideline. Think about it: entering someone's energetic field without their permission is what cult leaders do—it's energetic violation.

To do Reiki on someone without them knowing can destabilize the person. Imagine sensing a shift and not knowing what it is. I once experienced this very thing sitting on my sofa one fine Sunday afternoon and then, wazaam, I dropped into the one and only full-on panic attack of my life. Once I figured out what happened later that night, it was definitely a superb note-to-self moment—one I can thankfully never forget.

- How can you as a practitioner know that you are detached if you are so attached to doing a session?

- How can you know for sure that your ego is not invested in the results?

The best policy is to honour the sacred contract at all times. It's best for everyone, including you, because every time you violate someone's energetic field you jeopardize your integrity and lower your vibration. This leads nowhere pretty down the line.

THE TRANSFORMATIONAL POWER OF PRAYER

The good news is that your hands are not tied when a friend or family member is in crisis and cannot or does not give you their consent to do a distance Reiki session. Rather than step into a Reiki-motivated session calling in the Reiki symbols to access their energy field, assessing their state, and motivating changes in their energy fields, you pray for them.

Prep and pray:

a. Meditate to soften your energy fields out of worry mode and into the highest vibration of unconditional love and compassion you can muster by connecting to the earth, the sun, ascended masters, guides, and ancestors.

b. Conjure and bask in the light of your love for the distressed person.

c. Once fully concentrated and immersed in this energy, send love puffs to them posthaste.

d. Then add to this missive high-vibration emotions such as inner peace, trust, honesty, integrity, dignity and wisdom.

First, when you love someone and radiate your love on them while in a meditative state, you fortify their spirit. Because it's not just getting well that they need, it's the willingness and courage to delve into the root cause of their illness. As you know, this can be a scary prospect. Your love helps quell their fearful contraction by bathing them in the expansive energy of love, the antithesis of contracted fear.

Second, when you add other high-vibration emotions into the mix, you stimulate their connection to their innate high-vibration medicines and their Sacred Tree. This boost to their Sacred Tree ecology can reduce the influence of the whole host of low-vibration emotions they are likely experiencing and can stoke their resolve, fuel their curiosity, and ignite their intuition. In other words, when your prayer is so much more than begging for different circumstances or pleading for the evaporation of the challenges, it can help your loved one change their tide from disharmony to harmony from the root cause outward. In this sense, prayer, like Reiki, is powerful and active.

INSPIRING HARMONY

DISHARMONY ⟶ HARMONY

LOW-FREQUENCY EMOTIONS	HIGH-FREQUENCY EMOTIONS
OVERWHELM	COGNIZANCE
· Fear	· Love
· Anxiety/Shock	· Compassion
· Abandonment	· Inner Peace
· Shame	· Tranquility
· Horror	· Trust
· Powerlessness	· Honesty
· Heartache	· Integrity
· Worry	· Dignity
· Excessive Grief	· Wisdom

CHAPTER TWELVE

EXPLORING SACRED TREE ANATOMY: THE CYCLE

NATURE'S ANCIENT ELEMENTAL AND CYCLICAL WISDOM

For centuries, Chinese shamans and medical Qigong and traditional Chinese medicine (TCM) practitioners have elaborated on the interconnectivity of the human experience with all other living beings and the regenerative cycle of Nature. Their observations and insights are a vibrant reminder that harmony and well-being are not fixed ideals; they are ever-changing and evolving states you co-create with Nature and all living beings, including the earth and the sun. Their wisdom and flow charts help you remember the rhythm of Nature and your corresponding physical, emotional, mental, and spiritual tides. Harmony in summer, for instance, is very different than harmony in winter. At any given moment, harmony expresses itself as one flavour of equilibrium in the great enterprise of living well at a particular juncture in Nature's omnipresent and regenerative cycle.

HARMONY AND DISHARMONY

Chinese shamans and medical Qigong and TCM practitioners observe that all living beings are in a constant flux between harmony and disharmony or are sometimes navigating a virtual 50/50 blend. In light of this, harmony is never a *fait accompli*. At any given moment, you can experience harmony because you cultivate and support this balanced state, or conversely it can slip between your fingers because you neglect it. Thus, harmony is not interdependent with external circumstances deemed perfect, a privilege, a special aptitude, or a superior spiritual container. It is an innate and active alchemical agent you grow or neglect. In other words, if you water your innate Sacred Tree-ness, it grows; and if you neglect watering it, it withers.

Harmony expresses your innate alchemical capacity to align with your built-in orientation and life-sustaining flow with the earth and the sun.

Likewise, disharmony is never a given or fixed entity. For instance, it's not because you are slammed with adversity at a particular juncture that you are invariably plunged into disharmony. The state of disharmony is not interdependent with external circumstances deemed challenging, a built-in flaw, hard luck, or incompetence. Rather, it speaks of a fleeting or tenacious disorientation and confusion. Basically, you are in a state of disharmony when your requisite connection to the earth and the sun is ignored, disrupted, obstructed, and/or disengaged.

No matter what is happening or has happened to you, you remain a Sacred Tree and are connected to the rhythms of Nature. No amount of torment can disrupt your interconnectivity with Nature's primary orientation and progression. Although it feels like it sometimes, it's actually impossible to escape it. For example, when your spirit inhabits a physical body, this body will age and eventually die. Although this built-in underpinning can be unsettling, your Sacred Tree's impulse and capacity to grow and blossom is just as certain. In other words, all the subtle or grand manifestations of harmony are just as palpable and accessible as the seemingly unpreventable disharmony and suffering along the way.

Mercifully, you are a Sacred Tree and alchemical master no matter how extreme the circumstances. While harmony is not something you can take for granted once you experience it or achieve it, the same can be said of disharmony. You can always count on your innate capacity to transform unlove into love, even when it seems delirious to think so.

Consequently, Chinese shamans and medical Qigong and TCM practitioners gauge disharmony by measuring its variation from the ideal and harmonious midpoint. They describe the loss of harmony as a state of flux away from harmony. I choose to express the divergence from harmony as either explosive or implosive—it's either more explosive than harmony or more implosive than harmony. This dyad simply indicates in what direction the emotional, mental, or spiritual imbalance is going, from mildly explosive or implosive to excessively explosive or implosive. Please note that I do not itemize explosive or implosive physical disharmonies. A large body of information is available on hot and cold imbalances in TCM texts and other resources.

You are in a state of disharmony when you are not in sync with your innate Sacred Tree-ness and its fundamental orientation to the sun and the earth.

THE FIVE YIN-YANG ORGAN ALLIANCES

Your human experience is never static because you are always in the perpetual flow of wholesome or unwholesome input. Therefore, you are always somewhere in the continuum between harmony and disharmony. Harmony and well-being either grow or decline moment to moment. Likewise, disharmony and dis-ease either prosper or decrease moment to moment. Consequently, the harmony and health of your Sacred Tree ecology is synonymous with discernment, maintenance, and cleansing. For instance, when you don't clean your house regularly, you soon dwell in a chaotic, congested, unproductive, and unpleasant environment. It's unescapable. The same patent wisdom applies to your Sacred Tree.

Fortunately, your Sacred Tree ecology, alchemical fortitude, and resilience rest in the fact that you have a built-in cleansing and self-healing system. Your Sacred Tree is equipped with five specialized energetic orbs each including solid yin organs and hollow yang organs paired together in dynamic healing teams.

While your yin organs (namely the liver, heart, spleen/pancreas, lungs, and kidneys/brain/reproductive organs) do their extensively acknowledged biological work, they also work energetically on the physical, emotional, mental, and spiritual levels.

Your hollow yang organs are doing just as much physically and energetically. They process the food you eat, eliminate the unwholesome byproducts, and transform and later imbibe wholesome nutrients. They also facilitate the absorption and integration of all energy that is beneficial and nutritious as well as the elimination of all energy that is harmful and detrimental.

While some of these alliances seem logical, some may surprise you, especially if allopathic medicine has been your dominant template for health and healing.

    a. When you nurture and cleanse your gallbladder, you heal your liver. *Sure.*

    b. When you nurture and cleanse your small intestine, you heal your heart. *What?*

    c. When you nurture and cleanse your stomach, you heal your spleen and pancreas. *Okay.*

    d. When you nurture and cleanse your colon, you heal your lungs. *What?*

    e. When you nurture and cleanse your bladder, you heal your kidneys. *Sure.*

GENERATING CYCLE

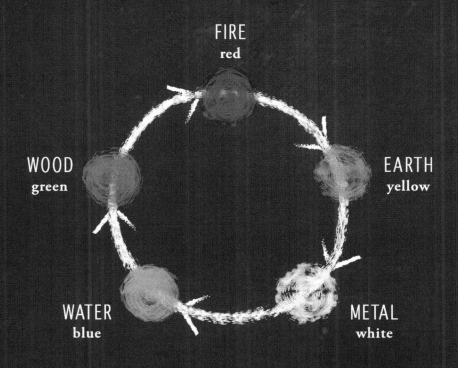

FIRE
red

WOOD
green

EARTH
yellow

WATER
blue

METAL
white

THE FIVE YIN-YANG ORGAN ALLIANCES

ELEMENT	WOOD 木	FIRE 火	EARTH 土	METAL 金	WATER 水
COLOUR	·Green	·Red	·Yellow	·White	·Blue
SEASON	·Spring	·Summer	·Late Summer	·Autumn	·Winter
YIN ORGANS	·Liver	·Heart	·Spleen ·Pancreas	·Lungs	·Kidneys ·Brain ·Reproductive Organs
YANG ORGANS	·Gallbladder	·Duodenum ·Small Intestine	·Stomach	·Colon	·Bladder ·Sea of Marrow
EXTERNAL ORGANS	·Eyes and Third Eye	·Tongue	·Mouth	·Nose	·Ears

THE FIVE ELEMENTAL ORBS

These five yin–yang organ alliances are the building blocks of the five energetic orbs in your Sacred Tree. The five energetic orbs are love's powerful processors synchronizing the elements, seasons, high-frequency vibrations, low-frequency vibrations, and a plethora of other cyclical wonders of living and thriving as a spirit in a human incarnation. They activate your evolutionary impulse at a specific juncture in Nature's cycle, and they work together in an eloquent and expressive sequence. While each energetic orb is a spoke in the wheel of life, love and compassion ignite the regenerative power of Nature's cycle, not unlike water in a water wheel.

Each yin–yang organ group and energetic orb is imprinted with a medley of physical, emotional, mental, and spiritual life-giving vibrations to process your suffering and transform it into wisdom. Reminiscent of your chakras and dantians, each yin–yang energetic orb in your Sacred Tree is a hospital, staffed with very dedicated, competent, and specialized doctors and personnel. As such, each energetic yin–yang orb in your Sacred Tree is a reliable source of high-frequency medicine and guidance.

    a. Your liver and gallbladder host love and compassion specialists.

    b. Your heart and small intestine host inner peace and tranquility specialists.

    c. Your spleen/pancreas and stomach host trust and honesty specialists.

    d. Your lungs and colon host dignity and generosity specialists.

    e. Your kidneys/brain/reproductive organs and bladder/sea of marrow host wisdom and clarity specialists.

Therefore, when adversity strikes, each energetic orb acts as a shock absorber for the energies in direct opposition to their optimal vibration and specialty. Despite your overwhelmingness and confusion, your energetic partners actually make sense of the chaos and host the low vibrations they are most equipped to re-integrate, transform, and heal. In other words, your Sacred Tree's energetic orbs absorb your suffering in their self-healing facilities to comfort and rehabilitate the traumatized astronauts and architects of survival. Thus, disharmony alchemically transforms into harmony—the fluid and innate expression of your Sacred Tree and spirit in action.

Your Sacred Tree's alchemical capacity is steadfast, unless your Sacred Tree ecology is consciously or unconsciously neglected, or overwhelmed, and faltering due to intensely traumatic experiences or unwholesome activities. If this is the case, the five yin–yang energetic orbs and organ alliances can become besieged hospitals with waiting rooms full of traumatized astronauts and architects of survival waiting for treatment from inundated personnel and doctors. The backlog crowding your hospital waiting rooms cumulatively decreases the effectiveness of your innate healers.

When a "hospital," orb or organ, hosts a backlog of untreated traumatized astronauts and architects of survival, it raises a white flag in the form of sensations and discomfort. If this message is not acknowledged, it produces more obvious imbalances and pain. And if again these stalwart emissaries are ignored, your Sacred Tree ecology will produce illnesses with as many bells and whistles as you need to heed their plea for your conscious and active engagement with neglected or suppressed low-frequency emotions.

This plot unfolds to ensure your growth and evolution. Unless you catch up with your abandoned traumatized astronauts and architects of survival as well as the love and life curriculum you are consciously or unconsciously overlooking, relief will only be temporary. In contrast, when you revitalize your overburdened teams with rest, nutritious food, meditation, self-inquiry, a physical practice unifying body–mind–spirit, and cleansing, your innate high-frequency emotions, teachers, and healers become accessible again. You then have the fuel you need to escort your traumatized astronauts and architects of survival back to love.

THE FIVE EXTERNAL ORGANS INCLUDED

This Chinese elemental system is vast. Your entire physical body, including all of its tissues, is mapped out on its grid. Although I decided to focus on the yin–yang internal organ groupings within each elemental orb, I discovered that if I also included the external sense organs, I opened up the template enough to uncover more clearly your mighty trauma healing matrix. These partnerships reveal very salient information about your experience and process in traumatic conditions and your corresponding capacity to heal:

> **a.** eyes, sight, and the liver/gallbladder;
>
> **b.** tongue, verbal expression, and the heart/duodenum/small intestine;
>
> **c.** mouth, consumption, and spleen/pancreas/stomach;
>
> **d.** nose, in-and-out exchange, and the lungs/colon; and
>
> **e.** ears, hearing, and the kidneys/bladder.

ELEMENTAL ORBS AND ORGANS

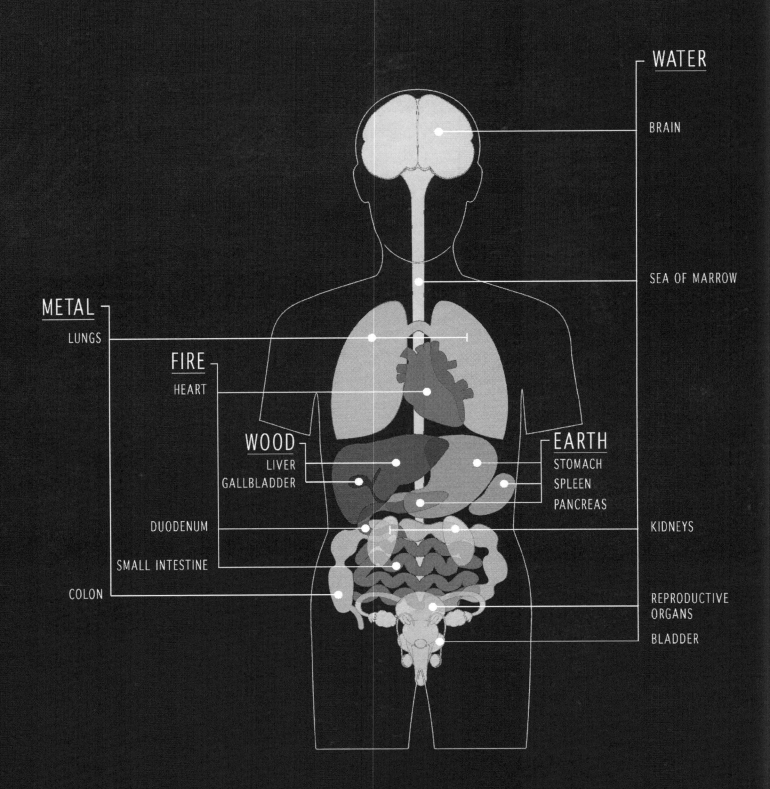

WATER

BRAIN

SEA OF MARROW

METAL

LUNGS

FIRE

HEART

WOOD

LIVER
GALLBLADDER

EARTH

STOMACH
SPLEEN
PANCREAS

DUODENUM

SMALL INTESTINE

COLON

KIDNEYS

REPRODUCTIVE
ORGANS

BLADDER

INNATE HEALERS: HIGH-FREQUENCY EMOTIONS

Emotional energetic currents have different vibrational rates, ranging from high-frequency emotional states to low-frequency emotional states. High-frequency emotions are the living expression of harmony. They not only raise the vibratory rate of your physical body and energetic orbs, but they are the innate and motivational forces bolstering the transformational and alchemical power of each orb in Nature's regenerative cycle. These spiritual teachers and guides, referred to as prenatal virtues in medical Qigong and TCM, are imprinted in your five energetic orbs before birth. Thus, harmony is always within reach because its imprint exists in your organs and orbs. They are the alchemical agents bolstering your capacity to transcend trauma, including sexual abuse. In other words, when you tune in to and nurture their power, you have access to the keys to unlock the gate and set yourself free.

TRAUMA: LOW-FREQUENCY EMOTIONS

When you avoid, suppress, or deny low-frequency emotions, they accumulate within your body and energy bodies, thereby creating disharmony. Thus, the stockpile of low-frequency emotions in your organs weakens your energetic fields and vice versa. Consequently, your life force contracts and flows incorrectly. Please note that the maelstrom of painful emotions experienced in traumatic circumstances in and of themselves do not set into motion disharmony, but it's the buildup of neglected low-frequency emotions that creates disharmony and illness. It's important to make this distinction. When flowing, all emotions create harmony, including the low-frequency ones. For example:

a. The fluid expression of anger can provoke the creation of healthy boundaries and motivate you to right some wrongs.

b. The fluid expression of excitement can foster happiness and relaxation.

c. The fluid expression of worry can instigate introspection, preparation, and change.

d. The fluid expression of sorrow can disperse grief, relieve distress, or instigate beneficent concern and action.

e. The fluid expression of fear can stimulate healthful vigilance and discerning self-protection.

ELEMENT	WOOD 木	FIRE 火
YIN ORGANS	· Liver	· Heart
YANG ORGANS	· Gallbladder	· Duodenum · Small Intestine
EXTERNAL ORGANS	· Eyes and Third Eye	· Tongue
HIGH-FREQUENCY EMOTIONS	· Love · Compassion · Benevolence · Kindness · Patience · Unselfish Actions	· Inner Peace · Order · Contentment · Pleasure · Courtesy · Forgiveness
EXPLOSIVE LOW-FREQUENCY EMOTIONS	· Anger · Rage · Intolerance · Hatred · Resentment · Stubbornness	· Agitation · Anxiety · Excitement · Restlessness · Mania · Arrogance
IMPLOSIVE LOW-FREQUENCY EMOTIONS	· Powerlessness · Hopelessness · Despair · Depression · Purposelessness · Addiction	· Heartache · Longing · Loneliness · Codependence · Self-Sacrifice · Dissociation

EARTH 土	METAL 金	WATER 水
· Spleen · Pancreas	· Lungs	· Kidneys · Reproductive Organs · Brain
· Stomach	· Colon	· Bladder · Sea of Marrow
· Mouth	· Nose	· Ears
· Trust · Honesty · Faith · Openness · Imagination · Stability	· Integrity · Honour · Justice · Dignity · Generosity · Social Responsibility	· Wisdom · Cognizance · Will Power · Quietude · Restfulness · Fluidity
· Abandonment · Obsessiveness · Workaholism · Competition · Covetousness · Instability	· Excess Grief · Guilt · Greed · Control · Affluence · Exploitation	· Fear · Terror · Panic · Horror · Victimization · Endangerment
· Worry · Regret · Self-Doubt · Remorse · Suspicion · Diversion	· Shame · Sorrow · Disappointment · Stinginess · Self-Pity · Pessimism	· Disorientation · Overwhelm · Stagnation · Aloneness · Insecurity · Paranoia

THE ELEMENTAL ORBS IN ACTION

WOOD ATTRIBUTES   green   SPRING PULSE

WOOD ATTRIBUTES	SPRING PULSE
· Manifestation of Genius and Life Purpose · Strategic Planning · Comprehension of the Past · Recognition of New Possibilities · Change, Transformation, and Evolution	· Capitalize on Nature's vivacious energy. · Be bold, despite growing pains. · Face uncertainties and risks. · Wake up, shake down, and grow. · Create, make things, do things, and begin again.

FIRE ATTRIBUTES   red   SUMMER PULSE

FIRE ATTRIBUTES	SUMMER PULSE
· Love and Self-Love · Inner Peace and Abundance · Sustainable Service · Fulfilment and Contentment · Enthusiasm and Laughter	· Drink in the sun. · Blossom and transmute your flowers into fruit. · Manifest your genius into service. · Be vibrant inside and out: sparkle, move, dance, run, and play.

EARTH ATTRIBUTES   yellow   LATE SUMMER PULSE

EARTH ATTRIBUTES	LATE SUMMER PULSE
· Unconditional Nurturing Embrace · Vitality and Revitalization · Stability, Clarity, and Strength · Interdependence with All Living Beings, including the Earth and the Sun	· Eat fresh foods to heal your body. · Burrow your roots in the earth. · Manifest your genius. · Hang out in Nature and receive its guidance.

METAL ATTRIBUTES   white   AUTUMN PULSE

METAL ATTRIBUTES	AUTUMN PULSE
· Dignity and Self-Worth · Recognition of Value Beyond Yourself · Global Consciousness and Social Responsibility · Generosity · Letting Go	· Open up to your essence and love. · Savour the fruits of your hard work. · Distribute what you have produced. · Sort, consolidate, and purge. · Prepare for winter and do not overexert.

WATER ATTRIBUTES   blue   WINTER PULSE

WATER ATTRIBUTES	WINTER PULSE
· Seedbed of All Life · Reservoir of Willpower and Manifestation Energy · Courage and Strength · Tidal Rhythms and Cycles · Fluidity and Adaptability · Path of Least Resistance	· Go inside to meet your unadorned essence. · Dedicate time to self-inquiry, introspection, reflection, meditation, and concentration. · Pay attention to your dreams and visions. · Restore energy and reserves. · Gather strength for the next cycle of growth.

DOING SELF-REIKI ON ELEMENTAL ORBS

While unconditional love is the one-size-fits-all fuel of well-being and all flavours of harmony are contained within it, narrowing in on specific expressions of this magnificent energy amplifies your self-awareness and self-healing potency. I invite you to create your own lists using the charts in this chapter to help you match up the flavours of disharmony you are experiencing with the particular flavours of harmony in direct relationship to them. When you focus your attention precisely on the innate high frequencies you need, including love, it's like going from 110 volts to 220 volts. Your self-Reiki and Reiki practice taps more efficiently into your or your client's innate treasure trove of medicine, hence motivating and activating your and your client's healing power house, the innate Sacred Tree.

HARMONY

If most of the harmonious vibrations you identified are in the same orb and element, these innate healers are the most accessible guides on your journey now. Inviting these high-frequency emotions into your self-Reiki and meditation practices enhances your capacity to blossom. Accordingly, the traumatized astronauts and architects of survival in this orb and organ grouping are the most readily healable. In other words, work with the teachers and innate healers who are already stoked to gain traction on your evolutionary journey.

DISHARMONY

If most of the disharmonious vibrations you identified are in the same element, the work ahead is clear. You are summoned by the foremost teacher of this orb. It is important for you to soften into this element's wisdom now. If the disharmonious vibrations encompass several elements, then all these elemental teachers reflect a piece of your self-healing puzzle.

If the season matches the season you are in, then follow this path wholeheartedly and live by its song. If the season does not match the season you are in, you are guided to a rhythm that will calibrate your spirit. For instance, if your winter pulse is out of balance in the middle of summer, you need to temper your fire by slowing down, looking inward, and resting. If the disharmonious vibrations you identified encompass several seasons, then all these dance teachers and rhythms reflect a piece of your self-healing puzzle.

If most of the disharmonious vibrations you identified are mostly explosive disharmonies, then this orb and organs, or several orbs and organs, need to be purged. You must release the excess energy in these orbs and organs. If most of the disharmonious vibrations you identified are implosive disharmonies, then this orb and organs, or several orbs and organs, need to be nourished. You must tonify these depleted orbs and organs. Either way, purging your overactivated orbs or/and nourishing your depleted orbs supports your besieged innate healers, thereby reactivating your powerful transformational and evolutionary matrix and self-healing capacity.

REIKI PLUS PLUS
LEVEL THREE

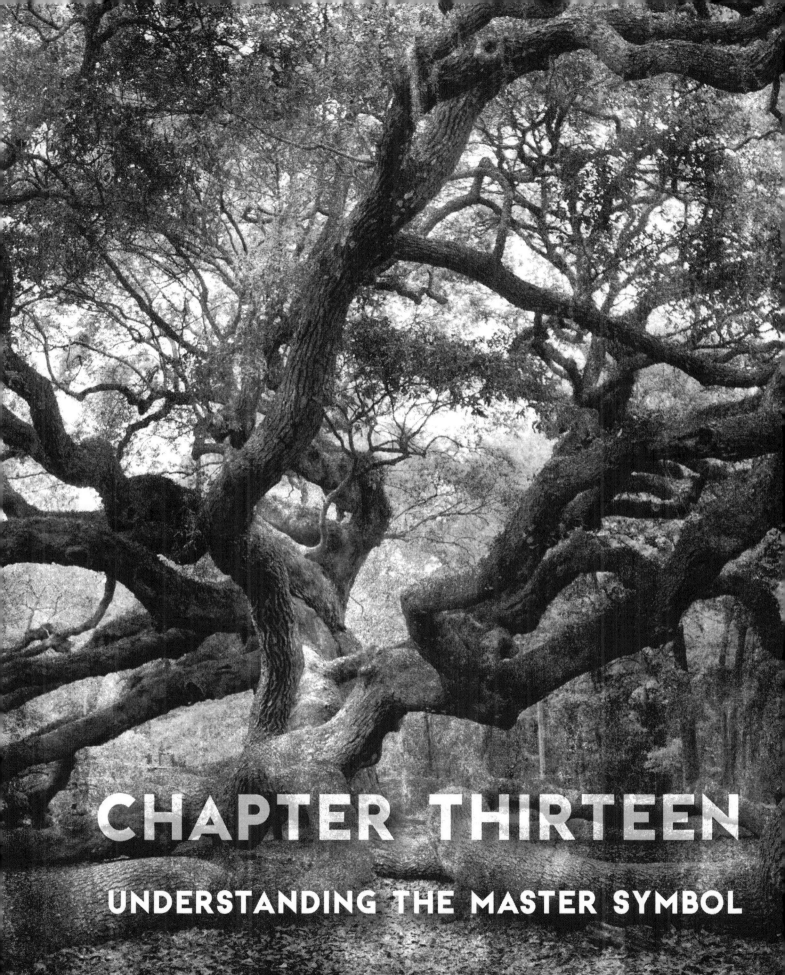

CHAPTER THIRTEEN

UNDERSTANDING THE MASTER SYMBOL

DAI-KO-MYO

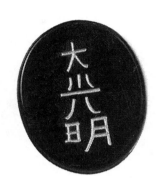

EMPOWERMENT AND UNITY SYMBOL

"Purify, illuminate, and inspire now!"

Concentrating on Dai-Ko-Myo

- Combines the power of all three symbols (Cho-Ku-Rei, Sei-He-Ki, and Hon-Sha-Ze-Sho-Nen).

- Stimulates a bright shining light. *Dai* means "great" or "big," *Ko* means "smooth" or "glossy," the word *Myo* means "bright light." As such, Dai-Ko-Myo fosters inner knowledge, truth, and enlightenment.

- Enhances connection to Universal Love and healing Reiki energy.

- Invites purification, cleansing, and awareness on all levels.

- Shines a powerful light on your genius and purpose. In so doing, it soothes and orients your spirit.

- Underlines the presence of spiritual contractions, including religious indoctrination, oppression, domination, overmanagement, colonization, self-sacrifice, depression, or creative blocks, and ignites your heart's wisdom and with it your self-worth, discernment, and personal power.

- Helps you recognize your "Buddha within" and your intact spiritual heart. It brings you closer to the power of your spiritual heart.

- Activates your intuitive perception and gratitude for your innate wisdom.

- Brings "light" into your life and helps eliminate blockages at all levels: physical, emotional, mental, spiritual, past, present, and future.

- Heartens and emboldens you to evolve, grow, change, and embrace transformation.

- Increases the energy flow throughout your being, thereby nourishing you on all levels.

- Inspires you to nurture yourself and do the same for others.

- Enhances the healing effects of self-Reiki and Reiki sessions by revealing the root cause of the dis-ease.

- Accelerates the connection between your spiritual heart and that of your client's.

- Enhances the healing properties of crystals, herbs, tinctures, and homeopathic remedies.

DAI-KO-MYO

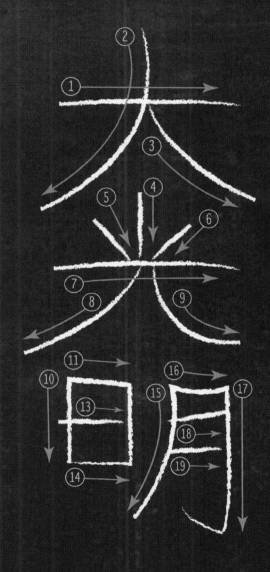

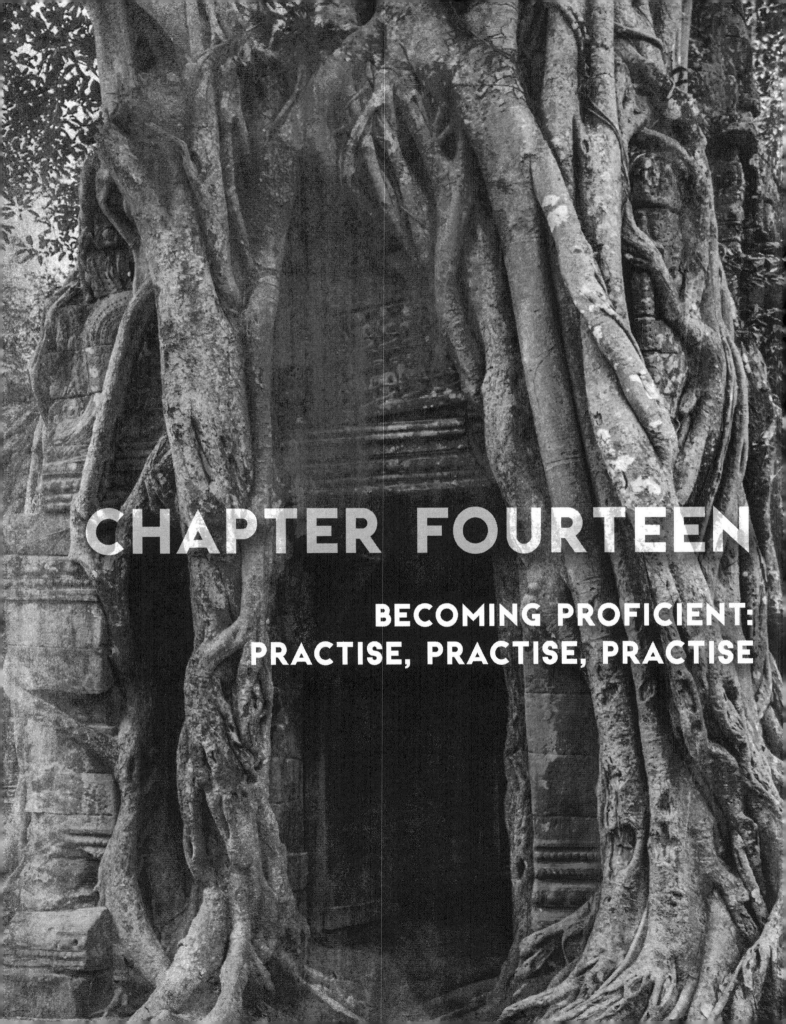

CHAPTER FOURTEEN

BECOMING PROFICIENT:
PRACTISE, PRACTISE, PRACTISE

THE MORE YOU DO IT, THE MORE YOU GAIN

This is the shortest chapter of all because I can't do it with you. The only way for you to become proficient at self-Reiki and Reiki Plus Plus is to do them as often as possible. It's simple: the more you do it, the more you gain traction. Let's face it, there is nothing new or foreign or unknown about any of this. Self-Reiki and Reiki simply prompt you to remember and induce an innate capacity into action. It's already there, but it's dusty because it's been left in the corner untouched for far too long. The only way around this problem is awareness and active engagement with this untapped potency. Self-Reiki and Reiki are about living this great human enterprise with all engines turned on all the time. It's a call to action. To be fully alive and thriving is a full-time, full-on, and full-throttle joy ride. As Diane Bruni would moan in my ear, at some key juncture in her yoga class when my energy was sagging, or when fear, impatience, judgment, self-doubt, or whatever else was surfacing: "Doooo it!" She was right. It always paid off.

*It's totally worth stepping over the hurdles,
no matter what they are,
to dust off who you really are.*

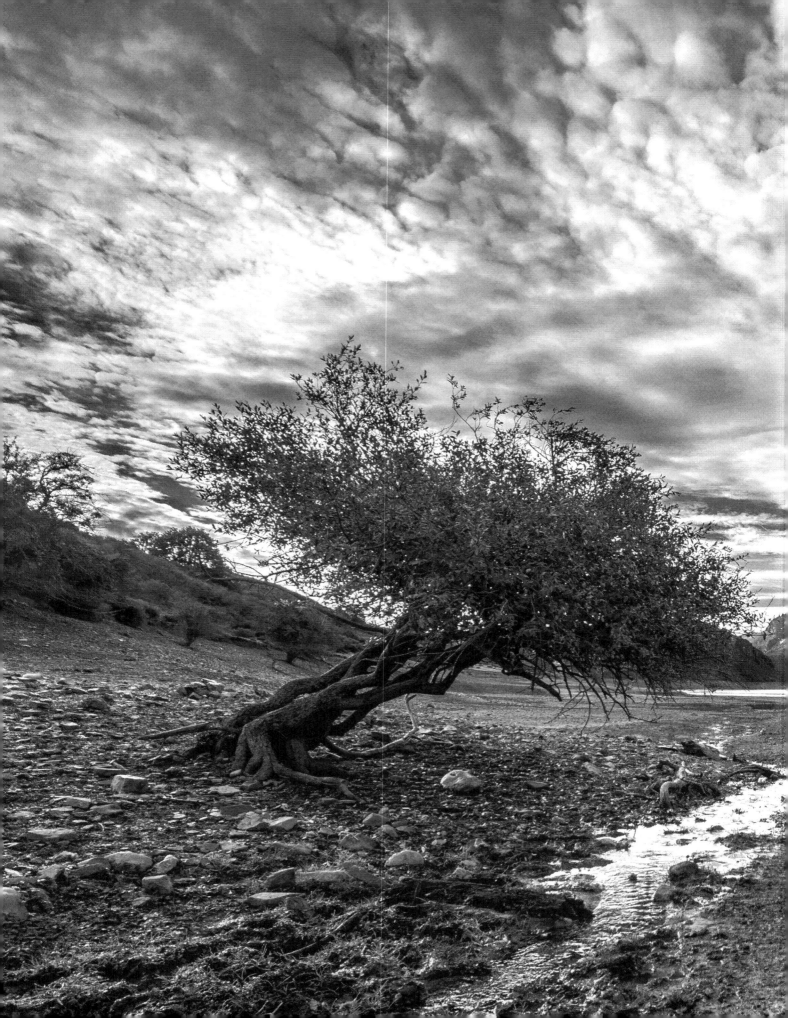

PART THREE

REIKI PLUS PLUS IN ACTION

MAKING THE INVISIBLE VISIBLE

My goal in this part is to make the ephemeral practice of Reiki Plus Plus as tangible as possible—to make the invisible visible. My hope is that you deepen your connection to your own innate wisdom and capacity to alchemically transform trauma by witnessing the patterns that emerge in these reconstituted sessions, when the violence of sexism runs amok, symptoms of victimization manifest, systems of survival cleverly develop, and eventually healing blossoms.

I present to you the journeys as they progress, with some of their twists and turns, cathartic realizations, releases, dramatic detox, stagnation, resistance, and fabulous breakthroughs. Each chapter begins when I meet the client and ends at a narrative juncture, not necessarily the last session. I do not recreate all the sessions but rather choose to focus on certain themes. The similarities that emerge—no matter how different the persons, the resources available to them, or their circumstances—speak of the logic of trauma, survival, and healing rather than the specifics of events, context, and culture.

The dialogue form conveys the process of self-discovery, release, and integration that occurs in a self-Reiki or Reiki Plus Plus session. It also allows me to describe a practice that is energetic and occurs in a linear time-and-space continuum. That said, the energy work per se occurs more slowly than the time it takes you to read the dialogue. Although the exchange and process may sometimes read as if it occurs instantaneously, each session lasts an hour and therefore the dialogue often does not take into account the time that transpires between actions and results. Please remember that each of the voices you read is just the whitecap on that client's big, beautiful wave of transformation.

CHAPTER FIFTEEN

ANJU
PART ONE

OCTOBER

Anju at age thirty-nine

ANJU   My naturopath recommended you. I have a lot going on: digestion issues, body pains, hormonal shifts, and skin rashes. I seem to get better and then I slide back again. My symptoms keep changing, and they get noticeably worse when I have contact with my family. She felt this kind of work might help find the underlying cause.

D   *I lay my hand over Anju's eyes.* Wow! The energy in your head is striking in its power and frequency. Your upper chakras are radiant with beautiful light. Your sixth chakra is active, and the flow of energy in your left-brain hemisphere is fluid. It's fantastic—I *sense* that you have an extremely strong desire to be part of the solution.

ANJU   I practise Kundalini yoga and I'm really into my career as a social worker and activist. I have fought for women's and girls' rights since my early twenties.

D   And you have done a lot of talk therapy.

ANJU   Yes, indeed.

D   Hmmm … *I float my hands above Anju's throat.* It's a really different story in your body. The fluidity radically cuts off at your neck. Your fifth chakra is very congested and depleted.

ANJU   Oh dear …

D   Yes, there certainly is a lot of contrast.

A few minutes later:

Hmmm … I *hear* you arguing with someone. Is it your mother?

ANJU   Oh yes!

D   I *sense* that the conflict and verbal arguments with your mother since early childhood have drained your creative energy. For all the verbal excess, your voice is nonetheless silenced.

ANJU   I love to sing … but I do it so rarely.

D   You're not singing and you're not speaking your truth either. There seems to be a significant disconnect here. The channel between your throat and heart chakras is blocked. *I slide my right hand to Anju's chest.* Your heart energy is extremely jumpy.

ANJU   I frequently experience heart palpitations. I feel like my heart chakra is closed.

D   Your whole chest is congested, not only your heart chakra.

A few minutes later:

Oh … Your liver is a big part of it. It is significantly compromised … The energy is stagnant and contracted. I *sense* that there is a long story written here with many chapters. You've been building this dam for a while.

ANJU   Yeah, well, my diet is really not what it should be.

D   We'll get back to all of this, but let's keep moving down so we get the sense of the whole picture. *My hands slide down to Anju's pelvis. The congestion gets even denser.*

A few minutes later:

Your pelvis is a block of ice. It's frozen more solid than the polar ice caps. You are very disconnected from this part of your body. The distance between your head and your pelvis is like Canada to Iceland. And unfortunately your cosmic underwear is damaged.

ANJU   Oh … what does that mean?

D   You have an etheric field close to your body. This energy field is basically a replica of your whole physical body. When healthy, it's a fluid blue fabric that resonates with love and compassion. In that sense, it's porous and absorbs nourishing beneficial energy. Yet it is also like a shield that repels unbeneficial energy, like water off a duck's back. In your case, your etheric field is virtually non-existent from navel to mid-thigh—that's the portion I refer to as your cosmic underwear. Life is much better—in fact, it's a whole other story— if your cosmic underwear is intact. This weakness in your field speaks of sexual trauma. Are you aware of any violation in your history?

ANJU   I have no memory of being sexually abused. No.

D   *My sense is that there is sexual abuse in Anju's history, but the memories are repressed. I choose not to mention it in this session.* Let's check your legs. Hmmm … The energy here is like molten lead. The congestion in your body significantly amplifies as I move down to your feet. Your connection to the earth is tenuous. It looks like you live in your head.

ANJU   That makes sense.

D   We've moved a lot of energy here today. I suggest you take an Epsom salts bath every day for at least a week. This will help you integrate this session and keep the flow moving. We need to thaw your body, especially your pelvis. We've just updated your self-healing to-do list by a lot. Your self-healing team is now awakened out of its status quo mode and is now deployed on various missions in the tissues of your physical body, as well as your emotional, mental, and spiritual bodies. The process of integration normally takes approximately three weeks, more or less one week for each level.

ANJU   Wow! I do feel different.

D Also, by boosting your ki energy and encouraging your openness to love and compassion, we create a climate that lends itself to cleansing and detoxing. Eat lots of green leafy vegetables—especially the bitter ones, like parsley, rapini, and dandelion leaf—drink lots of water with lemon, especially in the morning, and eat dinner no later than seven so that your liver can rest and flush through the night.

ANJU OK. I'll do that. Thanks.

D I look forward to witnessing your integration in the next session.

Namaste.

ANJU Namaste.

NOVEMBER

ANJU I don't feel so great. I've had a headache for the past four days. I've been nauseated too. I had a chest cold for seven days a week ago. It's been rough.

D I am loath to say it, but I think this is very good news. *I rest my hands on Anju's shins for a few minutes.*

Indeed, your liver has kicked into high gear. You are very open to change. Your headache and nausea, though, are indicating that your liver is having to work very hard. It needs support. As I mentioned in our last session, your toxicity levels are high. I recommend you do a liver cleanse supervised by your naturopathic doctor. In the meantime, eat light and green and keep drinking lots of water. In terms of the chest cold, my *sense* is that you are clearing your lungs. Do you smoke?

ANJU I stopped smoking ten years ago!

D Still, the energy flow in your lungs is quite stagnant. *I rest one hand on Anju's thigh and place the other on her floating ribs.* Some of the nicotine residue is still present and actively clearing. Once you get going on the liver cleanse, you will feel some relief. The liver is the main filter in the body. It will facilitate the detoxification process in all your organs and in your lymphatic system too.

ANJU Actually, my breasts have been extremely sore since the last session. Also, my menstrual cycle was super-short last month. My naturopathic doctor thinks that I didn't ovulate.

D   Now this is really good news: it means your pelvis and reproductive organs are thawing. You're responding really well to this work. It *is* progress, if you can believe it. You are moving out of numbness into sensation. Welcome the sensations. Nothing is more wrong or broken than it was a few weeks ago. The clearer and louder the voices are, the easier it will be to make the connections and clear the underlying causes. These voices let us know where to focus love and compassion.

ANJU Oh dear … is it going to hurt more?

D   In the long run, what could hurt more than the numbness? These voices are a blessing. Numbness hides your truth, and sensations speak it. *I'm delighted that Anju's shock and traumas are speaking already. It is clear that we are delving into submerged memories of sexual abuse and that they are emerging already. Anju's previous therapy, academic studies, and activism have paved the way. I again choose not to speak about this in this session.*

ANJU I see, it makes sense. My hands and feet have also been extremely sore for the past few weeks.

D   *I lay a hand on each hand.* Hmmm … I *sense* your mother's energy in your hands. Does your mother experience pain in her joints?

ANJU She does! My mother has arthritis in her hands and feet.

D   My *sense* is that you are hesitating to do something; something you know your mother will disapprove of.

ANJU Yes, I am! I'm thinking about quitting my job to become a freelance consultant. My mother disapproves of this idea vehemently.

D   I *sense* that she disapproves because she's scared. She is worried that you are throwing away your ticket to safety. What does your gut tell you?

ANJU It tells me that it's time. I can do this. I'm scared too, but it feels right. It's what I want to do. I've wanted to do it for so long. I think I just need to take the plunge.

D   I think you're right.

DECEMBER

Anju at age forty

D   What is winter solstice stirring for you, Anju?

ANJU   I'm not sure. What do you mean?

D   The winter and summer solstices as well as the vernal and fall equinoxes are particularly auspicious times for change, healing, and transformation. Nature's wheel is turning and taking you along with her into another incarnation of her power and abundance. It's like the riverbed in which the life force flows narrows by a quarter at equinox and by half on solstice. The power of this current propels you toward your truest expression of your genius and life purpose. On the two solstices especially, you are buoyed through the archetypal journeys of death and rebirth. I see great shifts in my friends, my clients, and myself at these junctures.

ANJU   Well, I've been on a liver detoxification program supervised by my naturopathic doctor for two weeks.

D   Fantastic news! I'm so delighted to hear this. Your liver and gallbladder orb is the instigator of growth and change. Let's see how you are responding.

     I hold Anju's head in my hands. Wow! … The energy in your throat is shifting dramatically. Your fifth chakra is much less congested. I *hear* a loud voice in there. Not the one actively in conflict with your mother; this is a voice that is closer to your heart. I *hear* "I'm so pissed off! No, no, and no!" Hmmm … It's a younger you rattling her cage. I *sense* that you're in your early teens.

ANJU   Oh, that makes sense.

D   It looks like you're not only meeting the part of you who was hurt and argued with your mom but also your courageous and angry teenager who created boundaries in whatever way she could. Think of her as an architect of your survival—these are your old friends and allies who stepped in and set up strategies of survival based on the resources you had at the time for whatever adversity or crisis you were experiencing. They're always really clever and often pretty tough—in this case, she's one angry young girl.

ANJU   Oh yes, I definitely was.

D   Let's check your liver. *I settle my left hand on Anju's liver and my right on her right thigh.* There's no doubt your liver cleanse has stirred this valiant architect out of her slumber.

A few minutes later:

Woo … There's nothing like an angry teenager. She's on a rampage. I *hear* "I want out, out, out! And I want to be drunk and stoned out of my mind!"

ANJU   Oh my God, I was so out of control. It was bad … really bad! I drank so much … all the time ... for a long time … for years … up into my thirties. It was really bad ...

D   I'm sure your liver is now releasing some of these physical toxins. But, was it really about being out of control and bad or was it a strategy to numb your pain?

ANJU   Huh?

D   It looks to me like you were numbing your body and mind using the resources you had at the time. I *sense* that it was a reasonable response to your circumstances. Yes, you drank and smoked a lot, and the toxic impact of these substances on your liver is not healed yet (that will take some time); yet it looks like you successfully created healthy boundaries. Although seemingly "out of control," I *sense* that you made sound choices.

ANJU   Well, I still had A's in school—and in university too.

D   So you created a framework and stuck to it. It doesn't look to me as though you were so out of control after all. Your architect created a perfectly successful system of survival. Your induced numbness was your much-needed balm and your sword, protest, and strength.

ANJU   Oh it was! I've never thought of it like that before.

D   Witness your fourteen-year-old architect of survival with compassion. See how brilliant she was. It's winter solstice today; we transition into winter, the season of inner awareness and introspection. It's the perfect day to welcome that young and misunderstood self into your heart. It's a sacred holiday and a potent time to reclaim aspects of yourself that have been long buried or, worse yet, exiled. There's no better time to celebrate your courage, resourcefulness, commitment, and beauty!

ANJU   Mmm …

D   I *sense* that you've been looking at yourself through your mother's eyes. Your mother, unfortunately, judged you rather than supported you. And in turn you judged and still judge yourself. The resourceful Anju who has surfaced today has been cast out into the doghouse for years. For years she has been criticized for being the "wild one," a troublemaker and a failure.

ANJU   Yes, she was a source of shame for the family.

D   There is no shame in surviving in whatever way you could. Compassionately embrace your wild one. Induct her into your hall for great women and girls. Honour your quest to survive and your Herculean effort to pull yourself out of your oppressive family dynamic.

ANJU   Absolutely!

D   Great job. Your wild one sure is enjoying the long-overdue respect and attention. She loves it. Your self-acceptance is like mega WD-40 in action throughout your body. Your ki energy is actively creating new pathways though old blocks to help you connect to the earth and the sun.

ANJU   She's so beautiful! *Anju shakes her head.* Wow … What she went through!

D   Indeed. And we only really know the half of it.

ANJU   So true. It's so long ago.

JANUARY

ANJU   I got together with my teenage best friend in my hometown over Christmas. She gave me a photograph of the two of us at age nineteen. We laughed and reminisced and told stories until the wee hours of the morning. It was amazing!

D   I *hear* lots of music.

ANJU   Oh … We used to sing and dance on my bed like crazy!

D   Cyndi Lauper fans perchance?

ANJU   For sure. Girls just want to have fun.

D   Hahahaha … It's such perfect timing … I can't think of a better time for you to reconnect with an old teenage friend. It's such a gift to actually share stories with someone who was there with you, an ally no less.

ANJU   Yeah, she reminded me of stuff I didn't remember. And vice versa. It was amazing to be immersed in that era of my life like that. It's all so much more tangible now. I was so beautiful. I'm totally in awe of what I did … of what I did to survive.

D   *I check in with Anju's liver.* You now honour your wild teenager, witness her, love her, see her through your own eyes, and celebrate your rebellion and your voice. This is fantastic. As a result, your liver is still in high gear clearing physical, emotional, mental, and spiritual toxicity. The released energy is floating through your energy field on its way out to the earth through your feet.

Anju quiets down and drops into a deep meditative state. She drinks ki energy for twenty minutes, voraciously quenching her thirst and surrendering to her release and integration. Once the loosened toxic debris is out of the way, Anju opens on a deeper level. Going back to your hometown and connecting with a teenage friend is serving you well. It looks like you retrieved a soul fragment left behind. You rescued a part of you who was still trapped in your childhood home. Let's help you welcome that part of you into your heart now. *Anju stays with the process. She is brave and focused.*

ANJU   Oooh … *Anju raises her hand to her heart. She experiences pain in her chest and left breast.*

D   Hmmm … I *sense* that someone is touching your breast. Yet you feel powerless rather than loved. I *sense* that you are unable to stop him. Do you see who it is?

ANJU   No.

D   Is it your brother?

ANJU   Oooh … I remember being alone in the house with my brother. I'm twelve years old. My shirt is off and my brother is touching my breasts with his hands and … and his mouth! Woah …

D   *Anju's distress lurches out in a sob. It's like a volcanic eruption. Anju's chest heaves as the scene plays itself out in her mind's eye. Her day-to-day consciousness is forging a new relationship with her submerged memories and traumatized astronaut.* It's OK, Anju … You have been running on parallel tracks for a long time. Now your knowing self and unknowing self are meeting. Isn't it strange how you can feel you knew without knowing all along?

ANJU   Yes … It is a very strange feeling. Yes, you're right … I've known all along. Oooh.

D   Stay with that knowing, Anju. This is soul-level knowing. You are dropping into a moment that you haven't acknowledged in your day-to-day consciousness for a while, maybe never. You've heard of dissociation—it's very effective. When you are too powerless to get out of a situation physically, your clever little architects find ways to get you out anyhow. So you were gone. But your knowing self is very powerful, bringing you to this moment. Connect with this energy. It's with love, and lots of it, that you're going to unlatch these painful memories from your tissues. *My hands channel love and compassion to every level of Anju's Sacred Tree. I affirm my presence as a guide and a compassionate witness. My steadiness and connection to the earth and the sun create the space for Anju to stay focused on her heart consciousness. I feel Anju's throat tighten. One of the ropes keeping the secret securely hidden is resisting the release.*

Ten minutes later:

Hmmm … Part of you is resisting the shift. I *sense* that your silence protected your brother too and that you are still trying to protect him.

ANJU   Yes, he's a victim too!

D   You are seeing your vulnerability, but you are vividly seeing his as well.

ANJU   Yes. It's unbelievable the danger we were both in every time we left that house. We were the only brown family in that small town in Alberta. We were so … vulnerable!

D   And allies too. *Anju sobs. Her anguish and sorrow are palpable.*

A few minutes later:

You were both in it together. Yet he hurt you too. It's a very powerful act to break the silence, and so hard to do if it feels like it is separating you from one of your allies. Allow yourself to soften into yourself, embrace yourself with as much love and compassion as you have for your brother. That's it! Hold both of you with compassion.

A few minutes later:

Your energy is shifting rapidly. Welcome back into your body and Sacred Tree, Anju! You are safe, loved, heard, and witnessed. Your energy is flowing in your legs and feet too. Hmmm … I *feel* you connect to the earth energy, but it's not here in Canada. The earth is extremely red. Are you connecting to the earth in India?

ANJU   At twenty-eight, I travelled in Kerala, a southwestern province on the Arabian Sea. The earth there is very red. I felt a deep sense of connection to the earth there. That's where my father was born and raised.

D   You were in India during your first Saturn return! That's a rather propitious time to set off on such a big adventure.

ANJU   Yes, I left my boyfriend and spent a year travelling and working in India.

D   Welcome home, Anju, welcome to your Sacred Tree rejuvenated by the beautiful red earth of Kerala and the sun.

ANJU   Ooouuuh … Hahahaha … It's amazing.

D   I suggest you follow the same protocol as last time. Epsom salts particularly support clearing this kind of trauma. Rest as much as possible and of course drink a lot of water and eat green. Your liver is going to continue clearing, so take care. Give yourself time to absorb and integrate the information that surfaced in the session. Soften into your rekindled connection with your twelve-year-old self. Listen hard for her whispers and love her to bits.

Namaste.

ANJU   I will. Namaste.

MID-FEBRUARY

ANJU   I have had horrible headaches! I'm nauseated all the time and I have a skin rash. And my hands have been sore all week.

D   Oh dear … Let's see … I *sense* that you're detoxifying big-time. *I settle my hands under Anju's head for a few minutes.* Lots of unbeneficial energy has been loosened out of your tissues, yet it still hangs heavy in your aura. You're only partly through the process of clearing it. Something is blocking your progress. Hmmm … The sympathy you feel for your brother's victimization clings to your breast tissue and chest. It's overriding your own sorrow and anguish. Compassion is a very powerful energy. But it's not heavy like this. Something is amiss.

ANJU   Oh?

D   Ah … A thick cloud of shame hangs over your left chest and shoulder. Let's see what your hands are saying. I *hear* "What if Mother finds out!" The plot thickens. Your hands are burdened by shame and culpability. You are still holding on to another aspect of the secret. This is a different architect of survival, one who has dedicated all her energy to maintaining this censorship 24/7 for over twenty-six years. *Anju's energy shifts dramatically. Her body sinks into the table. Her breath deepens.* The pressure to keep the secret is tangible. Do you feel that?

ANJU   It's awful.

D   The good news is that the secret's guardian is open to receiving our love and compassion. We're here for you. We love you.

ANJU   I so love you! *Anju closes her eyes and shifts her body. Her focus speaks of her years of therapy and her ability to be courageously present to do the work. She softens into compassionate witnessing.*

D   Little Anju is right here. Do you feel her? *Anju nods.* It's OK. We're here. We love you. I *sense* that you are rocked to and fro by ferocious waves. It feels like you are drowning. It's OK. Reach out; we're here.

    Five minutes later:

    Suddenly, Little Anju lurches forward and blurts out her secret. Here it comes, Anju, I *hear* "I'm having sex with my brother!" *Anju's chest visibly heaves.* Sweetie, it's OK. We can see that you are hurt. You've done nothing wrong. Through her tears, I *hear* Little Anju saying: "But I touched my brother's genitals!"

ANJU   Ugh …

D   You believe you've done something really bad. You're afraid of being punished, so your architect of survival is keeping the secret to avoid being reprimanded and rejected. You are hurt, Little Anju. You need to be rescued, loved, and cared for. This is not sex, it's abuse. Your shame and guilt are submerging your truth. Your brother sexually abused you.

ANJU   It's so confusing … and scary.

D   You store this shame and guilt deep in your bones, Anju. You felt utterly condemned. *Anju shivers from head to toe.* That's it, Anju, you are letting the vibration of love touch this part of you.

A few minutes later:

The cells and molecules in your bones and marrow are releasing this unbeneficial and traumatic charge. Dignity is flooding back into your spiritual, mental, emotional, and physical energy bodies. Thankfully, you only think you have lost your dignity. On a soul level, you always know your truth. It's only on the other levels that you suffer the perceived loss of dignity. The shift is profound, Anju. You hear your wisdom and witness your experience.

Five minutes later:

Ah … Your ki energy is travelling up to reach the sun and down your legs to embrace the beautiful red earth of Kerala. That's the taste of integration.

ANJU   Oh my God … That was intense. That was buried so deep.

D   Take your time, Anju; lie still for at least five minutes. Give yourself time to integrate. The rest will give your energy bodies the chance to reset and regroup before you have to deal with all the usual effort and stresses of daily life.

ANJU   I'm going straight home. More Epsom salts baths, that's for sure. Words fail me. Thank you.

D   It's a lot of information to embrace in an hour. Just stay with the love. Place your hands on your heart while you bathe. And hold on to Little Anju. She's one brave and beautiful girl!

ANJU   She is. I had no idea.

LATE FEBRUARY

ANJU   I've had headaches again … STILL! I have a looming deadline though, and my long work hours are probably contributing. I am really exhausted.

D   *I slip my hands under Anju's head for a few minutes.* I can feel that you're tired, yet the energy in your head is unusually blocked. These headaches are not like your previous headaches either; they're not due to your liver detoxification. The congestion is more on the left.

ANJU   Yes, I feel that.

D Normally, your head is quite clear energetically and your body is blocked. Hmmm … Releasing the secret embedded in your body seems to have dislodged a deep-seated belief. I *sense* that you have been imprisoned in a duality that's causing a profound rift in your being: you perceive your spirit as beautiful and pure and your body as ugly and dirty.

ANJU Oh yes, that sounds very familiar.

D Yes—a familiar and helpful architect of survival for a while. Yet this mind–body split is not working for you anymore. A big part of you knows you've done nothing bad, so you don't need to reinforce that split anymore. Let's make sure your twelve-year-old is on board with the rest of you now. *I shift my hands to Anju's abdomen.*

Five minutes later:

Refreshing, fluid energy pulses through newfound pathways in her pelvis. That's it, Anju, more unknowing is melting and with it old self-loathing. You've done nothing wrong or dirty. And you're not dirty or impure because someone has violated you. You so know this on an intellectual and political level. Your therapy, studies, and activism amplify the potency of your release. Now let the knowledge drop into your heart.

A few minutes later:

That's it, Anju! Your energy is clearing in your biological heart. *I shift one hand to Anju's chest.* Breathe in your beauty, strength, and dignity! Let self-love flourish in your heart and lungs. Release the hot disharmony of shame from your lungs. You are so there, Anju. Fantastic! How are you feeling?

ANJU Better, but my head is still sore.

D OK … let me check in again. Hmmm … Even though you are opening up to your truth in your day-to-day consciousness and are willing to know more if necessary, your denial machine is still clunking along, reinforcing that mind–body split. Architects of survival are die-hards. They hang on until they are absolutely certain that you are safe. Yet the pain in your head is also evidence that you are aware that the system is old, that it doesn't serve you anymore.

A few minutes later:

That's it, you're doing great! The whirring machine of denial in your left-brain hemisphere is grinding to a halt. That's it, continue to forge an even deeper connection with Little Anju. Welcome her into your heart and Sacred Tree!

ANJU I see you, Little Anju, I really do. I love you. I'm here for you.

D   Anju is your primary caregiver now. She loves you and cares for you. You're safe. You've done nothing wrong. I can see that there are still more memories locked in your pelvis. It's OK. You're in a process, one piece at a time, little one. You don't have to keep the denial machine going in order to release, safely and in their own time, the memories. You can be at peace with the process of self-healing and trust its timing. It's OK. You're OK. You can soften and be safe. We love you.

A few minutes later:

Channels of energy open in Anju's pelvis like a web of melting paths through an iceberg. Receive.

ANJU   OK, more baths. Same routine. I am going straight home again. Woo, it's intense. Good, but intense.

MARCH

ANJU   I hate men right now! I mean, really. This thought never leaves my mind! I'm not sure about my boyfriend either. I'm exhausted. I'm just so exhausted! I decided to go back on the liver cleanse.

D   *I slip my hands under Anju's head for a few minutes.* Hmmm ... I sense that you are working with Kali energy.

ANJU   Yes, I am.

D   Are you meditating regularly?

ANJU   Yes, I am.

D   You are calling in big energy. It's bound to stir things up. After all, it's Kali, the Goddess of death and transformation, we are talking about here.

ANJU   Hahahaha ... Yes, it is. She's rather potent.

D   And that's still an understatement. The good news is that you're detoxifying. You have a long way to go though, so the process is exhausting. In addition to Kali's fire, the wood energy of spring and the vernal equinox is also accelerating and amplifying the magnitude of your liver cleansing. This is the prime time of year to clear the liver. It's unfortunately hard to pull off this kind of spring-driven growth and clearing without some physical discomfort. You're stirring up a lot of emotional toxins too. Among other things, you are clearing rage.

ANJU   Oh yes, that's an understatement. Hahaha … I'm fuming.

D   Yes, it is infiltrating your present. Listen carefully; with practice you will learn to distinguish the old from the new. All that said, there is something more going on this week. Let's check in here. You're exhausted, yes … but I *sense* that you also feel overwhelmed, powerless, and out of body.

ANJU   Yes, I do. It's true, I don't just feel tired.

D   Exactly. It's the weight of this emotional state that is dragging you down. It's exhausting to feel oppressed. The weight of these emotions bears down on your chest and mouth. *My left hand shifts from Anju's liver to her chest and my right works on her field above her mouth.* Is there something more specific going on with your boyfriend? It seems to me you were triggered earlier this week. Something to do with his mouth … Does your boyfriend have a beard? Did he shave it?

ANJU   Oh … yes, he did. Oh … Oh, now I remember … I went totally out-of-body when he kissed me, especially when he touched my breasts. Now that I think about it, I was totally freaked out.

D   His smooth, hairless skin triggered you. You know, your brother didn't have facial hair when he abused you.

ANJU   He still doesn't! Oh my God, I've always dated men with facial hair!

D   You've been unconsciously yet very cleverly avoiding this sensation and trigger for years. As painful as the trigger is right now, it's extremely useful. It's a clear signal that a part of you is still in distress.

ANJU   Ugh …

D   I know … it is excruciating while you are in it, but in the long run triggers are fantastic tools. Let's reach out to your little one. Let's make sure she knows it's all over. Invite your twelve-year-old traumatized astronaut here now. Let her know that she's lovingly sheltered in your heart.

        Five minutes later:

        That's it, allow the sensations you experienced while your brother kissed you surface. You'll feel edgy for a few minutes and might be uncomfortable for bit.

ANJU   It is uncomfortable. But I want to do it.

D   Remember it's just you; your brother is not here. You are inviting yourself at age twelve, thirteen, and fourteen to be present—without him or anyone else who hurt you—just your beautiful self.

A few minutes later:

That's it … hold your young teenage self while she tells you her story. Let her cry in your arms if she needs to. Soothe her. Embrace her. Let her know she's safe and that it's over. Acknowledge how bewildered and confused she is. Like a big sister, explain things to her. She's not alone anymore. You're her caregiver now.

Ten minutes later:

Yes! You're doing great, Anju. You are compassionately witnessing your younger self. Your love is loosening the roots of your outrage, disgust, powerlessness, helplessness, shame, shock, and trauma. Encourage your love to swell even more. Feel a wave of compassion build over your chest and mouth. Feel the wave heave, so much so that the pressure in your chest dissipates.

A few minutes later:

That's it. Feel the flow burst onto the shore at your feet. Hear the resonant crash celebrating your release from your pain. Acknowledge both the trauma and the love as they travel down through your pelvis, legs, and feet. Let it all release in the earth through the soles of your feet. That's it. Clear. Clear. Clear. Honour your grace and power. Feel gratitude flow in your being. In turn, receive the regenerative energy of spring in the earth and the sun.

Receive. Receive. Receive.

A few minutes later:

There you are, you're reconnecting to Kali's fire, and the red, red earth of Kerala. You are in harmony with the earth and the sun. Oh … Little Anju is fast asleep in your heart. It's a long-awaited reprieve. Receive.

ANJU   She *is* fast asleep! I have such a hard time resting. Oh … I don't want to wake her up.

D   Take your time—there's no rush. Take the time to integrate. Soak in this harmonious state without my presence in your field. Imprint the sensations and know that you can be in this state without my guidance. Drink quietly. Lie still for a bit.

APRIL

ANJU   I'm feeling really challenged right now. I'm tired. My hands hurt and my uterus too! My skin is breaking out again! My relationship is collapsing … I'm totally terrified of being alone!

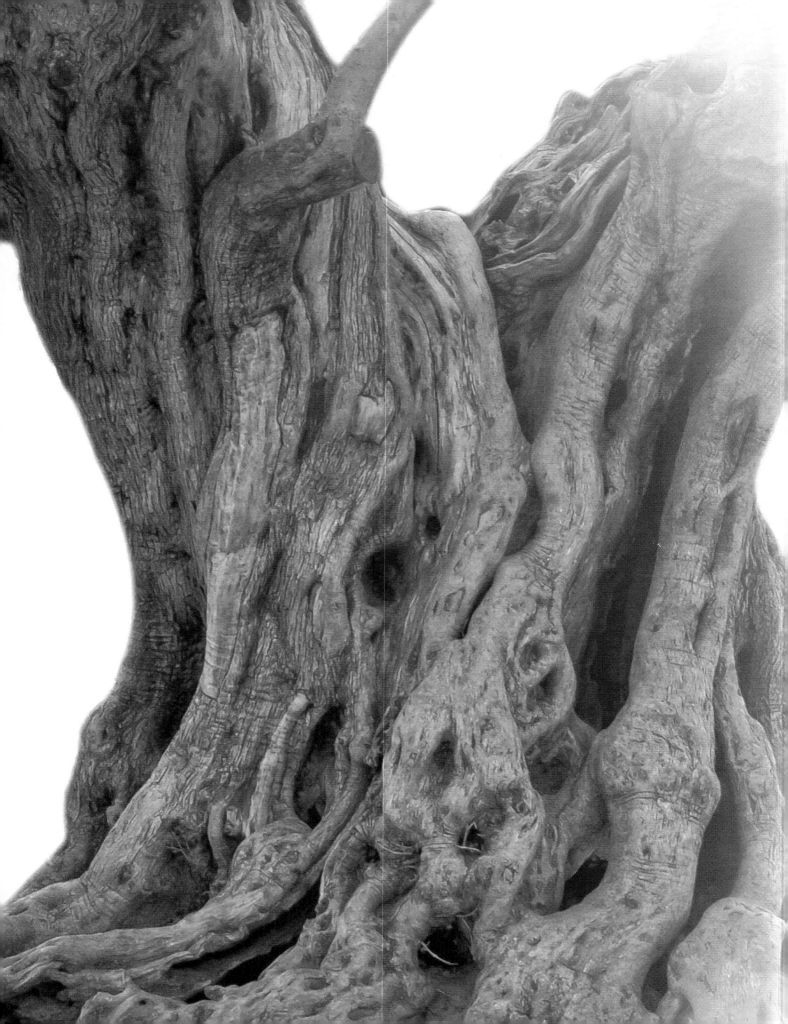

D *I slip my hands under Anju's head for a few minutes.* Hmmm … Your fear is really strong. So much so that your upper chakras are rather shut down. That's very unusual for you.

A few minutes later:

When you say that your relationship is collapsing, are you saying that your boyfriend is distancing himself from you or is it rather that you are distancing yourself from him?

ANJU I guess I'm the one really.

D Are you more aware of your dissatisfaction?

ANJU Yes, there's all kinds of stuff coming up for me.

D We are in the spring thaw now. You're moving a great deal of energy and growing on many levels. Your perception of yourself is shifting. It's often part of the healing process to see your family, friends, and lover differently, and they you. You're a different person than you were when you met this man. It makes sense that he feels different to you now. Your needs are changing. Do you think he is willing to change with you?

ANJU Oh God no. He's not the therapy type. He doesn't look at his stuff, ever.

D If he's not changing with you, are you then willing to wait for him? Do you think this could actually work?

ANJU No, not really. I'm committed to my healing. It's a priority for me.

D You don't want to be alone though. This fear really has a grip on you right now. It's more than that though. Hmmm … I *sense* that you don't want to find yourself without a caregiver again. Is your boyfriend really a viable caregiver?

ANJU No …

D Caregiving is a contract that reaches far beyond the sexist construct that your man be your provider and protector. Caregiving is soul work. None of your younger selves should be reliant on the man in your life for care, love, and safety. You are taking care of your teenage self, and my sense is that you are also willing to be present for all parts of yourself that may still be in distress. You are your own most capable and loving caregiver.

ANJU I am! Yes, absolutely.

D So no part of you is truly alone then. All young Anjus can count on you all the time. In light of this, you can go beyond shifting this old dynamic with your boyfriend; you can liberate yourself from your parents too. You don't need them now like you did when you were a child and teenager. Even on that front, you can shift the dynamic. You truly are your own primary caregiver now.

ANJU   Absolutely, yes.

D   *Kali's fire blows into Anju's sixth and seventh chakras and from there through to her entire body. Energetic debris floats through Anju's body toward the earth through her feet.* There you go, old caregiver contracts are toppling down. It's a big spring thaw!

A few minutes later:

Oh and your kidneys and adrenal glands are releasing fear. Kali's healing flame is warming your kidneys and softening your cold fear of loneliness. You so know that you are the most reliable and trustworthy caregiver you could ever wish for.

ANJU   I am!

D   OK, so in the same way you are never alone on a spiritual level either. That old familiar loneliness and fear of solitude fundamentally speaks of your disconnection with your competent caregiver self—your Sacred Tree, high self, soul, inner wisdom or the Buddha within, or whatever you want to call it.

ANJU   They're the same thing?

D   Yes. And your competent caregiver is a most important aspect of your reliable triumvirate: Sacred Tree, the earth, and the sun. So to make matters more intense, trauma often amplifies this disconnection by also uprooting your Sacred Tree and destabilizing its connection to the earth and the sun. This is the core issue at play when you are in the grip of such intense fear. In other words, the feelings you are experiencing are more akin to a spiritual crisis than feelings rooted in the collapse of your romantic relationship.

ANJU   It makes so much sense. I feel this absence deep within me. No wonder if felt so big.

D   You got it! *Anju's energy shifts dramatically. Love and compassion from the earth and the sun flood in.* You're plugging in! Acknowledge the harmony within your Sacred Tree. Feel your legs strongly connected to your pelvis and firmly rooted in the earth. Land in your tracks. See your path. Feel your head and arms reaching for the sun and drinking its energy. Witness your strength, beauty, and purpose. Now, invite Kali energy. Welcome her fire. Open to your wisdom, clarity, and inner knowing. From this place … decide what needs to be done. From this place … listen to your uterus. What is she saying?

ANJU   Hmmm … You mean listen rather than run around like a chicken with my head cut off. Yeah … right … That sounds like a good plan.

D   Yes, basically that summarizes it. Plug in, hang out in your Sacred Tree, and take the time to listen. Receive. Namaste.

ANJU   Namaste.

MAY

ANJU   It's over with my boyfriend! I'm done.

D   You listened to your uterus?

ANJU   I did! It was so clear once I calmed down and listened.

D   *My right hand cradles Anju's sacrum and the other rests on Anju's chest.* It's definitely a breakthrough, but a burden is bearing down on your chest. Are you feeling good?

ANJU   Not really. I'm relieved, but I'm still really anxious.

D   Yeah … I *sense* that you feel disempowered. Although you are in control and have made the decision to leave your boyfriend, and you know this is for the best, I *sense* that you are still seized by fear. You see clearly enough to do what is best for you, but not so clearly as to be securely in the flow of love and compassion. Your connection with your Sacred Tree, the earth, and the sun comes in and out.

A few minutes later:

Hmmm … It looks like it's hard for you to trust that everything will be OK.

ANJU   Exactly, I took the plunge, but I just don't feel safe.

D   Give the breakup time to play itself out. Patiently move through the emotions that come up, without fear or trepidation. Grieve, clean your apartment, rest, reconnect with friends, and remember to connect daily with your most powerful allies: your Sacred Tree, the earth, and the sun. Meditate and call Kali's fire.

A few minutes later:

When you think of it, the breakup with your boyfriend is more potently a reunification with your Sacred Tree, the earth, and the sun than a separation from him. In time, the feeling of relief will be stronger than the disorientation and sorrow.

ANJU   It's such a relief actually. I know it's the right decision. I know I'm on track. I just have to settle into the process.

D   Exactly. Soften into it rather than contract. You are not only strengthening your connection to your Sacred Tree, but you are also coming into alignment with your personal power!

A few minutes later:

You're not victimized by a breakup; you're actually setting yourself up to manifest your genius and life purpose.

ANJU   I am. I so am.

A WEEK LATER

ANJU   I'm really concerned. I'm still not feeling good. I went for tests. I have mononucleosis. It's a liver disease … figures!

D   *My right hand cradles Anju's sacrum and my left rests on her liver for a few minutes.* Your liver is screaming. Yet you've been cleansing your liver on and off for months now. This is really old stuff trying to emerge. It feels more like a traffic jam rather than stagnation, dis-ease rather than disease. The impulse to shed is there, yet something is stuck. What are you holding on to?

ANJU   I don't know.

D   *My right hand shifts to Anju's pelvis and my right to her chest.* Hmmm … You're holding on to it tightly. I *hear* "If I let go, who knows what will come out? My secret? My shame? All of it? Everything?" It's OK, Anju. There's another layer, that's all, just another layer. You have cleared so many already. You know how do it.

ANJU   OK. I'm ready.

D   Ah … A dense energy has been dislodged from your left breast. It's hovering in your aura. So something is shifting. *I place one hand above Anju's left breast and one immediately under.* There's a particularly potent and tightly packed density clogging your left nipple.

ANJU   Oh dear …

D   Invite love and compassion and call on Kali's fire to penetrate your seventh chakra. Welcome the bright golden light. Surrender to its nourishing flow throughout your body. Encourage the density in your nipple to yield to this flow.

A few minutes later:

That's it; you're doing it. The blockage is softening. I'm *hearing* a charged silence. A young Anju is surfacing. Let's greet her with love and gentleness.

ANJU I love you.

D Hmmm … It's a young Anju around eleven to thirteen years old. We're here to support you, little one. We love you and respect you. You've done nothing wrong. You're hurt. We can feel that. Let us know what we can do for you. We're here for you.

A few minutes later:

Young Anju is extremely distressed. Hug her, Anju. Give her lots of love. I *hear* "Look at this horrible thing I did! Look at all the horrible and shameful things I did!"

ANJU Oh, we're back there again. Geez …

D We are. It's OK. Let's listen and give a lot of love. Hmmm … I *sense* arousal in your nipple. It's erect. It looks like you felt aroused when your brother stimulated your nipples. It's OK, Little Anju. You're not doing anything wrong. You're reaching for love in whatever form is available to you, and your body is reacting to stimuli. It doesn't mean that you are participating in a consensual, mature, or loving sexual interaction. You're a child looking for love. Your brother's contaminated attention is the closest available facsimile to the love and care you crave so much.

ANJU Ugh …

D *I hear an even more charged silence.* That's it, Anju. Stay present. Let the sensations surface. There you go … *A bolt of stinging, electrical energy shoots through Anju's being.*

ANJU Whoa … What's that?

D It looks like you experienced orgasms when your brother touched and kissed your breasts.

ANJU Oh? Ouuuh … My breast really hurts … Ouch.

D You're doing great. Stay with it if you can. We so love this little one. What's happening, little one? We're here with you. You've done nothing wrong. It's hurting. We feel that.

A few minutes later:

I *hear* "There's an even bigger secret." It's OK. We love you no matter what. We're here to help. We love you so much. You're safe now.

ANJU I see it! I held my breast! I presented it to my brother for more touching and kissing! Ouuuh …

D   *A tidal wave of shame and guilt cracks open and pours from Anju's breast, through her chest, and down through her pelvis, legs, and feet.* That's it, let it out through your feet. The earth is there to receive the energy and compost it. Stay with it, you've done most of the work. Let it move through you so that you clear these fierce untruths. Your interpretation of your actions and physical sensations cannot successfully reframe the abuse as consensual sex. This is not proof of anything about you. You are blaming yourself for acts of violence perpetrated against you. He manipulated you and took advantage of you. You were looking for love. This is not love. Feel your sensations. This is pain, not pleasure.

ANJU   Whoa … This is so intense.

D   It is. Orgasms can mask intense pain. I believe it's a survival strategy. Unfortunately, they also amplify the feelings of culpability and shame. It so often hooks in the trauma because your orgasms are used as proof that you are a bad girl doing something disgustingly wrong.

ANJU   That's such a different way of looking at it.

D   It is. And so often these masking orgasms are the crux of the matter. Soothe your little one. Let her know she's done nothing wrong or dirty. Release her from her brother's manipulative grip. Witness her confusion and bewilderment. See her anguish and distress. This is hardly a feel-good operation here. The orgasmic charge ripped through your being. Witness your blown circuits. Feel how out-of-body you are and how detached you are from your soul. If it really was an orgasm, in the true sense of the experience, then it would feel rather different from what you are remembering right now.

     A few minutes later:

     Let your brother carry the weight of his actions. Let him be accountable.

ANJU   Oh … She's on my lap. I can feel her hair, her hands … all of her … her whole body. She's suddenly so real.

D   Hold her tightly in your arms. Fill your heart with unconditional love. Unite and integrate her into your heart and Sacred Tree. What does she need to settle in?

ANJU   You're so beautiful. You're so sacred. I really see you. I love you.

D   *Now in a meditative state, Anju witnesses the horror, pain, fear, terror, and confusion that choked her young traumatized astronaut as her physical body biologically responded to the sexual stimulation within an abusive context. She also experiences the powerfully efficient survival system her body used to mask her pain. She is witnessing these moments from the inside. She is making the profound distinction between a physical orgasmic response during abuse and orgasmic pleasure that transcends the biological response and blossoms into the emotional, mental, and spiritual bodies. She suffers the split … sees it … feels it … and understands it …*

Fifteen minutes later:

Whoa … You're doing great! Your liver is releasing the charge too. Your wild one has just rolled in, you know, that plucky architect of survival we met in our first couple sessions. I *hear* "Madonna wears black! I wear black. And I have a best friend and she wears black too!"

ANJU   Oh! It was the era of *Desperately Seeking Susan*! Remember … the black leather jacket and leggings!

D   Your booming voice howls "Like a Virgin" … Wow! You're so brilliant. You sang your innocence! You *were* a virgin. The sexual abuse was not your sexual awakening. This is so great! Witness your clarity, cleverness, courage, and chutzpah! *Anju laughs and cries simultaneously.*

It couldn't be sweeter! So many teenage girls belted out this song at the top of their lungs. Obnoxious, irritating, disempowering, sexy, or fun, whatever you think of it, in the mouth of a sexually abused girl, the lyrics articulate a profound truth. It is a most beautiful, inspiring, and powerful anthem of salvation.

ANJU   It is! It's so powerful.

D   And beautiful. Namaste.

JUNE

ANJU   I moved into a larger apartment so that I can host my parents in Toronto. It's awful. Everything is wrong! It's just awful. I loved my sweet nest with all its humble quirks, even my funny little fridge. I so regret my decision. I just rushed into it.

D   *I rest my hands on Anju's shins for a few minutes.* Ouch … You're frozen … You're not in your body and Sacred Tree at all. You have no sweet home. This is a powerful trigger for you.

A few minutes later:

Your distress is rather intense. Your response, however, feels greater than the situation warrants. I feel your mother's energy. What does she have to do with this?

ANJU   I'm not sure. I did move so I could host my parents in Toronto.

D   Hmmm … I *see* you wringing your hands like she does. You are sinking in fear, helplessness, and powerlessness like she does. Your resourcefulness has been hijacked. I *sense* that the loss of your home-sweet-home has awakened a very old trauma.

ANJU   I'm feeling really awful. My anxiety is through the roof.

D   *I rest my left hand on Anju's heart and my right on her right thigh.* Hmmm … I *see* a living room. It's evening. There are very few lights on. You are quite young. Maybe five years old. Your mother picks up the phone. After uttering a few misshapen words, she collapses on the sofa.

ANJU   Oh … this must be when my mother found out that her brother was dead. She mothered him, you know. He committed suicide!

D   Ah … Upon hearing this news, your mother passed out. The shock constricted her being and blackened her universe. In a fraction of a second the world changed in your house in that small town in Alberta: your mother found out that her dear brother died, but not only that, you thought your ama was dead. You stood there, paralyzed by terror. I *hear* "Ama's gone! She's dead." Piercing grief flooded your little being.

ANJU   Ouf … *Anju's chest heaves under the burden of this core abandonment trauma.*

D   Yes, you suffered an intense loss. And of course, she was not physically dead, you realized that after a while, but you felt abandoned nonetheless. She was never the same after that. She was traumatized and frozen emotionally. *Anju's hands throb. I embrace her right hand.*

ANJU   My ama never really came back after that!

D   The sudden loss of your emotional connection with your mother is at the core of everything. This profound experience of abandonment is when the connection with your Sacred Tree started disintegrating.

ANJU   You know, my mother didn't fly home to India to attend the funeral.

D   Your hands throb with your mother's regret. I *sense* that her arthritic inflammation is a physical manifestation of this trauma. Your mother's hands, the hands that tenderly embraced her brother, that lovingly cared for her younger sibling, that once loved—now grieve in silence and regret.

ANJU   She was so powerless. We all were. Oh God, that house … that town. What were we doing there?

D   Yes—from having a home with a loving mother, you ended up in a house without a loving caregiver at the helm. And now, you ask yourself the same question: What am I doing in this apartment? What am I going to do without a safe haven? At forty years old, you're not alone, abandoned, helpless, or powerless like you were at five years old. You have access to far more resources, especially now that the trigger's charge is conscious. Your little five-year-old Anju is safely tucked into your heart. She has a beautiful home and a most devoted Ama—you! In time, you will create a lovely home for yourself.

ANJU I will. I will.

A DAY LATER

ANJU The new apartment ... It's not working ... I still feel awful. I barely slept last night. It's awful, just awful.

D *I rest my hands on Anju's heart for a few minutes.* Hmmm ... There's more to the night of the phone call. Let's keep working through this. You'll feel so much better when the trigger's charge is diffused.

ANJU OK. Let's do it.

D *I drop back in to that dark winter night.* Ah ... I *see* that your father and brother were also present in the living room. Your father also entered a state of shock. Oh ... Your father, too, collapsed on the sofa. Helpless, lost, and overwhelmed, he focused on his wife. You watched in silence. No one supported you—neither one paid attention to you. You felt abandoned by both your parents.

ANJU It was so desolate all of a sudden.

D Yes, by a lot. All of you were even more isolated now, even more scared in Canada's glacial landscape and culture. Your hearts, more than ever, feared, ached, and throbbed with searing aloneness.

A few minutes later:

All of you were, then more than ever, trapped in that living room in that small northern town. You were the only East Indian family, the only brown-skinned family, the only clan of otherness in 1970s rural Alberta.

ANJU That's just it. All of us, alone together, scared and utterly isolated. Why didn't they go back to India for the funeral? It's so crazy!

Five minutes later:

Anju wrings her hands. Oh ... my father was scared of losing his job. He didn't ask for a leave of absence from work so they could attend the funeral. I guess he didn't think he could ask! He was scared to even take that chance! To be that powerless ... that scared ... Oh God ... *Anju shakes her head.*

A few minutes later:

You know, my mother did not return to India for eleven years after that. It's so sad. *Anju raises her hands to her face.*

D   I *sense* that to this day Ama wrings her hands and relives that moment and their decision. Her arthritis screams her sorrow, helplessness, and regret. Hold your little one, Anju. Mourn together the emotional collapse of your ama ... of your beloved ama!

ANJU   My mother was never the same after that. It's so true! Nothing was ever the same after that.

D   Bathe your traumatized astronaut with the reassurance that you are there for her. You will be her caregiver no matter what. Help her settle in the safety of your love, the new home-sweet-home you will create, as well as the energy of the earth and the sun.

ANJU   Ah ... I felt so scared and I felt so alone after that. I really did.

D   Take as much time as you can to rest and take care of yourself over the next few weeks. You are witnessing an aspect of your core wound. Soften into it and call in love and compassion. Soften into their embrace. You were never abandoned by earth and source. Divine Mother's fire, Kali, is there for you, all aspects of you, even all your little ones.

ANJU   Wow! I feel that. Thank you.

D   Happy summer solstice! Yeah, you're right on schedule for a death and rebirth initiation. Welcome to the season of the heart!

ANJU   Oh yeah ... of course. Wow! Intense.

D   Summer solstice is like riding a bucking horse. Just hold on and trust the momentum. Your wood is feeding your fire; it's undeniably helping you shift into a higher vibration.

ANJU   Thank you. Happy solstice, Dany.

SEPTEMBER

ANJU   My parents came and went and all of that, but I can't settle down. I'm experiencing pain in my abdomen. I'm afraid to say I'm still a mess.

D   *My hands settle on Anju's shins for a few minutes.* Hmm ... You're eating wheat again. That's guaranteed to wreak havoc, especially in late summer. Dampness is at an all-time high in this season. Ideal conditions for intestinal yeast. It's a double whammy.

ANJU   Makes sense.

D   *My left hand shifts to Anju's liver while my right rests on her right thigh for a few minutes.* Yikes! Under that wet candida blanket, you're fuming something fierce and mean business. Your liver is crashing its heels on the floor like a flamenco dancer determined to exterminate an army of killer ants. I *hear* "FUCK YOU ALL!" Whoa … Your wild one has screeched back on the scene.

ANJU   I'm angry?

D   It's a smouldering cauldron in there. Let's drop into this.

        A few minutes later:

        Hmmm … The role of daughter strangles you.

ANJU   Oh *that*—for sure—I'm furious.

D   I *sense* that you spit at the systemic sexism drenching your parents' words and gestures when they compulsively celebrate their son.

ANJU   That's putting it mildly.

D   You're choked by the silence your familial contract imposes on you.

        A few minutes later:

        I *see* you lurch around your apartment from chair to table to kitchen, where the fumes of your brother's presence linger and stick. You are and were repulsed by your brother's presence in your home. You are incensed by his entitlement, obliviousness, and power.

ANJU   One month! A whole month!

D   Of course, it wasn't only your parents' visit. It was your brother's visit too. He was there most of the time!

ANJU   That's the most time my brother has ever spent in my home.

D   And there you all were at the table again and again. Now that your brother is not coming over anytime soon, it's safe to feel more now. That's it, Anju, breathe deeply. Drop in.

        A few minutes later:

        I *sense* that when you joined them at the table to share meals, you were present enough and aware enough to acknowledge that you were sharing a meal with your abuser.

ANJU   Exactly.

D Yes, isn't that the end all and be all of it all? I know that feeling all too well. You are expected to share meals as though nothing disruptive or violent has ever occurred. You eat together as if it's totally normal for you to share a "pleasant" meal with a man who has sexually abused you.

ANJU It's what we've been doing for twenty-six years!

D Every time you sit down for a meal together, you silently accept your parents' terms of engagement, namely, that it is your responsibility to maintain the peace at all costs. It's your job to create the illusion that you are a happy family. You have unconsciously agreed to this all-inclusive self-sacrifice. This contract essentially absolves your brother of his culpability and your parents of their responsibility to protect you. Not only that, they are utterly oblivious, eating their bloody sweets and stuffing their faces. Meanwhile, you are expected to stuff your truth down your throat again!

ANJU The pain is excruciating … watching them bond with him … it's awful.

D You now witness your silence and you see the role it has in maintaining your family's status quo. You also witness your role as a Good South Asian Daughter. That contract stipulates that you must acquiesce to the needs of the elders and the son. You are at the bottom of the pecking order.

ANJU Yes, and how!

D Whoa … Not just the left ovary but the energy in your whole left body is jammed.

A few minutes later:

Your denial machine kicked back into gear enough so that you could make it all happen for your mother and father: the perfect visit and the perfect happy family. You participated in the daily ritualistic performance of "happiness" and "familial love." You made it all happen for your mother and father and by default for your brother! *Anju's left body throbs with numbing violence from head to toe. She witnesses the link between her explosive and painful congestion and the denial of her truth to maintain the family peace.*

Fifteen minutes later:

ANJU I don't think I can do this again! Not in that way! And not for him! Part 2 of my healing process is going to include me at the table (or not). I will be fully present, honoured, respected, and loved or not present at all!

D Sun, red earth energy, and Kali's fire just ignited in all your chakras. Denial has many tendrils. It's generally hooked in on many different levels. It takes time, chutzpah, and patience to untangle the mess. This architect of survival was useful, you must remember that, but when it's time for an additional denial contract to topple, go for it! You have everything to gain by dismantling it. Besides, we are heading into the fall. The equinox and change of season spike your capacity for growth and evolution. You have good timing, as always!

ANJU   It's big.

D   It sure is. Take care in the next few weeks. Make sure to rest. And try to cut back on wheat. You will have more reliable access to your resources and your energy will be so much more fluid and strong if you do.

OCTOBER

D   What did the fall equinox stir up for you, Anju? You look like you've been through something.

ANJU   It's been unbelievably wild! I had a flu, fever, congestion, the whole nine yards. I had the worst yeast infection ever. It was so intense ... Basically I lay in bed reviewing my entire sexual history. I mean, everything! I realized that whenever a man expresses sexual desire, I respond; I get on the train without really considering whether this is something I really want. This is huge! Everything feels different!

D   Major fall detoxification of your lungs is underway! The fumes are thick! Grief, the cold disharmony of the lungs, is releasing by the bushel. And shame as well, the hot disharmony of the lungs. Your genitals are having a clear-out sale too. Some of this is linked to the painful physical orgasms you experienced with your brother as well as pleasure you experienced during out-of-body sex in your late teens, twenties, and thirties.

ANJU   I've always been out-of-body ... OMG! *Anju bursts into tears.* It's so painfully true.

D   You mourn the contamination of your sexual awakening and sexuality. You are mourning it and clearing it out simultaneously. This is not a "poor me" moment. You are doing a hard-drive cleanse of your whole man file, with Kali in attendance, no less.

ANJU   The whole thing ... Everything ... I'm bringing you all in to my heart. I love you all! The Goddess has as many arms as there are me's to hug, hold, protect, and celebrate!

D   I can *sense* that you're also turning your compassionate gaze to other women.

ANJU   ... so M-A-N-Y women in my life and career. We're all in the same boat!

D   Yes, we are. *We both soften into a deep meditative state. Anju drinks in the energy of the earth and the sun. Love and compassion nourish her parched Sacred Tree. She opens up enough to experience her body and Sacred Tree anew.*

Fifteen minutes later:

You may find that some of your intellectual, political, and academic beliefs shift in the next while. When you shift to a higher vibration, its wisdom is not contained in your personal life exclusively. Wisdom runs deeper and further than intellectual knowledge. Let it spread and let yourself evolve on all levels and in all aspects of your life. Eventually you will come together as one. The old "the personal is political" statement is a profound spiritual statement of unity and oneness.

ANJU   Of course. Yes, of course it is.

NOVEMBER

ANJU   I am so out of it! I came this close to jumping in bed with a close friend!

D   Hmmm … *My hands settle on Anju's shins for a few minutes.* That statement does not seem to jive with the energy you are presenting. Rather, I *feel* you are worn out after a long battle with your old pattern of responding to sexual interest without questioning if it's something you actually want. I *sense* that the drama was a messy affair: spit flying, nostrils flaring, and horns thrusting forth.

ANJU   Oh?

D   You are not out of it, you lie here victoriously exhausted. You literally took the bull by the horns and flipped it on its back and lashed its hooves. You're so not out of it, you won!

ANJU   For Pete's sake! You're absolutely right! I maintained my boundaries for the first time in my life!

D   Exactly! You won the battle with the horny bull. *My left hand rests on Anju's abdomen and my right rests on her thigh for five minutes.* It's OK to be exhausted and feel a little bruised and out of it. It's a fair price for a little more wisdom. Nothing a little self-love and yoga can't fix. The timing is uncanny. Think of the realizations we discussed in the last session. You received a perfect opportunity to manifest and integrate your newfound wisdom.

ANJU   OK! Wow! I see it now. That's a big step!

D   It's huge! And it's such a blessing!

A few minutes later:

You met your friend's sexual energy and transformed your usual pattern and response. No matter the struggle and messiness of it all, you ultimately created healthy boundaries and stoked your personal power. It's all good, really, really good! Take the time now to drink the earth's energy and bathe in the light from the sun.

A few minutes later:

Drink it up! Receive.

ANJU   I'm so tired.

D   Just keep drinking to replenish your stores. This is what so many spiritual teachers refer to when they suggest that you must thank your petty tyrants. You were given the perfect opportunity to manifest your newfound connection with your Sacred Tree and wisdom. It's such a perfect example. It's a blessing! This is love and compassion in action. That's what that looks and feels like. Go home and rest! Take the weekend off. Celebrate!

ANJU   Ahahaha. I will!

D   Congratulations!

ANJU   Thank you.

DECEMBER

Anju at age forty-one

ANJU   I think I'm having new memories! I think there's other abuse! I'm scared … to think there might be more … others!

D   OK, let's see what the energy of winter solstice is digging up. *I rest my hands on Anju's shins.* An unbeneficial energy coats your head like a balaclava; it's over rather than through your head. *My hands rest on Anju's abdomen for a few minutes.* I *hear* "I hate my hair! I hate my face!" I *sense* that this dates back to your teenage years. Did you torture your hair to change its appearance?

ANJU   I sure did! It was crazy. I tried everything …

D   You also wore thick makeup.

ANJU   Oh yes, dark kohl under my eyes. It was quite the thing.

D   That mask speaks of your internalized racism. Hmmm … Your entire body is wrapped in a toxic layer of unbeneficial energy.

A few minutes later:

Memories are surfacing, you're right. Hmmm … I *sense* that it's at school. I *see* a tall, swank, totally full of himself, sleazy male teacher.

ANJU   Oh I know who that is! He was the vice principal of the high school too!

D   Did he wear extremely tight-fitting, brown plaid pants (balls-to-the-left tight)?

ANJU   Hahaha … Yes, he did. That's him for sure! He undressed me with his eyes all the time!

D   You were the exotic one!

ANJU   I was the only girl who belonged to a visible minority ethnic group!

D   And you were the wild one to boot! I see you in his office.

ANJU   Oh yes … I remember him confronting me one day. He said he knew I was stoned!

D   I *see* you sinking into the floorboards … you in your see-through black leather jacket and leggings. Your clothing felt like nothing more than frail mesh.

ANJU   He always undressed me with his eyes. It was awful.

D   That's bad enough, but I think there is more to it than that. I *sense* a glacial tide seize the blood in your veins. It seems to me that you were also triggered. A dormant terror choked you deep in your being. I *hear* "He knows! He knows that I'm a bad girl!" You were still in denial then. You still believed that you were doing bad things with your brother.

ANJU   Of course …

D   Your perceived guilt uncorked and splattered across the room. I *hear* "He knows! He knows I'm having sex! He knows I'm having sex with my brother! He knows I'm a really bad girl!"

ANJU   Of course it would all jumble in on top of one another.

D   And then you are victimized again … more. You're not only dealing with a teacher with X-ray vision; you are reliving your trauma. Sleaze Balls is sticking to your unresolved trauma and guilt, penetrating your pain, and tearing the secret open. Not to mention the fact that your history of abuse, not only your exoticized flesh, attracts Sleaze Balls like the most powerful Velcro ever devised by DuPont. Unconsciously, he knows and smells your vulnerability and isolation. He's like an animal hunting for its prey. Every cell and molecule of your terrified "dark" being betrays you. He fetishizes your dark skin and mars your flesh with his "voracious sexual appetite"—the very thing he projects onto you. You're cornered. You're the perfect target for sexual harassment.

ANJU   He was quite the operator in our small town! I found out later.

D   Oooh he smells bad … He has quite the history … It looks like he does not take no for an answer. When he wants it, he gets it. He thinks he knows what women need! The political climate of the early 1980s is part of it—you would hope he wouldn't get away with that these days …

ANJU   Uuugh … He does smell real bad! Uuugh. It's awful! Uuugh.

D   You're untangling Sleaze Balls's intrusive gaze from every fibre of your being. His X-ray vision was abusive. He did not have to touch you to violate you. Your auric field is shedding his inappropriate sexual charge, his racism, and a layer of your own internalized racism. A soothing balm heals your skin and strengthens your etheric field. You are released from the floorboards in his office.

Five minutes later:

That's it, Anju, let love and compassion swell over your chest and let the wave of respect dissipate the hurtful charge through your pelvis, legs, and feet.

A few minutes later:

That's it; let it out the soles of your feet. Ride the wave, Anju, ride the wave!

ANJU   Wow! I'm so relieved. It was abuse, but I thought it was much worse. I can see how doubly vulnerable I was because of my brother's abuse.

D   Yes, the fact that it piggybacks on your brother's abuse amplifies the levels at which you were implicated and hurt. You're so on it though. You softened into winter's gift of self-knowledge and awareness. You let it flow. Although you *sensed* your traumatized astronaut's intense pain, you stayed in your Sacred Tree. You stayed the course enough to receive the gift of transformation, on solstice no less!

ANJU   Thank you. I'm so relieved.

JANUARY

ANJU   I'm feeling really rough. Over the holidays, my brother convinced my parents to move to Toronto! He totally bullied me on the phone! My left breast is really sore again!

D   *My hands settle on Anju's shins for a few minutes.* I *sense* that you are triggered. The daughter/sister contract has reared its ugly head again. Your brother's energy and his actions are reminding you that you are their daughter, his sister; that he is the son so you must listen, not ask questions or challenge his authority.

ANJU   Yikes!

D *My left hand settles on Anju's abdomen and my right hand on her thigh for a few minutes.* Hmmm … My *sense* is that you tried to go into denial. It looks like you tried to play the game by their rules like you did it in the past, but it isn't really working, is it?

ANJU No!

D No, not really. I *sense* that you refuse to be shoved back into the dark. No matter how much your sense of obligation tugs at you, denial is not really an option. Your memories flood your chest.

ANJU Ouuuh … It's extremely painful!

D Your heart and left breast scream to remind you of your abuse. It's a no-go, Anju. You cannot be in denial and abandon that part of yourself anymore. You have the right to refuse to adhere to the terms of their contract.

ANJU It's easier said than done.

D I *sense* that you're making yourself smaller to fulfill the role your parents and brother want you to excel at: the Good South Asian Daughter.

A few minutes later:

I *see* you standing there at nine years old: a girl in a short pink dress with your hair in braids.

ANJU Oh my God … that dress. I so see her … her hair!

D She's the good Indian girl who will grow up to be the good Indian wife.

ANJU Of course she is. Oh dear …

D Furthermore, you must be obedient to all members of your birth family: father, mother, and brother. Eventually you will be inferior to your husband, and as a daughter-in-law, you will be subservient to your husband's father, mother, and sons. The tyranny is endless!

ANJU It is endless.

D And as a second-generation South Asian–Canadian woman, you must be subservient and yet you are also free, simultaneously!

ANJU Oh, come on over here. You're so done with all that.

D That's it; liberate her from the confines of all these contracts, demands, expectations, and contradictions. You don't have to obey anyone! And let your little one wear what she wants.

ANJU   Jeans, a T-shirt, and a short 'do, for sure!

D   And give her lots of space to grow, to expand her horizons and reinvent herself as many times as she wants.

        A few minutes later:

        It just so happens that you're wearing a T-shirt with a print of a little girl wearing a short dress, playing an electric guitar with one victorious arm in the air!

ANJU   It's my favourite T-shirt! I bought it at Lilith Fair years ago! The little girl in the dress! I've always loved this T-shirt. I never made the link with the little girl in the pink dress and braids.

D   She's unleashed. Twaaang! Shed your old skin! Align with your capacity to be reborn now. Align with the young girl on the T-shirt with her arm in the air! Let love win!

ANJU   Yes! *Anju raises her right arm in the air.*

JULY

ANJU   I had a terrible nightmare last night: my brother was shacked up in the tool shed. His bed was there. I was there with him. He tried to touch me! And then later my mother tells me, "Oh, the tool shed is your brother's favourite place!"

D   Did he touch you?

ANJU   No, he didn't! I said no. I pushed him away.

D   This is a breakthrough dream. You successfully pushed your brother away. You said no to him for the first time! *I settle my hands on Anju's shins for a few minutes.*

ANJU   Yes, I did! Actually, earlier today I showed him the apartment I rented for our parents. He freaked out. I said, "Tough! This *is* the apartment."

D   You actually said no to your brother in waking life too! Wow! Nothing like a little summer solstice action! This is fantastic! And all of this is riding on your no to the horny bull and all the men in your man file. The season of the heart and fire element is so much about healthy your "yes" and healthy "no." It's all about order and the likelihood of inner peace when healthy boundaries are created. You are cooking with propane!

ANJU   I am … I hadn't put it all together.

D   Your head is tilting to the right shoulder though.

ANJU Oh … I wasn't aware.

D *I slip my hands under Anju's head for a few minutes.* Hmmm … I *sense* that it's a physical manifestation of an emotional state. It seems to me that your head tilts this way when you go out-of-body. Hmmm … You turned your head this way when your brother abused you. Your head is turned in a silent scream, your silent no.

ANJU Uuugh … I always looked toward the door … in my bedroom (*sobs*) … in his bedroom (*sobs*) … Oh and in the living room too (sobs) … I still lean my head that way during sex! (*sobs*)

D *Now in a deep meditative state, Anju releases the intense pain of being out-of-body—the shock of it … the numbness of it … the intensity of the sorrow that results when there is a deep split in the mind, body, and soul. Grounding energy flushes in as Anju sheds another layer of shock and trauma. She feels heavier, more solid, more present, and more grounded than in any other session.*

 Twenty minutes later:

 That's it, Anju. You are dropping into your body and Sacred Tree on a whole new level. Drink it in. Enjoy! It's a huge transition.

ANJU It really is.

D HUGE. It's such an honour to be one of your witnesses. Namaste.

ANJU Namaste.

SEPTEMBER

ANJU My parents now live in Toronto! I'm a wreck! It's totally crazy.

D *I rest my hands on Anju's shins for a few minutes.* Oh dear, you're right, you are an out-of-body wreck! And your father's energy is attached to your left body and your mother's energy is attached on your right. Yikes! They're both getting under your skin.

ANJU I am totally caught between the two of them.

D And my *sense* is that you're running like a chicken with her head cut off. The Good South Asian Daughter contract is unfortunately still in effect. It looks like you are seeing your parents at all hours of the day and night. You respond to all their requests and attend to all their needs to ensure that they are settling into their new home with ease. You're going out of your way to help them acclimatize to Toronto.

ANJU Yes, while my brother is venerated, adored, and doted on by my mother! They're so lenient with him. In fact, he's doing nothing. Nothing! And they don't expect him to. And now he's sulking too. I pick up the slack and then he sulks because I've made the decisions. "Sure," he says. "You made the decisions—then go ahead, do everything!"

D You're exhausted. *My hands shift to Anju's kidneys and adrenals for a few minutes.* Hmmm … It looks like the Good South Asian Daughter is running on sugar and coffee.

ANJU And even then I'm barely able to keep up!

D And my *sense* is that you're neglecting yourself, abandoning healthy and nourishing rituals … Your food plan is out the window, along with your yoga and meditation practices.

ANJU I know, I know—all this bullshit "giving my all" is not working. It's not working.

D No. It's reinforcing the self-sacrifice aspect of the Good South Asian Daughter contract. I *sense* that whenever your mother or father faces discomfort, you dutifully assist them with household responsibilities. They're experiencing the challenges one would expect when making such a big transition. It's OK. It's hard to move. Look what you went through last summer. You cannot and are not obligated to relieve them of the experiences that come as a result of a decision they made. They'll settle in. It takes time.

ANJU I'm exhausted.

D Exhausted and neglected! *I shift my left hand to Anju's right shoulder and my right to her chest for a few minutes.* The Good South Asian Daughter is also sitting uncomfortably in her home office chair, leaning to the right, madly clicking the mouse, and breathlessly pushing through her work. You're barely taking the time to breathe.

ANJU I am uncomfortable at my desk. I just sit there trying to do everything as quickly as humanly possible.

D Exactly. While you focus on speed and efficiency, you're neglectful of your posture and strain your body. I also *sense* that you are working at all hours of the night to meet deadlines and professional expectations. Your schedule is totally mangled because you are devoting too much time to your parents' welfare. There's nothing efficient about this schedule.

ANJU It's so true. I'm behind on all my deadlines!

D You're "on call" 24/7. I *see* you scramble to your feet and float down the elevator shaft and into your car to rush to the scene; all their scenes.

ANJU I do! You can't imagine. It's out of control. I'm killing myself to keep up.

D *Keep up what? And why?* are the questions. Do you realize that it's over, Anju? The Alberta chapter is over; that house in that small town and all that came with it has come to a close.

ANJU Oh my God. I hadn't thought of it that way. Wow!

D And you have the resources now to set new boundaries, draw up a new contract. The Toronto chapter, this chapter in *your* city, offers the opportunity to create a new framework.

ANJU That's so true.

D You have the power to create a new family dynamic that includes your well-being and emancipation. You have the power to manifest this. You have the resources to create a dynamic in which you can maintain your equilibrium and live in alignment with your life purpose. The door is open, Anju. Walk through it!

ANJU It's so true … the Alberta chapter … that small town … that house … it's over. It's so true! It's all over! *Anju sighs.*

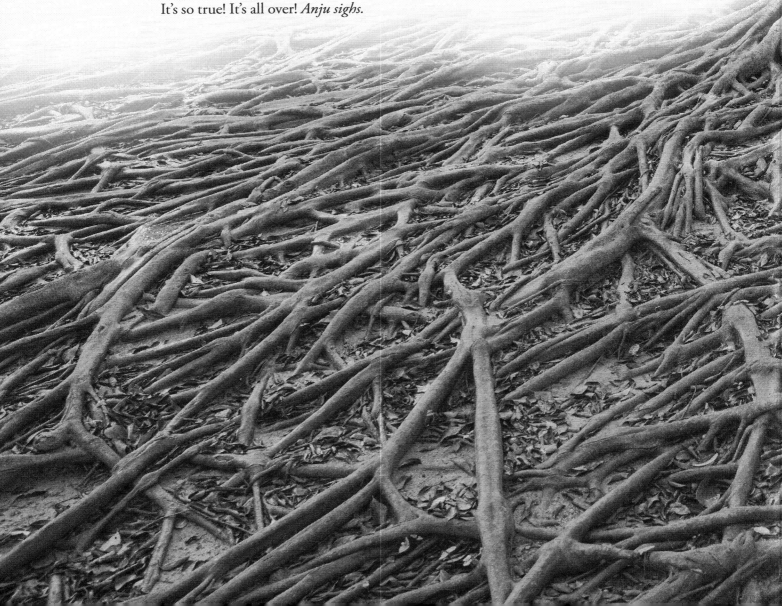

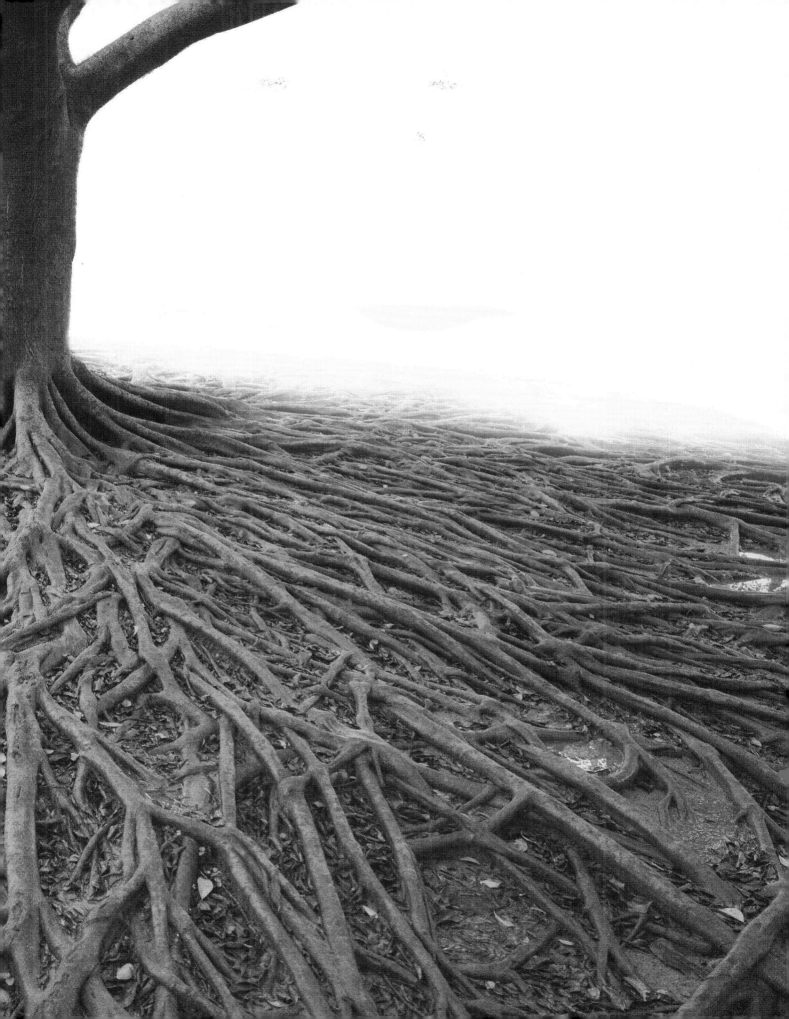

CHAPTER SIXTEEN

NAOMI

EARLY AUGUST

Naomi at age eighteen

Something bad is going to happen today. I don't know why I say that. It's nuts. There's no reason for me to panic, but ...

NAOMI   I finished high school with a very low grade point average. I scraped through all my classes.

All the bad feelings of the morning rush in again. The panic, the dread, and with it the certainty that something awful is going to happen.

D   It seems to me that you have been especially despondent for about two years. Were you scraping by only for two years or for all your years of high school?

NAOMI   For most of high school, I think. I don't want to go to university, and I don't want to get a job either. My parents are driving me crazy. They're insisting I go to university or at least try.

I could feel it; something really was peering down at me. I caught sight of the dark bird sitting still in the branches. I tried to tell myself that this was ridiculous, but somehow I knew that it was watching me. It was the biggest bird I had ever seen, plump and ominous with gasoline rainbows shining in its black feathers. I could see every detail of it clearly: the greedy dark claws, the sharp beak, the glittering and piercing eyes.

D   *I tune in with the home station.* I *hear* "Do something! Get out of bed now! Clean your room! Don't talk to me like that! You're lazy! Get off your butt! Do something with yourself!" Hmmm ... Your parents sound totally desperate. It sounds like they're really frustrated and angry at you. Do you guys fight a lot?

NAOMI   All the time.

D   I *sense* that your sleep is erratic. Do you sleep a lot some days and not so much on other days?

NAOMI   Yeah.

D   Do you have a boyfriend?

NAOMI   Yeah.

D   I *sense* that you hang out with him a lot, have sex, and party with friends.

NAOMI   Yeah.

D   It looks to me like you're having a good time!

NAOMI   Yeah, I guess.

D   *I shift my hands to Naomi's pelvis.* Yet you have big swirls of anxiety in your energetic field. You feel nervous, unsettled, restless—but also stagnant. Your energy system is so frenetic it's motionless! Parents aside, it's not all a good time. What's up?

NAOMI   I don't know. I just feel stressed all the time.

D   Your mother tells me that you've been different since you got back from summer camp a couple years ago. She says that she noticed a change then.

         He was still ogling me, undressing me with his eyes. Those blue eyes narrowing, going black with desire. I had the sudden feeling that he might yank me to him. I'm playing with fire, with something I can't control, I thought suddenly. And in that instant I realized I was terrified. My heart began to pound violently. It was as if those blue eyes spoke to some part of me and that part was screaming "danger" at me. Some instinct much older than me was telling me to get the hell out of there.

D   So even though you do have sex with your boyfriend these days, your pelvis is a solid block of trapped energy. Did something happen at that camp maybe? I sense a relationship gone wrong. Did a boyfriend hurt you?

         She couldn't contain her shudder. "Poor sweetie, she's cold. Got to get her warmed up," he said. I tried to push him away, but he was too strong, his fierce grip pulling me against him.
         "I want to go; I want to go right now …"
         "Sure, baby, we'll go," he said. "But we've got to get you warm first. Gosh, you're cold."

NAOMI   No one knows. He wasn't my boyfriend.

         "Stop," I said. "Stop now. Please!" His arms around me were only annoying at first, then restricting, but then with a sense of terror I felt his hands groping at my clothes to get to bare skin. Never in my life had I been in a situation like this, far away from any help … "Take your hands off me."

D   Do you want to talk about what happened?

NAOMI   I drank too much.

         "C'mon, get with it; I just want to warm you up all over …"
         "Let me go," I choked out as I tried to wrench myself away from him. He stumbled, and then his weight crushed me to the ground. "I mean it. Get off me."

D   I *sense* that you couldn't stop what was happening.

> *He tried rolling off me, giggling, totally oblivious to my distress. He was so drunk that his legs were heavy and uncoordinated, but not enough to weaken his resolve or strength. "Aw, c'mon, don't be like that. I was just warmin' you up, baby. The ice queen warmin' up … You're getting warm now, aren't you?" Then he pushed his hot, wet mouth on my face. I was pinned beneath him, and the next thing I knew his tongue was down my throat. And then I heard my skirt tear.*

NAOMI   I tried to. We were in the woods and everyone else was really far away.

> *I saw the full moon over his shoulder. It was strangely fitting that it would be the last thing I would ever see. My screams were stuck in my throat, choked off by fear. "Get off me," I whimpered, my unacknowledged prayer and my hope.*

D   He didn't listen to you?

NAOMI   No.

D   I *sense* that he really did not take no for an answer.

NAOMI   I don't know … I was drunk.

D   Nonetheless, I *sense* that your no was quite clear. He had no right to ignore that because you were drunk. No is no. It's clear that he didn't respect your verbal no. Hmmm … It feels to me like you tried to push him away too.

NAOMI   Yeah, I did.

D   Uh oh—it seems that your physical expression of no didn't work either. *Tears trickle down from Naomi's eyes into her ears and onto the pillow.* It's OK, Naomi, you are not the one to blame. Drunk or not drunk, you did nothing wrong. He's the one who did something very, very wrong. You were raped that night in the woods, weren't you?

NAOMI   I guess.

D   That's such a painful experience … and on top of that I keep *hearing* an inner voice repeating over and over again "No one listens to me! No one listens to me!" I *sense* that not only were you very hurt that night, but you're extremely angry at your father because of all the hurtful things he said when you got back from camp. Your father did not witness you. He doesn't understand you.

NAOMI   No, that's for sure. We argue all the time, but when I got back from camp that time he was constantly on my case about getting up too late—being late for school—sleeping in late on weekends too—living in a pigsty—partying and drinking too much—coming home late—not studying or doing my homework, and my low marks of course. I don't want to go to university anyway!

D   Sounds intense.

NAOMI   Yes, very intense. He accused me of not appreciating all the hard work and money that had gone into raising me and providing for me. Said he made sure I had everything—yeah, right!

D   Everything including getting raped at camp that summer.

NAOMI   Awesome, eh?

D   He was judging you instead of seeing you or witnessing your experience. He didn't notice how much you'd changed after summer camp that year. He jumped to conclusions instead of trying to figure out what was really happening.

NAOMI   Well, yeah … He never listens to me.

D   Did you try talking about what happened?

NAOMI   No, not really.

D   You were different though, and your mom noticed, but her concern couldn't compensate for your father's outbursts. Mind you, I *sense* she got on his bandwagon sometimes too.

NAOMI   Oh sure, both of them get on my case about marks.

D   You're furious and so you should be. I'd feel resentful too, and your congested liver tells that story. *I shift my left hand to Naomi's liver.* Aside from sleeping in late because you are out late, do you feel low energy in the morning, even when you go to bed earlier?

NAOMI   I can't get up in the morning. I felt pain on my right side. And I went for tests, but they found nothing wrong with my liver.

D   Yet I *hear* another silent scream. I *hear* "It's my fault. I let it happen. I'm to blame. I drank too much. It's my own fucking fault and I have to live with it for the rest of my life!" Whoa, that's pretty intense. It sounds like you are judging yourself too. It's not only that you are angry at them, but you're angry at yourself too! *As more tears flow, Naomi's exhaustion is palpable under the weight of her self-recrimination.*

           It's OK, it's not your fault. Drunk or not drunk, it's date rape. That guy is the one who screwed up big-time. You did nothing wrong. You trusted him. Nothing's wrong with that. He should have been trustworthy. He should have done the right thing by respecting your clear no. He went way too far … way too far.

NAOMI   I guess he did.

D   Yes, *he* did—not you! *Naomi's liver heaves the stored recrimination and self-loathing out, like a spontaneous torrent in a monsoon.*

A few minutes later:

That's it, Naomi, let your rage leave your liver, let it soften in your body. See your pain and witness your experience with compassion. This guy hurt you. Let all that pain soften up too. Let's call in a tidal wave of love and gentleness to wash off all those feelings down through your pelvis, liberating your genitals, and freeing your legs. Let it all out through your feet. That's it, Naomi, let it all wash off of you, your pain, your anger, and that guy's energy. We are clearing him off you now. *Naomi's energy shifts drastically.*

A few minutes later:

Wow! You are one brave young woman. You did that like a pro. *Naomi opens her eyes and the tell-tale sparkle of healing greets me.* Make sure you rest today and go to bed early tonight. Spend time in bed, relax, sleep, loaf around without guilt, and take a long, luxurious Epsom salts bath, then tuck yourself in for the night. And if you feel like crying, let the tears flow. You'll feel relieved—like a huge weight is coming off your chest. How do you feel now?

NAOMI   I feel calm and relaxed. I feel quite good. Thanks.

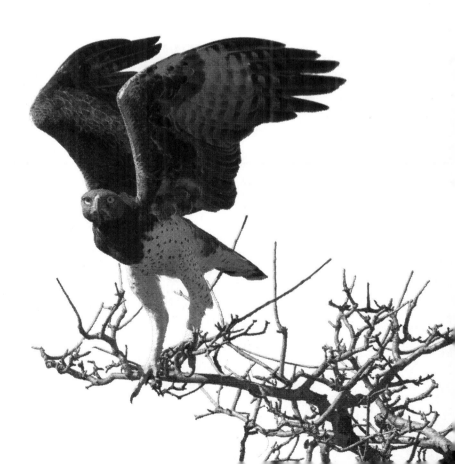

MID-AUGUST

D   How are you feeling?

NAOMI Good. I felt a lot better after the last time.

D   *I settle my hand on Naomi's shins for a few minutes.* Hmmm ... You're not quite present in your physical body though. Something else is up. Hmmm ... I *sense* that you've been feeling like this a long time ... high school and grade school too. Were you nervous about school?

NAOMI Well, my father is extremely demanding academically. He expected me to have high marks in everything.

D   I *sense* that you were extremely anxious and nervous about underperforming. It feels as though both your parents were concerned, your mother too, and I *sense* other adults' concern too. Did your parents and teachers talk about you?

NAOMI Ugh—I felt judged all the time.

D   *I shift my hands to Naomi's skull for a few minutes.* Did they develop all sorts of theories as to why you had difficulty in school?

NAOMI Yeah, I was diagnosed with ADD in high school because I had such a hard time concentrating.

D   I *sense* that they talked about you but didn't ask you what you thought or how you felt.

NAOMI No—they always had meetings without me.

D   I *sense* that you felt very vulnerable, exposed, and resentful.

NAOMI Yes, very—they never included me.

D   The bones in your skull, namely your frontal and your right temporal bones, are quite stuck. That sure as hell can't help concentration. The parietal bones at the top of your head are releasing easily. Hmmm ... It feels to me like you lean your head on your right arm often.

NAOMI Yeah, I do that all the time.

D   This posture exerts a lot of pressure on your temporal bone. I *sense* that you do it more when you get overwhelmed by information you feel like you can't absorb.

NAOMI I do it a lot in school or when I do homework. Actually, my mom always wonders how come my right eye looks smaller sometimes. It twitches sometimes too.

D   The pressure and stuckness in your skull would account for that. There's more to it though. *I shift my fingers to the base of Naomi's skull and neck for a few minutes.* Your atlas, the top vertebra in your neck, and the third and fourth vertebrae are out of alignment.

A few minutes later:

Overall, the compression in your neck is significant and your tissues are extremely guarded. You have a hard time thinking clearly, I'm so sure! Your atlas feels like it's been locked for years, Naomi. This physical injury has made it very hard for you in school.

NAOMI   Oh?

D   When people have the top vertebra out of alignment, they can't think their way out of a brown paper bag. This condition would make it virtually impossible for you to concentrate on what a teacher is saying or absorb new information while reading. Also, when the atlas is off, one tends to be trapped in a perpetual state of overwhelm.

NAOMI   Sounds like my life.

D   *Waves of energy start coming through. An intense claustrophobia and panic swells a few minutes later. I sense that Naomi is stuck in the birth canal. She fears for her life.* Well, Naomi, it seems that you have experienced these blocks your whole life. This compression is linked to your birth. How are you feeling?

NAOMI   A little strange, but OK.

D   I'm going to start clearing some of this shock. ADD is so often linked to adversity during birth. As you can imagine, it's quite the feat to get the skull through the birth canal. My sense is that your mother was encouraged to push too early on. So you were pushed down but had nowhere to go. You were stuck and mortal fear set in.

A few minutes later:

Oh … I *see*—your neck was torqued to the right. The intense asymmetrical pressure on your neck caused the injury and with it even more threat and danger.

NAOMI   Makes sense, like, stuck and squeezed down a tube, that's me—I always feel really claustrophobic emotionally. I always feel pressured to make decisions or to perform.

D   And when you feel trapped emotionally, anxiety floods your being. This is a powerful trigger igniting the fear of death that marked your nervous system when you were stuck in your mom's birth canal. Feeling pressured is intense anyway, but even more intense when it's life or death trauma that underlies your response. And now, beyond the physical and emotional injury, we are realizing that you were judged, misdiagnosed, and mislabelled. On that front, I *sense* that you felt silenced.

NAOMI   I did!

D   It follows that your self-esteem collapsed under your parents' and teachers' pressure, disappointment, and frustration. The injustice has worn you down, Naomi. You are very intelligent, and nothing is wrong with your brain or your innate desire to learn. You *could not* focus and absorb—not while your craniosacral rhythm, the bones of your skull and neck, and your dural membrane were so thrown off by your birth trauma.

NAOMI   Wow! That's such a different story.

D   You are very smart, Naomi. It's virtually impossible to concentrate when there is a loud rock band rehearsing in the room next door. You have been trapped in circumstances that have made it very hard for you to perform at school.

NAOMI   Ugh …

D   We have achieved a significant release in both your neck and head. It's such a relief to know there was a structural problem. You are very intelligent, Naomi. You haven't had the chance to taste your own mental capacities. You should notice a significant shift. Rest. Let it all heal. I'll mention it to your mother that you will need to sleep more in the next few days.

NAOMI   OK. Thanks. I'm going to have to think about all of this. It's so different.

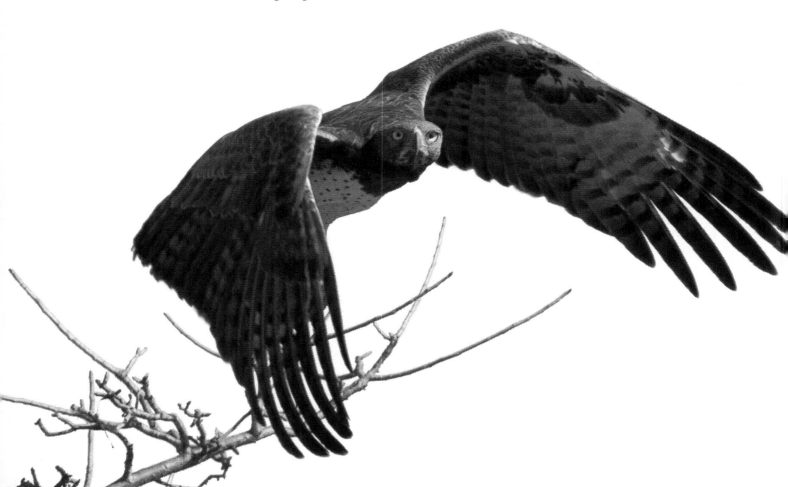

LATE AUGUST

D   How did you feel after the last session?

NAOMI   I felt great—I cleaned my room. I feel more relaxed and able to spend time alone. I like hanging out in my room and resting. I'm laughing more. I feel happier.

D   Yay! I am delighted to hear you feel some relief! Thank the Goddess for that! You so deserve a break. *I settle my hands on Naomi's shins for a few minutes.* You still feel tense though. A part of you still feels powerless. You store this energy in your left knee. *I shift my right hand to her left knee for a few minutes.* Hmmm … Are you nervous when you have exams?

NAOMI   Totally. I'm extremely nervous before exams, singing performances, and confrontations. I often puke, I'm so nervous.

D   I *sense* that you expect to fail a lot and the weight of that threat is unbearable.

NAOMI   Two years ago I had a nervous breakdown before an exam.

D   It's really intense because with the threat of failure in an exam comes the fear of losing your parents' love and respect.

NAOMI   Oh, that makes sense.

D   And not only that, you also anticipate harsh judgment from your teachers and peers too. All of that adds up. Unsurprisingly, you choke under pressure.

NAOMI   I basically feel nervous and scared all the time.

D   It's been building up over the years. All the perceived little failures and perceived bigger failures add up. The weight is mind-numbing and it's pounding your self-confidence and personal power to a pulp.

NAOMI   I always think I'm going to fail.

D   Yes, and you have been keeping track. I *see* that you have set up a bulletin board in your mind and every time you or someone else perceives that you fail, you add a Post-it note with all the pertinent details to your board. It's full by now. My sense is that you constantly bear the weight of perceived past and future failures, and with it feel despair.

NAOMI   Yeah, I feel really sad sometimes. Even though I started this session saying things were better—they are—but … I don't know. And I still have this stupid kink in my neck.

D   The third, fourth, and fifth cervical vertebrae are still compressed. Have you strained your voice sometimes?

NAOMI   I used to sing soprano really loudly in the school choir.

D   Hmmm … You hurt your vocal cords. Did you love singing?

NAOMI   I loved it, but I don't do it anymore.

D   Do you have a sense why?

NAOMI   My feelings are hurt.

D   Ah … The cumulative impact of the critical and judgmental attitudes at school and in your home has smothered your voice and expressive channels. *I place my hands on Naomi's ears for a few minutes.* Imagine that my hands are like magnets drawing out all the criticisms that are untrue—they are pulling out all the judgmental and disrespectful comments that hurt your feelings. That's it. Let it all out. Free yourself of everything that has been said about you that is untrue. There's lots of it.

A few minutes later:

That's it, deep inside, you know what is untrue. Let it all out!

NAOMI   That feels great!

D   Yeah … It's like relief after a massive indigestion … We chew and chew on the crappy untruths, then swallow it all, and then it all gets stuck in there and creates total havoc. Yet deep inside we actually know what is true or untrue.

Ten minutes later:

Hmmm … Your right temporal bones are still compressed. This is the bone directly behind and above your ears. Even though your dural membrane has released and your sphenoid, frontal, and parietal bones are more fluid, the assertion that you are intelligent is still shaky. Ah … We've hit the nail on the head, pardon the pun. Now your craniosacral rhythm is expressing its force. That's right, Naomi, you are not stupid. Far from it, you are a very intelligent young woman.

NAOMI   Yeah, I guess.

SEPTEMBER

NAOMI   My room is still clean! I even split off from some friends who are not supportive. I feel calmer—and I read a whole book this week!

D   Did you enjoy it?

NAOMI   I did. It's a good book.

D   *I settle my hands on Naomi's shins for a few minutes.* Oh … Your energy is much more fluid. I *sense* that your feelings of trepidation are diminishing. You don't walk around worrying that you are going to fail at everything anymore. Your left knee is releasing your dread.

NAOMI   I feel so much better.

D   You see yourself more accurately and compassionately. You respect yourself more. I don't *hear* so much negative talk anymore. The itty bitty shitty committee is on strike!

NAOMI   Hahaha!

D   You have turned things around rather quickly. You are renarrativizing your childhood and adolescence through this new lens we've been talking about—and it's your lens, not anyone else's.

NAOMI   Yeah … And I'm thinking of going to school in September. I'm thinking of studying literature.

D   Wow! … I love literature too.

NAOMI   I talked to one of my old English teachers.

D   Your relationship to yourself is shifting big-time. You are reframing and re-examining everything. You are reclaiming your dignity, self-worth, and well-being. Hooray!

NAOMI   Yeah, I feel so much more relaxed. Phew …

D   It's not like it's all magically gone, but let's just say that you are taking a stab at turning the ship around.

NAOMI   I hope so.

Before I realized what I was doing, I dropped my backpack and picked up a rock … "get out of here, you spectre," and the shaking anger in my voice echoed the shivers running up and down my spine. "Go away!" And with the last word, I threw the rock as hard as I could. Untouched, the large bird soared up in a loud kerfuffle of feathers and leaves. Its wings were so huge that I crouched, suddenly panicked as it flapped directly over my head, the wind of its wings ruffling my hair. But it swooped up again and circled, a black silhouette against the cloudy sky. Then, with one harsh screech, it wheeled away toward the wood—for the time being, anyway.

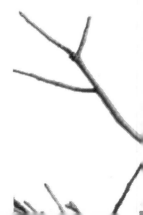

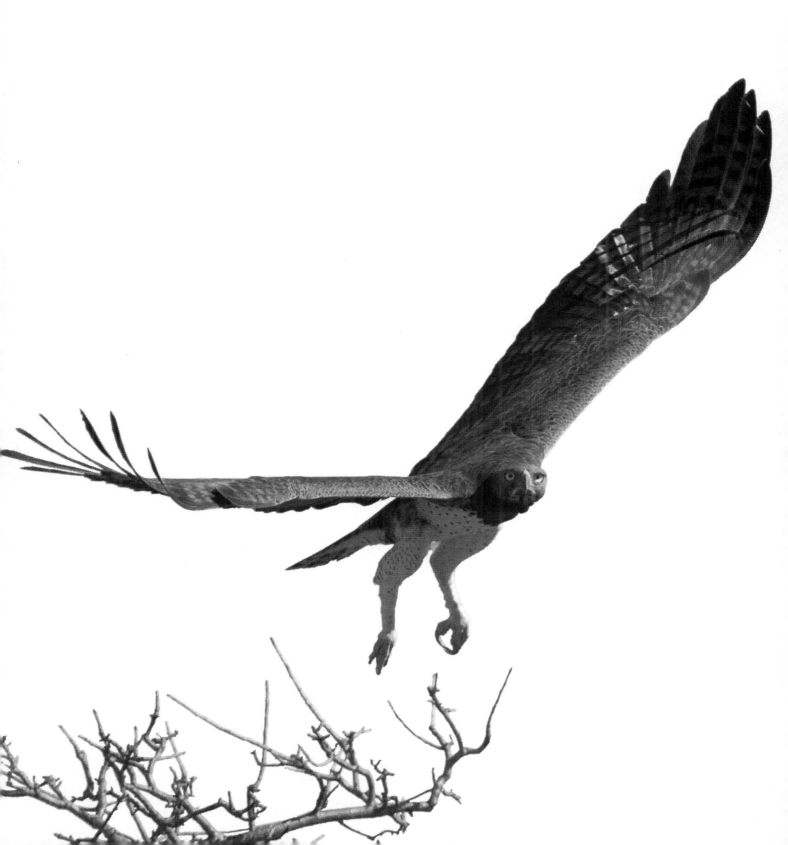

CHAPTER SEVENTEEN

SARAH

JANUARY

Sarah at age thirty-seven

SARAH   I have a huge deadline coming up. I have an opening at an art gallery SOON. I'm a mess. Ha! Actually, I'm feeling rather crazed at the moment. I'm really getting desperate.

D   *My hands settle on Sarah's shins for a few minutes.* I *sense* that you are out-of-body. This looming deadline has clearly destabilized you. You feel triggered.

A few minutes later:

I *sense* that there is more to it than a deadline; this anxiety is piggybacking on something else. You're hanging on the ceiling fan whirling at high speed.

A few minutes later:

Ah … I *hear* "One day, everything will fuck up and maybe it's NOW!" It sounds like this abysmal internal dialogue torments you day and night.

SARAH   I wake up totally startled in the middle of the night!

D   *I settle my left hand on Sarah's left kidney while resting my forearm on her right kidney for a few minutes.* You feel anxious, that's one aspect of it, you feel dread; however, above and beyond that (as if that's not enough) an overwhelming sense of doom paralyzes you.

SARAH   Well … I *have* to get going! I'm scared shitless that I won't make it this time.

D   So you drink lots of coffee and eat lots of sugar. Hmmm … Are you drinking Coke?

SARAH   Yup. It's really bad right now.

D   Even better, right—lots of caffeine and sugar all in one shot! You want the jolt, now. You are resorting to an alluring mix of stimulants.

SARAH   I need it.

D   Unfortunately, this cocktail is not really stimulating your creativity; it's feeding and amplifying your fear. This combo is lethal—you're sinking deeper into your paralyzed frenzy with every hit.

SARAH   I just can't stop right now.

D   Your cravings are very stubborn and nagging, I can feel that. And your doom-and-gloom internal dialogue is persistent and loud. It's quite the combo: lots of sugar, caffeine, and bullshit. I'm calling it bullshit because it's patently untrue. You don't need it.

SARAH   I wish I didn't.

D   My *sense* is that you are triggered. Let's try to find out what all of this is tied into because it sure as hell ain't an accurate weather report on your life and resources now. *I rest my left hand on Sarah's thigh and my right on her shin. Right legs usually tell me what's up in terms of career. It's in this part of the body that I receive most reliably the story that reveals the person's level of connection and ease with manifesting their life purpose.*

     A few minutes later:

     Hmmm ... I *sense* that you had a creative block in university.

SARAH   Oh yeah ... that was a disaster.

D   Hell on wheels, that's for sure! I *sense* it was a very difficult time for you. I realize you knew that much at the time and still do, but something about that experience is more complex and layered than you currently fathom. First, it looks like you decided at that time—and my *sense* is that you still think this now—that your attempt at being an artist was a failure.

SARAH   Well, it was.

D   My *sense* is that you feel that you failed to be good enough (in that academic context anyway). And you are convinced that you are about to do a repeat performance.

SARAH   For sure.

D   Second, my *sense* is that this all sits on a rather nasty untruth about you around age sixteen.

SARAH   Uuurgh ... high school! It was awful.

D   Yeah ... that whole thang. I *sense* that you judge your sixteen-year-old self very harshly too. You don't like her very much. Yet it looks like you were suffering and buckling under a lot of pressure. I *sense* that you felt extremely isolated and stressed out.

SARAH   It was really awful.

D   You're not kidding! Let's give a lot of love and compassion to your sixteen-year-old traumatized astronaut. You were suffering.

A few minutes later:

It looks like that era of your life was marked by the cumulative impact of social pressure and artistic and academic demands. Were you locked out of the creative and artistic clique?

SARAH   Oh sure … I wasn't cool enough for them.

D   It's even worse than that though … Dare I say you actually fit in with the nerds?

SARAH   Eeek! My nemesis.

D   *A jolt of static energy flashes through Sarah's being. I check in with her left thigh for a few minutes.* Your left thigh speaks of an even more intense fear. *I feel a terrified nine-year-old Sarah. I chose not to open this file at the end of this session.* You are trapped in the fight–flight–freeze survival response and you have been for a very long time. *My hands shift back to Sarah's adrenal glands for a few minutes.* This state has been your baseline since childhood. This survival state is not exactly conducive to the ecstatic expression of your creative self. It is necessary to unwind this old survival habit. The best thing to do right now is to try to reduce your intake of caffeine and sugar. You're exhausted. You need to let yourself crash and sleep for a few days. I'm having a little conversation with your adrenals right now. They're with us here. Your production of stress hormones can be reduced if you do not encourage its secretion with stimulants. Rest. Succumb to your exhaustion. Nourish yourself. Eat lots of vegetables and brown rice. Watch an inspiring film. Read some literature. Feed yourself on all levels. The world will be a different place after a few days on this regimen.

SARAH   It's so hard for me to trust that.

D   For one thing, once rested, you'll find the wherewithal to put one foot methodically in front of the other. This soothing interlude will be the most productive you have been in weeks. It will create a window for your creativity to flow. That's true productivity: first things first.

SARAH   Actually, I do feel so much saner than when I walked in here.

D   You'll see, there's nothing like having your feet on the ground and being fully present in your body. Are you on board with the rest and relaxation program?

SARAH   I'll try.

D   It'll work! The energy cleared in this session will support you. Just stay with it. The ceiling fan has stopped spinning and your feet are on the ground. Your job is to go with it and trust it.

FEBRUARY

SARAH   I felt so much better. I did rest, and my ideas did flow for a while. I feel stuck again though. I'm starting to go a little loopy again.

D   *I rest my hands on Sarah's shins for a few minutes.* You are getting tense again. Your left-brain hemisphere is really fired up, yet creativity is a state that flourishes in the right-brain hemisphere. It appears that you are lost in a detour just now.

SARAH   Yes, one of my many detours.

D   First, it looks like your left-brain intelligence is hooked in as a defence mechanism. My *sense* is that your keen left-brain intelligence has been a reliable source of external validation.

SARAH   Oh sure.

D   It's hard to say no to validation or feel safe while taking a walk on the wild side. Left-brain intelligence is unfortunately far more celebrated and rewarded in our culture than expansive right-brain creativity.

SARAH   Yes, isn't it?

D   You are caught in an alarming pattern I have witnessed in so many artists in my practice: you have an overdeveloped connection to your art and practice in your left brain. This imbalance is in part due to the fact that you, like so many contemporary artists in Canada, are required to write grant proposals before you actually produce your work. You wrote a grant about this project, right?

SARAH   Yep.

D   So the first manifestation of your creative impulse was in academic language, and not only that, it was thrown to the dogs in a juried and competitive grant application environment.

SARAH   Oh, the stories I have about that. They're all peers too! The whole thing is a bomb waiting to happen.

D   The assault is two-fold. On the one hand, this process accelerates the concretization of the idea in a non-creative language. It causes an imbalance and an unbeneficial left-brain focus in what is meant to be a creative and imaginative journey. Your creative impulse would mature completely differently if given the opportunity to do so in a private exploration in its appropriate medium and brain hemisphere.

SARAH   I so get that. I try to get myself out of my left brain all the time. It's so hard.

D   Yeah … It's like trying to get yourself out of your head, literally. Plus, the other pesky problem with this whole thing is that the grant application exposes the seed of your creative impulse to a jury and external committee. Yikes … Your work, in its embryonic state, is presented to an audience. So you spin the idea for that audience of peers—how could you not?—before it even has a chance to mature in your artist's soul! Your creative impulse was pushed out into the world too soon. This forced birthing can become an abortive process very quickly and block your creativity on so many levels.

SARAH   Oh God … it's happened more times than I care to think about.

D   I'm so sure. Plus, do you work as an arts administrator?

SARAH   Yes, I'm a freelance consultant.

D   That's another problematic aspect of the art world in North America. So many artists, like yourself, work on art councils, or as art administrators in different cultural institutions, or as curators, or professors in academic institutions, and even as critics to financially support their creative ventures. Daily, and often for more hours than you can engage in your creative activity, you focus your energy on left-brain activity, and in turn you are more readily celebrated and rewarded for it. Since this external validation is more easily cultivated, your professional development and growth can easily become skewed.

SARAH   I've been struggling with this balance, or rather imbalance, for years.

D   The sad truth is that time in the "art world" becomes time away from your art and your priorities get all blurry. This is a harsh reality to recognize and rectify.

SARAH   It's a curse, actually.

D   I couldn't agree with you more … but we are getting somewhere here. We've been shifting your energy to your right-brain hemisphere throughout this session. It's all nice and warm. It's glowing with your intent to express yourself and create art. You are on fire still, but in the right-brain hemisphere rather than your left. Plus, the flow expresses itself in your sixth chakra, throat chakra, and heart. You are glowing with your passion to create.

SARAH   Oh good … It's like my wires get crossed.

D   Quite literally, yes.

SARAH   Are they better now?

D   Absolutely. Both brain hemispheres are fired up, along with a nice juicy flow between them. You'll have a good time test-driving this new equilibrium.

A week later:

SARAH   I'm on a roll with my project.

D   Fantastic. Delighted to hear that your creativity is flowing. *I decide to check in with Sarah's left thigh again. After a few minutes my hand is drawn to Sarah's left knee.* Hmmm … I'm connecting with a Little Sarah, at age nine. I encountered her two sessions ago but did not explore her experience. Ah … She's very present today. Do you feel her?

SARAH   Yes—I feel her anxiety.

D   Do you wish to connect with her?

SARAH   Yes, I do.

D   Indeed, she is helpless and frightened. Let's see what's going on. It's OK, little one. We're here. We love you. I *see* you.

Five minutes later:

Hmmm … I *see* that you're wearing a short skirt and knee-highs—it's not your choice by a long shot. What year is this, anyway?

SARAH   Grrr … That was my parents' idea of proper school attire.

D   The other girls mostly wore jeans. This unfortunate dress code is making you extremely vulnerable. I *sense* that you were constantly bullied in school.

SARAH   Yeah, I was smart, brown, and I wore a short, goofy skirt!

D   This is a serious liability in the Canadian school system: you were unequivocally pigeon-holed as a nerd. And let me guess, you're not a nerd, you're an artist.

SARAH   Exactly!

D   That all started rather young. Wow! At age nine you were already fighting that battle. Your innate genius and life purpose were stifled by your peers' reaction to the colour of your skin, your parent-enforced fashion crimes, and academic performance. Some pretty weighty labels buried the artistic you. You were smart, brown, and an artist. It's rather insulting, isn't it? Why shouldn't those three things go together? And how could any one of them be a liability?

SARAH   It's a curse.

D   You keep saying that, and it sure is—but it gets worse! I *sense* that you were not only a brown fashion victim with an embattled identity as an artist; you were being shoved into a misogynist mould of girl and woman. Hmmm … Are both your parents sexist?

SARAH   Absolutely.

D   It looks like your parents shoved this sexist bullshit down your throat in more ways than one. So you were disempowered at home *and* at school. This is very unfortunate, especially because it's all coming to a head at a key juncture in your growth. For girls, gender construction is at its most pivotal point at around age nine. It is generally around age twelve for boys. You're getting a rather big dose of sexism. Geez Louise, talk about bringing it on with a bulldozer! *Five mintues later, Sarah's energy jolts. My right hand shifts to her left shoulder and my right remains on her left knee.*

SARAH   Ugh … I was attacked by a teenage boy when I was nine!

D   Oh dear … indeed. I'm with you now. You are trapped in the moment, the specific instant when you felt you lost the battle.

SARAH   He groped around and tore my blouse!

D   You were terrified. It's OK, little one. We're here. We love you. We're here to help you. You're not alone anymore. Let's shift this energy here: a thick wall separates your left breast from your chest. *I shift my right hand and rest it above Sarah's left breast and my right hand rests immediately below for a few minutes.* You have energetically detached your breast tissue from your body. You rejected the flesh that the bully touched.

SARAH   I feel that. It makes so much sense.

D   It's the glorious work of an architect of survival you created during the attack. That clever Sarah blocked the bully's energy out as efficiently as possible. However, the problem now is that this barricade does not allow beneficial energy to nourish and cleanse this area of your body to this day. Let's kick out the bully's energy fully and forever. *My right hand sweeps the bully's invasive hands off Sarah's chest.*

Ten minutes later, the density in Sarah's field dissipates and a gentle glow of love warms her breast.

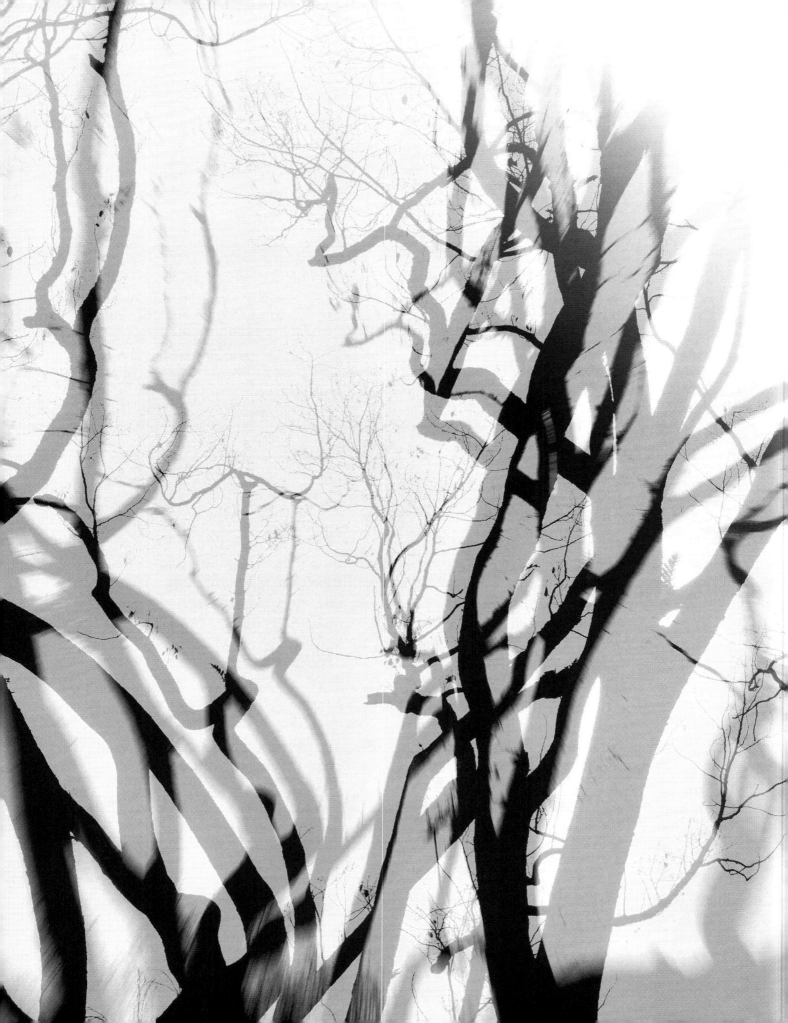

SARAH   It's such a relief to clear that off me.

D   We need to do more work though. His brutal touch tore your etheric field, an energetic field that replicates your whole physical body. We now invite your etheric field to heal all the rips or tears. *The fingers of my right hand feed the severed fibres with love and compassion. I gently wiggle my fingers to activate Sarah's etheric field and awaken her self-healing system.*

Ten minutes later:

That's it, Sarah—your field is regaining its vitality and filling in the gaps.

My right hand shifts to Sarah's heart chakra while my left hand still rests below her breast. She is now in a deep meditative state. I now encourage you to reintegrate this sacred pound of flesh into your body, mind, and soul. No need to throw the baby out with the bathwater. You expulsed your attacker's energy but now reclaim this part of your body. *Sarah opens her heart and shares its magnificent energy with her whole torso.*

Fifteen minutes later:

There you go … Your breast is now attached to your chest. Not only that, but your chest is one glorious unit, including your heart.

SARAH   Wow! I really feel that.

D   It's such a relief, I find, to have a chest rather than breasts. There's so much stuff attached to breasts in our breast-obsessed culture. As primary sexual ornaments, your breasts are like lightning rods for sexism. It's a little much for a few pounds of flesh to carry.

SARAH   Ouf … That was intense. I'm exhausted.

D   Yes; tomorrow is another day. For now, you're done. *Sarah's eyes bulge out of her head.*

SARAH   I have so much to do!

D   Trust it, Sarah. Go home and rest. Whatever you thought you would get done today will get done in spades tomorrow. You'll wake up revitalized. Are you kidding, with all of this off your chest, you're going to fly.

A week later:

SARAH   I'm still moving forward but also still waking up anxious in the middle of the night.

D   *I place my hands on Sarah's shins for a few minutes.* Hmmm … It looks like we're picking up right where we left off in the last session. It sounds like your nine-year-old has more to say. Are you OK with that?

SARAH   Yeah, let's do it.

D   *My left hand settles on Sarah's left shoulder and my right to her left thigh for a few minutes.* Talk about coming out ahead if you face sexism with your whole body rather than let your breasts carry the brunt of it! There's energy here you haven't acknowledged yet. I feel strength, power, chutzpah, and victory. That's quite a different tune …

      A few minutes later:

      Wait a second here … You kicked off your attacker! In fact … *I quickly check in with Sarah's cosmic underwear and—sure enough—it's intact!* You successfully kicked that guy off of you!

SARAH   Hmmm … I guess so.

D   I *sense* that the bully's intention was to rape you. His violent intent is marked on your flesh. Yet you harnessed your strength and determination. You were strong enough to kick him off! Oh my Goddess, Sarah, this is amazing. I don't get good news like this very often: you lost the battle, but you won the war!

SARAH   I guess I did.

D   For crying out loud, your victory has been buried under the girl-victim paradigm all this time. All that victim stuff is truly bullshit. You won! Do you realize how rare this is? The "I was attacked story" implies that you were raped. This narrative fits in with the misogynist, dominant narrative: women as victims. And it was most likely amplified by racism.

SARAH   My mother hangs on to this story quite well.

D   Yet you won that day. You were not raped. You need to hear this story too—we all do! Basically, you were attacked not only by a bully but also by the racist and sexist victim narrative. Your mother's internalized racism and sexism reinforced this story. The impact of this is far-reaching. Your identity was truly hijacked.

      Now in a deep meditative state, Sarah rekindles her connection with the true "attack" story.

      Fifteen minutes later:

      Your mother's words sizzle to smouldering ashes. Ha! Your true strong and resourceful self rises like a phoenix out of the flames! Your emotional, mental, and physical bodies reconnect with the truth. You have always known in your heart and soul that you avoided rape. It's your day-to-day consciousness that is catching up. The true story celebrates your personal power and spirit.

SARAH   Wow! … That's so different. I'm furious!

D   And so you should be. That was quite the onslaught of racist, sexist bullshit.

SARAH   I am strong. That's just it. I feel that inside. I just have never been able to live it.

D   I think that's about to change.

A week later:

SARAH   I am on track with my projects, both the art and my consulting, but I still feel frustrated and anxious.

D   *My hands rest on Sarah's shins for a few minutes.* Woowee—you are clearing your mother's internalized sexism. It penetrated your field through your left ear. Good riddance, I say.

SARAH   You're not kidding. I'm so done with it.

D   Internalized sexism is so pernicious. *I sit behind Sarah's head and cup both her ears for a few minutes.* Hmmm … I *sense* that you also had to obey your mother and do what she said to the letter.

SARAH   I sure did. I had to toe the line.

D   Your mother's rulebook is still in your left ear. Imagine that my hands are magnets. Let them draw out all the rules and untruths.

A few minutes later:

That's it, Sarah. Hmmm … That's not the end of it. You created an architect of survival who strategized constantly to gain her approval and love.

SARAH   I still do!

D   And to do so, you suppress your capacity to think for yourself. You try to think what she would think rather than trust your own wisdom. It worked for you when you really needed your mother to be there for you and protect you, but it's not really working for you now. We thank this hard-working Sarah, yet we invite this architect of survival to soften into a luxurious bubble bath. Her job is well done and complete.

SARAH   It's such a nasty cycle.

D   Indeed, especially because it creates even more havoc. I *sense* that based on your perceived failure to deserve your mother's love you concluded that you are unlovable. Not only that, but you are especially unlovable when you are in alignment with your personal power. In other words, it looks like you must be disempowered to deserve your mother's love.

SARAH   Fuck.

D   Fuck is right … and let's not forget your father. His energy seems to be attached to your left ankle. *I move on down to place my hands on Sarah's left shin and ankle for a few minutes.* It looks like your father's sexist beliefs metaphorically broke your ankle.

SARAH   That ankle is often swollen and sore. I've had problems for years.

D   The irony is that he disempowers you, expects you to remain disempowered, and then says, "See, you can't walk! You're a girl—of course you can't walk!" In other words, you learned that you do not have the means to live your life fully, walk your walk, provide for your needs, care for yourself, or honour your life's sacred purpose.

SARAH   As if!

D   That's it, Sarah. Your centre of gravity is lowering and your first chakra is opening! You are welcoming fire energy in the traditionally male-dominated spheres of safety, home, and money. That's it, you alone own your chakras! Your energy pattern is shifting to a non-traditional, non-sexist model of strength and clarity.

SARAH   Ouf! *Sarah's hand reaches for her heart.*

D   Of course your heart is wounded. *I shift my right hand to Sarah's heart and my left hand on her left thigh.* Your caregivers drowned their love with conditions. It feels horrible to receive care and safety only when you act a certain way. You experienced abandonment.

SARAH   It's so sad.

D   It sure is. It's extremely painful. And in your case, you were then stuck in the helpless girl role. In other words, you had to internalize your parents' sexism, and in the process you also lost yourself. You had to abandon yourself to seek their love.

SARAH   I'm still trying to deserve my mother's love.

D   It's not working, is it?

SARAH   Nothing I do seems to make a difference.

D   It's not only a never-ending cycle within your familial relationships, but it's a cycle of disconnect within yourself too. The constant yearning for your parents' love and the constant negotiation within yourself to do what you think they would approve of steers you away from your Sacred Tree. The helpless girl is an architect of survival. As you are painfully aware, it's a good way to survive but sure as hell is no way to thrive.

SARAH   Hell no.

D   In the long run, the consequences are serious. Rather than thrive in your Sacred Tree, you perpetually run around it and are therefore cut off from the earth and the sun. If you are not in your roots to connect to the earth to draw her nutrients, and you are not in your branches to reach for the sky to receive energy from the sun either, then you are cut off from your innate wisdom, peace, and stillness. It hurts to be stuck outside your tree. In fact, it hurts more to be out of your tree than it does to be cut off from your parents' conditional love; because, ultimately, if you are cut off from your tree, you are cut off from the life-sustaining energies of love and compassion.

SARAH   That's a whole other way of looking at it.

D   It's OK to drop into yourself, Sarah. In the end, it will be far more fulfilling. The mantras for your new ethos that I recommend are: I walk my walk. I provide for myself, and I live to my full and sacred potential.

MARCH

SARAH   Wow! My art project is launched! I'm on a roll!

D   Yay! Your right-brain hemisphere is buzzing with activity. You are really on fire now! Fantastic! *I settle my hands on Sarah's shins for a few minutes.* Hmmm … Meanwhile, back at the ranch, your sixteen-year-old Sarah still seems to be trapped in her nasty high school experience. I *sense* that your sadness and shyness are a miserable combination and that school is a daily grind. What haven't we tapped into yet? We haven't acknowledged an aspect of that experience yet. Let's send young Sarah lots of love and invite her to speak.

SARAH   OK.

D   I *hear* "I don't like HER!" Whoa, that feeling runs deep. Who is that?

SARAH   Oh, that must be my best friend. She was white, popular, beautiful (she had great clothes!), and she was super-articulate!

D   I *hear* "I will never be like her!" Yikes! That's a pretty intense belief to live with: you're not like her in high school and you will never be successful, popular, beautiful, desirable, or articulate.

SARAH   Oh yeah, she had a beautiful future ahead of her. I knew that.

D   And not you! I *hear* "Not me … I will NEVER be happy!"

SARAH   That sounds familiar.

D   It sounds like you were trapped in your self-imposed victim identity, and the victim narrative was unfolding as it should. Your perceived plight buried your sense of self in an abyss of hopelessness, judgment, and self-loathing … and self-silencing.

SARAH   I'm always worried of saying the wrong thing! Public speaking is still a nightmare.

D   Of course it is—if you believe you have no hope of being liked and you are unattractive and dress badly and you are inarticulate and you have no future ahead of you and you will never be happy—it's likely going to jinx the odds. My knees are buckling under me just saying it—you're living in that ethos every day and every time you speak.

SARAH   Oh geez.

D   It's an intense disharmony in your mental energy body. Basically, every time you open your mouth, you project onto your audience your expectation of rejection and judgment. You think you know the ending before you have even begun.

SARAH   It's awful.

D   It sure is. Plus, you get more proof every time the story plays itself out: "See! There's the proof again." And then this event, which you are giving power to by letting it prove to you that you are worthless, becomes your "truth." And then your truth is that you are a victim (here we are again) and this is the narrative of your life. It is your life, period. Quadruple yikes! It's a nasty cycle.

Sarah softens in a deep meditative state for fifteen minutes. Her heart opens and Little Sarah bathes in its warm light. That's it—you are witnessing your daily emotional strain and realize that your shyness is a symptom of your pernicious beliefs. They fuel nothing less than powerlessness, despair, and self-loathing. It's not who you are, Sarah. The warmth of your inner gaze nourishes Little Sarah. That's it. Your younger self is unfurling into her true expansive self. It's so clear that you are smart and have the ability to express complex ideas verbally as well as on the page.

A few minutes later:

That's it, let your self-confidence blossom and with it unleash your power to speak. That's it … Unleash your power to create not only art but your life.

APRIL

SARAH   I'm moving to London for six months on June first! I'm so inspired and really productive still!

D   It's great news on all counts! And both your brain hemispheres are humming in fabulous harmony. It's a huge and fantastic shift! *I check in with Sarah's right shin for a few minutes.* I *see* young Sarah, the teenage art student, grinning from ear to ear. She is content and loving your creative process and new ventures. She's coming along for the ride. Yippee!

SARAH   My show is opening in a month.

D   *I check in with Sarah's right foot for a few minutes.* You are more connected to the earth than ever. Even with such an imminent adventure and all the preparation it entails. You are on track in a major way.

SARAH   I'm practising Prana yoga several times a week and doing breathing exercises. My self-care program is in full gear!

D   You are eating well too.

SARAH   Oh yeah, kefir, the works. Protein-balanced meals. Everything. I'm on it.

D   The base of your spine, your sacrum, is trying to shift. Your posture of defeat, insecurity, and shyness is, by now, an old distortion. You have been clearing so much on the emotional, mental, and spiritual plane that now your body needs some help to express your new, improved relationship with yourself. The old "I'm not good enough" bullshit is ready to shift out of your skeletal structure.

Ten minutes later:

That's it, soften into it. Breathe. There you go … Your pelvis is more fluid and your sacrum is shifting into greater alignment. Feel that?

SARAH   I do!

D   Your sacrum and first chakra are dancing!

A few minutes later:

That's it, Sarah. Ki energy is flowing upward through your spine. Your dural membrane is releasing, and the cerebrospinal flow and pulse is expressing itself more fully all the way up into your head and upward to the sun. And now ki energy is flushing down both legs and to the earth. Taste your freedom! Your whole skeletal structure is adapting to your new baseline.

A few minutes later:

You're even more in your legs now, even more connected to the earth and the sun than when you walked in today. You are ready to step out into the world, to live and express your life purpose. You are walking your walk, Sarah. I'm so happy for you. It's an honour. Namaste.

SARAH   Thanks so much. I am so excited.

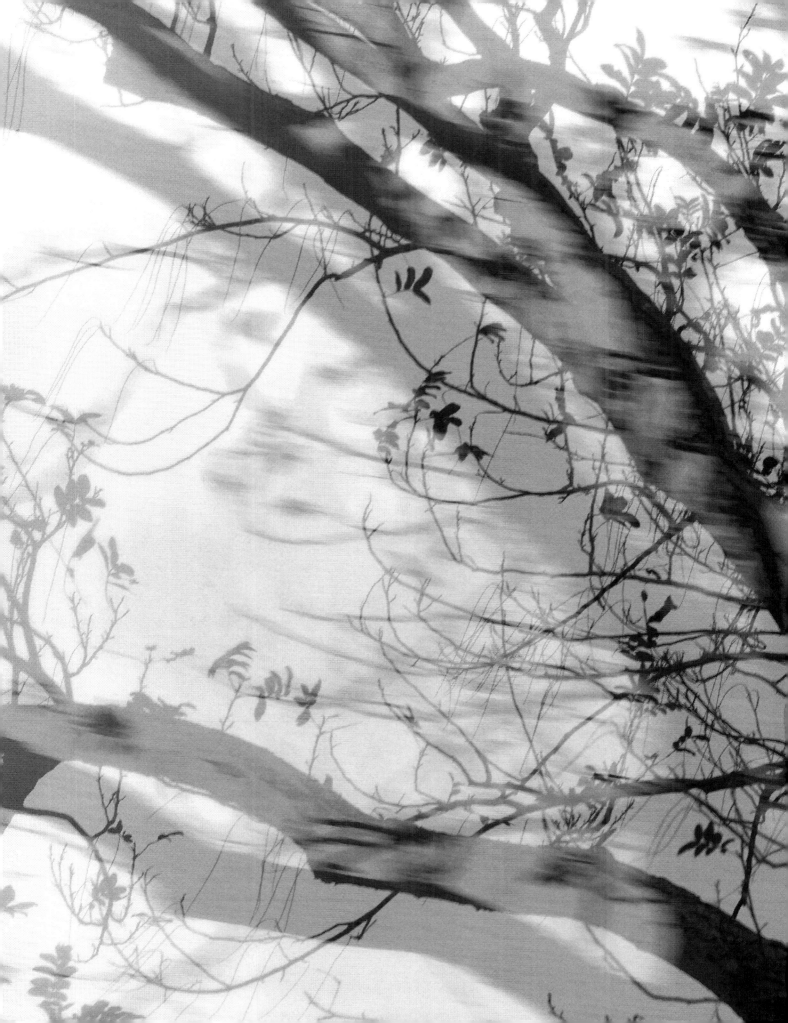

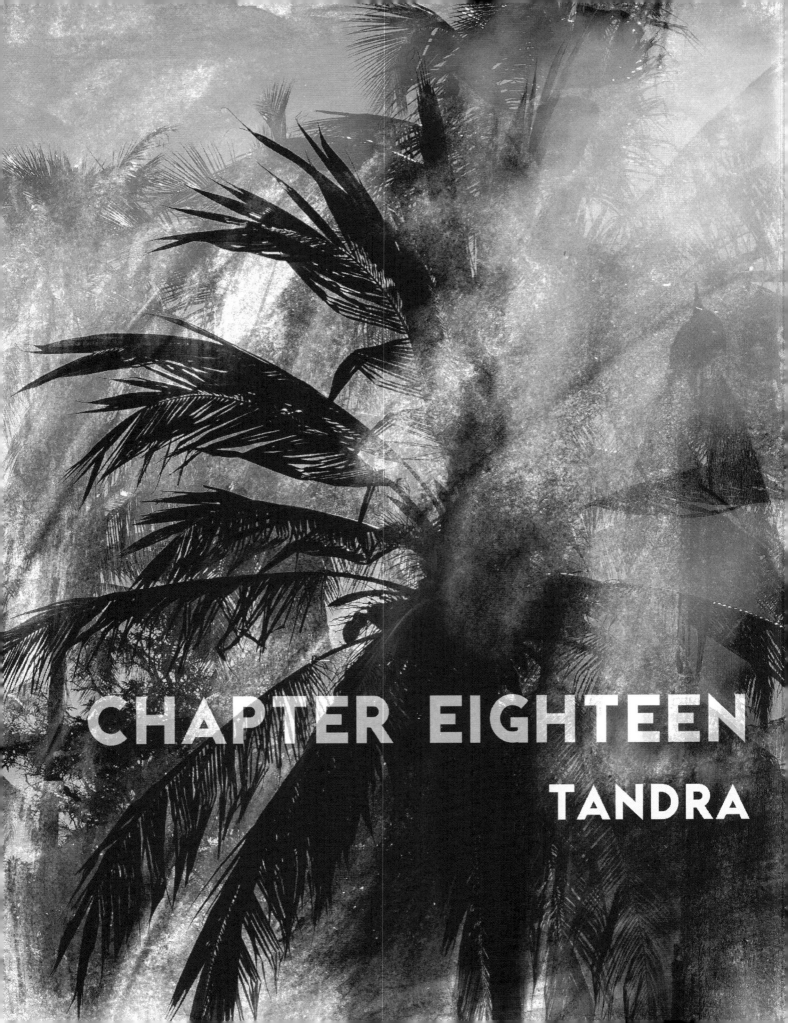

CHAPTER EIGHTEEN

TANDRA

MID-AUGUST

Tandra at age fifty

TANDRA I've been working with a naturopath who recommended you because I have a hormonal imbalance that is not resolving with the usual treatment. I also have a low libido and depleted adrenals.

D *I settle my hands on Tandra's shins for a few minutes.* Hmmm … A shield guards your pelvis. This armour speaks of sexual trauma. Are you aware of any violation in your history?

TANDRA That's specifically why my naturopath recommended you. I was sexually abused by my brother from ages six to thirteen.

D Thank you for sharing … Hmmm … This armour compensates for the fact that your etheric field is very faint from waist to mid-thigh. I refer to the luminous and fluid energetic membrane around the pelvis as cosmic underwear. They're long gone unfortunately! I also *see* that you're suffocating in this armour. You are fearful and sexually dissatisfied.

TANDRA Actually, I want nothing to do with sex. No, sister, I'm d-o-n-e! He hasn't had any for a long time. He just has to cope.

D Hmmm… Four or so years ago, I *sense* that you were in a different place. You were extremely terrified to lose your husband. You gave your husband sexual pleasure hoping that this would keep your marriage going.

TANDRA Oh sure, I got the lingerie and I put on a show. I didn't know what else to do.

D I *sense* that your body cringed away from his touch and caresses: "Don't touch me, I'll touch you." This approach worked but only to a point. You nonetheless felt pressure to perform—to give out.

TANDRA I'm married, for God's sake. He needed it once in a while, didn't he?

D This pressure weighs on you still, yet now you are willing to face the consequences if you say no.

TANDRA Yes, to a point.

D *My hands shift to Tandra's kidneys for a few minutes.* Acute fear emanates from your right kidney. Oooh … Your kidney is one tired puppy! It is strained and congested.

TANDRA I had a bladder infection recently.

D It's more than that, you have terror stored here. This vibration dates back to your abuse.

A few minutes later:

Hmmm … It seems to me that you experienced orgasms when your brother violated you.

TANDRA Ugh!

D The zing of orgasms detached from emotional, mental, and spiritual joy and connection really stings. I *hear* "I did this! I didn't say no!" Oh dear, you blame yourself.

TANDRA Well, I had an orgasm, didn't I?

D You are not at fault because your body responded as it would if your hand landed on a hot stove.

TANDRA I am to blame, aren't I?

D When an orgasm is divorced from all other aspects of your being, it's like a lightning bolt that pierces right through you. On one hand, it is a shocking and traumatic charge that overwhelms your circuits. And on the other, it masks your pain. It temporarily serves you. But in the long run, it distorts your interpretation of the events.

Tandra absorbs this information and drops into a very deep meditative state for ten minutes. Reach out to that rejected and punished girl and teenager who has been in the doghouse for years. *Tandra sighs.*

Let's make sure your brother is in the doghouse and not you. Allow him to bear the weight of his invasive and violent actions. That's it, open your heart and welcome young and bewildered Tandra into your heart.

TANDRA Come on over here, little sister.

D That's it, become a big sister for this little one; make it clear to her that it's not her fault. You didn't understand, little one. No one was there to help you. Your secret has weighed on you for so long. Let her know that you love her so much, care for her so much, and adore her so so much. Hold her. Hug her. See her beauty and let her know it's over.

TANDRA *Tandra whispers.* She's asleep. She's so tired … so tired.

D *We end the session whispering.* Allow the energy of life to replenish you both. Enjoy your nascent unconditional love and acceptance. The more your cells harmonize with love and compassion, the more the two of you will integrate into one big beautiful being, emanating love and compassion. *Gentle tears leak out of the corners of Tandra's eyes. She lies still. Grace infuses her being.*

TANDRA Thank you. Thank you.

D Namaste.

LATE AUGUST

D How did you feel after the last treatment?

TANDRA I rested all weekend. I was able to relax and take it easy.

D I'm delighted to hear you rested. *I rest my hands on Tandra's shins for a few minutes.* Hmmm … Your right adrenal gland is running full speed ahead on high-octane fuel. *My hands shift to Tandra's kidneys and adrenal glands for a few minutes. I hear* "I have things to do and places to go!" Where do you need to go?

TANDRA Actually, I've been running for my whole life, ever since I can remember.

D Yes, fear has governed your adolescent and adult life. Potent anxiety and apprehension present a daunting hurdle. I *hear* a twenty-something Tandra speak up: "My life is ruined! What a mess! What am I going to do?" Oh dear, you were totally freaked out in your early twenties!

TANDRA Oh yeah?

D I *sense* that the distress was linked to your brother's abusive attacks.

TANDRA Probably. It all is. Isn't it?

D Hopelessness sprawled from your past to the present and your future. Your flesh is still marked by it. I *hear* "I'm not a virgin." Shame soaks your cells. I *hear* "I'm sullied and useless." You did not see a future free from it. *Tandra's heart spontaneously opens to greet herself as a young woman. She's a quick study.*

TANDRA   Uh-huh. Come on in here, little sister, enough of that already. There's plenty of lovin' here. Right here. Don't you go worrying about them out there anymore. You're with me now. Let's give you a nice, long hug!

D   *Boooing!* Whoa, who's here? Hello! We just woke up an architect of survival. She just bounced up like a jack-in-the-box. *I slip my left hand under Tandra's right kidney and slide the right on top for a few minutes.* I *hear* "You got past me last time; not this time, honey. I'm in charge around here. I run this show."

TANDRA   Sounds like me all right.

D   A rather plucky four-alarm eight-year-old architect of survival stands before us, hands on her hips with her mouth resolute and her eyes blazing. She wants to make sure we know: "Danger lurks around every corner around here. Vigilance is mandatory 24/7."

We're delighted to meet you. It's rather intense in here.

A few minutes later:

The house of fear, this kidney, is not really a place for you to live. You've been in here for years. It's the least expensive unit on the ground floor, with traffic zooming by twenty-four hours a day and car exhaust choking the air. It's really not a place to live, is it? Would a penthouse suite work better for you? There's one available up here in Tandra's heart. You can move up in the world!

A few minutes later:

"Up, yes—penthouse no. I want the large corner office with the floor-to-ceiling windows!" she states emphatically. *Tandra's heart morphs instantly into prime CEO real estate.* Ha! Your plucky eight-year-old just hopped into the leather chair behind the largest desk *ever.* I *hear* "I can keep an eye on things from here real good … ha!"

TANDRA   She's liking this. The corner office! That works.

D   Never mind, it's top-of-the-line Eau de Love Puff that scents the air. This office is blessed with a top-of-the-line air purification system: unconditional love and compassion twenty-four hours a day. She'll relax soon enough. One step at a time.

TANDRA   Uh-huh. Thank you.

D   It's an honour. Namaste.

TANDRA   Namaste.

SEPTEMBER

D   How are you feeling?

TANDRA   I feel calm. Things are good.

D   *My hands rest on Tandra's shins for a few minutes.* You've had an oil change: less fear and way more love. You are integrating the work with ease and your cells are harmonizing with the earth and the sun.

A few minutes later:

You're doing great. However, though you experience well-being, I *see* tumultuous energy swirling around your head and neck. *I leave her shins to settle in with my hands under Tandra's head.* A protective shield guards your temporal bone while a turbulent energy gurgles under it. A memory of abuse is stirring. Your self-healing system is aligning with the portal the fall equinox is presenting. Are you feeling up to it?

TANDRA   I'm good. I'm going home after this!

D   *I pause to drop into the vortex of energy around Tandra's head and neck for a few minutes.* Do you remember being forced to perform oral sex on your brother?

TANDRA   No. It wouldn't surprise me though. I don't remember anything specific. I just know. *Hatred and rage float across Tandra's face. This expression is so entirely different than the Tandra I know. Her face normally radiates joy, gratefulness, and loving kindness.*

D   I *see* you kneeling before your brother as he drives your head on his penis. His grip was relentless. The more you resisted, the more forcefully he pressed down on you. Are you OK?

TANDRA   Uh-huh, I'm OK. I welcome the clarity.

D   The energy is flowing. Your upper chakras are opening and your skull is more fluid. Let's bring in the love big-time!

A few minutes later:

Welcome this younger self into your heart. Let her know that you do not judge her and that you love her very much. She so needs your gentleness and affection. She's been alone with all of this for decades.

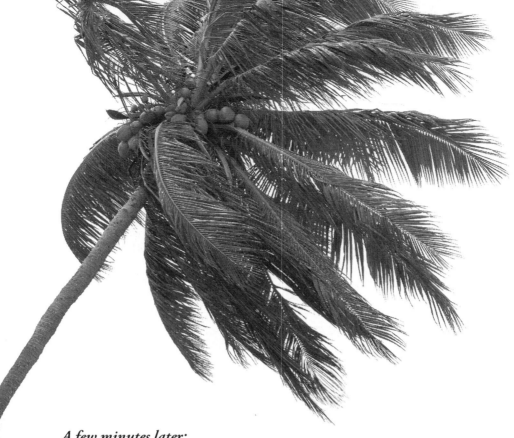

A few minutes later:

Hmmm … Then one day your brother was more insistent, violent, and fierce than he had ever been. You were trapped in his grip. The strain on your neck was excruciating. Your face, mouth, and throat were crushed in his frenzied quest to come. I *hear* "I can't breathe! I'm choking!" Panic and shock overwhelmed you. Are your feet numb?

TANDRA   Yes, like cement.

D   OK, good, the shock and trauma are leaving your body. Allow the wave to crest above your heart. Let the lightning bolts of anguish travel through. Allow the huge wave of love push through every cell from head to toe.

A few minutes later:

That's it … Let the energy dissipate into the earth. Do you feel that hot/cold feeling, like Tiger Balm?

TANDRA   Yes, I'm hot and very cold at the same time.

D   The heat is love and compassion in action, and the cold is the shock and trauma flushing out through to your feet and the earth.

TANDRA   It feels so cleansing.

D   Hmmm … There is more to this story.

A few minutes later:

It's a heart wound too. You are not only crushed by his grip; when smeared with semen and shame, your heart sinks into hopelessness. I *hear* "I'm condemned. Now, I'm really done for! Look at what I've done!" Darn, your brother is once again instantly exonerated. You reproach yourself for "giving him head."

TANDRA   Enough of *that*! You are out of the doghouse, girl!

D   Let's free you, little one. Let's be clear: you were brutally enslaved and attacked. Although you accused yourself of bad behaviour at the time, you can now compassionately witness your traumatic experience. Excellent, your energy is shifting. Love is bathing your despairing heart and soothing your kidney.

TANDRA   Enough of *that*! I get it! We're together now. We're on the same page.

D   That's it, Tandra, your open heart welcomes the humiliated and horrified Little Tandra.

TANDRA   Come on over here! Just cuddle in here, honey. It's over. Trust me. It's all over.

D   Oh! You-know-who is stirring. I *hear* "I'm in the corner office and don't you forget it. It's over! Ha!" she squawks into the intercom mic. Her voice resounds loud and clear in every floor of the office tower. She needs more Eau de Love Puff too—twenty-four hours a day for the next few weeks. It's OK, Tandra is listening.

TANDRA   It's all OK, little sister … all OK! Thank you.

D   Namaste.

TANDRA   Namaste.

OCTOBER

D   How did you feel after the last treatment?

TANDRA   I had a wild weekend. My God, it was intense! I wasn't able to swallow. It was so painful. My esophagus constricted, and my stomach bloated so much that I looked six months' pregnant. I figured it had something to do with all this stuff. It all calmed down after a couple days. But oh my God I couldn't believe the size of my stomach.

D   It sounds like you were able to stay with it and trust the process.

TANDRA   I did. I didn't panic. I rested and took care of myself. I was number one.

D   Hmmm… That's a strong reaction. Let's check in case there is another layer. *I place my left hand on Tandra's biological heart and my right on her right kidney for a few minutes.* Your heart still feels shattered. I *hear* "I could die and he won't care!" *My left hand shifts to Tandra's throat. I float my hand above the base of her neck and throat chakra and then rest it on her upper chest for a few minutes.* I *sense* that you were in a massive bind. You had to breathe, but you did not want to swallow your brother's semen. Yet if you swallowed, you knew that you would be able to catch your breath. You were caught in a major catch-22. "Do I swallow this gross fluid and die inside, or do I choke and really die?" Is this really a choice you would want your eight-year-old to face? You swallowed. *My hand shifts to Tandra's stomach for a few minutes. Tandra convulses as a sudden cramp bolts across her midsection.* Your brother's slime penetrated your body.

TANDRA   He's inside of me, INSIDE of me. He's everywhere! He's in me, in every part of me!

D   You were overwhelmed with dread. Your flesh, organs, and blood felt sullied and contaminated. Not only were you assaulted, you felt invaded and infested through and through.

TANDRA   There was nothing left of me that was left untouched.

D   Exactly. You felt defiled inside and out. I *hear* "I am unlovable by God, by everyone, by anyone." You felt cast out of the Garden of Eden! Yikes, you were also propelled in a monumental spiritual crisis.

TANDRA   I felt fatally flawed in the eyes of God!

D   All of this because you had to swallow so you could breathe, so you could live?

TANDRA   Ugh!

D   Your whole body is expelling this energy. Your digestive tract is clearing every last drop of your brother's seed. You are ingesting love and compassion instead.

TANDRA   I am loved! I love myself.

D   And your eight-year-old CEO observes from her high perch. Eau de Love Puff suffuses her office and pores. She's slumped in her chair, relaxed and nourished. A gentle smile on her face.

TANDRA   Yes. She is watching … but smiling. We all feel so much better. Namaste.

D   Namaste.

Email from Tandra

Hello Dany,

I wanted to let you know how much better I'm feeling after last Thursday's session.

My belly feels like it belongs to me. I keep looking at my flat (well ... almost flat!) belly! The last two sessions raised and resolved issues that were unconscious to my mind but very evident in my physical body. I'm really pleased about this level of healing. I felt detached from my belly, like I had no control over it and that it was an energy/entity unto itself. I also don't have that horrible constriction in my esophagus anymore, thank God.

I went to my chiropractor for my bi-monthly tune-up (three weeks due to holiday) and he knew my energy was completely different before he started the network entrainment (I said nothing). After, he said that I was completely different and had really opened up my energy.

Amazing ... but not unexpected.

Dany, thank you very much for being a powerful intuitive healer and for providing me with a much-needed healing experience.

I look forward to continuing the work.

With sincere thanks,
Tandra

....

MARCH

TANDRA I'm taking a Reiki course. I'm taking a step toward a long-overdue career change!

D *I check in with Tandra's right leg for a few minutes.* In sharp contrast with your enthusiasm about your course, your energy is shut down. You have one angry, fired-up architect of survival on your hands. With her eyes blazing, she pounds her desk: "Forget the peaceful revolution. It's all-out war!" What's going on?

TANDRA Oh ... my employer overlooked me. I didn't get a bonus this year! Well ... actually ... I got one ... an insulting amount. He blithely ignored all my overtime. I talked to him, but he did not change his decision. I'm working to rule now. Nothing more. I'm also saying no to my husband. I don't have my heart on my sleeve anymore. I'm going about my business. And with friends too!

D   But let's see here. Your energy is too stagnant to fuel an efficient revolution. It's not "like you" to say no all the time.

TANDRA   But I want to set my boundaries. Enough is enough!

D   You are in the grip of an anger-fuelled rampage that is going too far in the other direction. You are moving away from unconditional love rather than toward it. Anger often ignites; it's a fantastic catalyst, but love is the ideal fuel for evolution.

TANDRA   Hmmm ....

D   I *sense* there is more to this lockdown. *My left hand drifts up to Tandra's solar plexus and third chakra for a few minutes.* I *hear* "No one is taking care of me, so I will!" Words are very powerful. We have to be careful how we express our intentions. This statement obliterates your cooperation with the earth and the sun. Trusting the earth and the sun is like riding a horse bareback. You need to relax to feel the subtle shifts in the animal's pace, its emotional states, and to develop a heart connection with the magnificent beast who is graciously welcoming you on its back.

TANDRA   AH ... I get it.

D   Breathe deeply. Allow your breath to reach your heart chakra.

        A few minutes later:

        Oh good, here we go: unconditional love and compassion infuses your whole being. Slowly, your rage mellows and your focus is shifting away from the people at work and home.

        A few minutes later:

        That's it, the conversation is between you, the earth, and the sun. No one else is invited to the meeting.

        A few minutes later:

        That's it. You are yielding to the dance of the earth and the sun. Feel the power and gentleness of the life force working with you. Feel its love and openness.

TANDRA   I do! That feels so much better.

D   Yes, you are softening out of the contraction of adversity and of survival. To help you maintain this state, I recommend a wheat-free food plan, yin yoga, and some fresh air. Honour the vernal equinox by setting yourself up to blossom with her.

TANDRA   Well, I'm going to visit my parents in St. Lucia. My husband may or may not come. He hasn't decided yet.

EARLY JUNE

TANDRA My husband joined me in St. Lucia! We had a great time! Who knew?

D You radiate with light and love. *I rest my hands on Tandra's shins for a few minutes.* Your right leg is detoxing. Particles are floating in every direction. New pathways are being carved. You have had a huge breakthrough!

A few minutes later:

I *sense* that you have reconnected with your husband. You were sexual for the first time in a long time.

TANDRA It just happened. We eased into it without a fuss. It just happened, several times over the course of the two weeks!

D The sun and warmth of the island infused your spirit with clarity and well-being.

TANDRA I felt so relaxed the whole time I was there. I felt strong. We had such good talks. He's getting it. Who knew?

D And now back in Toronto you maintain your clarity still. You are releasing the bitter "I have to do everything myself or else nothing gets done" indispensability routine.

TANDRA I'm much clearer about what I need to do for myself and what others need to do for themselves. I don't need to feel indispensable anymore.

D You are letting go of your need for external validation.

TANDRA I know my worth. Love is good. I'll take that. Enough of that other stuff. Owww, my right foot is completely numb! I can't move it.

D Whoa … Your self-assertion and sexual awakening has stirred another younger traumatized astronaut out of a long, frozen slumber.

A few minutes later:

Wow, you just dropped right in. I *sense* that you are out-of-body and in the midst of being attacked. Hmmm … It's the first time your brother rapes you and it's your first time dissociating. You have no idea where you are or what is happening. I *hear* "Is this death?" You are floating in a blank space devoid of structure, logic, or love. You are alone and have lost all your points of reference. You can't make sense of your experience. I *hear* "If this is not death and this is what is in store for me, I might as well be dead!"

TANDRA   Ugh …

D   That younger self is awakening here in my studio today. She is painfully panicked and dazed. She's peeling one eye open and then the other. She's been in a traumatized, disembodied state for over forty years! It's big news to find out she is alive and well! She has been cut off from all communication, floating outside of your soul's vessel for decades. "I'm not dead?" She can barely utter the thought. She feels encased in concrete, she is so stiffened by fragmentation and dissociation.

TANDRA   Ugh. *Tandra holds her gut. Excruciating cramps shoot through her abdomen. She feels frantic.*

D   The memory of your physical anguish pierces the hymen of time. As the ordeal unfolds, terror and horror intermingle. The world as you knew it spun into a chaotic hurricane of panic. Your guts feel shredded.

TANDRA   It feels like nothing's left down there but a huge bloody, mangled mess.

D   I *hear* "Nothing's left! I'm dead. The world as I knew it is dead. It's all gone."

TANDRA   For forty years part of me thought I was dead? For *forty years* part of me *was* dead. I've always thought that the penalties should be the same! *Tandra fires up in a superbly calm rage. Her younger self basks in Tandra's kick-ass rant about rape and murder being on par. Her younger self feels sheltered in the lush haven of Tandra's open heart.* You are alive! I love you! You're not alone. I'm here. Welcome to our life here and now! Rest here, cuddle right in, I'll never leave you.

D   Blessings, dearest Tandra. Welcome back!

TANDRA   Thank you.

D   Namaste.

LATE JUNE

TANDRA   I have experienced more pain in the past ten days than during childbirth. I couldn't move my left arm. It was completely numb. I had two massages, acupuncture twice, and saw my chiropractor too! I've been living on Advil and ice packs.

D   Oh dear … Let's see who is screaming to high heaven hoping to be heard—on summer solstice no less.

TANDRA   Oh, yeah … I hadn't made the link.

D   *I settle on Tandra's right thigh for a few minutes. I hear* "I don't want to be forgotten! I want to heal too!" Your thirteen-year-old self is howling in a desperate attempt to be acknowledged and cared for. She feels unloved.

A few minutes later:

Hmmm … There are two currents surfacing simultaneously today. There is also potent shift in your personal power. Crisis aside, you're having sex with your husband and staying in your body the whole time! That's a huge shift.

TANDRA Sex is not such a bad idea after all! *Tandra says this smiling.* I'm on it! I tell him immediately when I do not like something. For years I did not make demands or express my needs. I'm clear and I'm speaking up!

D OK, so what is not being spoken or heard? What do you want to say, thirteen-year-old Tandra? *Sure enough, the four-alarm bells ring in Tandra's left shoulder.* That's the hot spot. I *hear* "Well, that's all good, but I hate my body!"

TANDRA I have had poor body image issues since age thirteen! I guess it's time to make a change in that department too.

D Yes, your emerging sexual desire has turned the light on in that room too.

TANDRA I was thinking that in the fall …

D Young Tandra pounces. I *hear* "The fall? How about now!" The summer solstice energy is letting you know it's time to really take care of yourself physically. It's time for more yoga, exercise, a new food plan, and the whole program! In other words, it's time to love yourself fully, body included!

Ten minutes later:

The heart meridian runs through both shoulders and arms. And the left arm is directly connected to the biological heart. Your self-loathing and poor body image are stored here. You get the picture?

TANDRA Oh yes. It's time for self-love.

D Summer is the season of the heart after all!

A few minutes later:

Woowee, young Tandra means business. Hating your body has taken its toll. Your heart chakra is connected to your upper chakras—but it's not connected to the chakras in your body. Yep, it's time to get on with the full program.

TANDRA I hear her. I'll make changes this summer.

D   She's so powerful, full of verve and determination. She is your potent ally, not your foe. She's going to be an insightful guide. I don't think she will let you get away with anything though. She's on it!

TANDRA   And so am I! I really have to face myself and get on with the body love program.

D   Namaste.

TANDRA   Namaste.

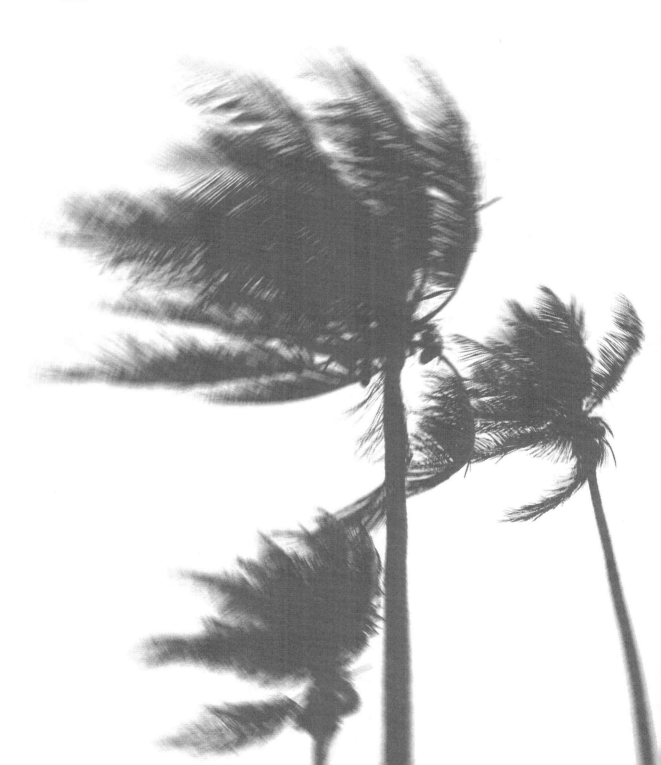

Email from Tandra

Om Shanti,

Dany, I trust you are enjoying lovely holiday time. As for me, I spent a lovely day with the Brahma Kumaris on Saturday in a seminar called the Four Faces of Woman. On Sunday I attended a Full Moon Circle where I spoke words to this effect: I release into the fire the behaviour that I do as a duty to others and I claim from the fire the behaviour/activity that is my life purpose.

I came home and placed my crystals/minerals in the moonlight overnight. Today I went to work and was let go from my job.

I'd say I'm one powerful woman!

I was in shock at first, but I'll get over it! I've never been fired. I worked very hard, contributed to the enterprise, and was well liked. I was replaced by someone with more experience in tax. Alrighty then! Still I got myself fired, which indicates that all is as it should be.

Can't wait to see what's next. Just had to share! We can talk at my next appointment!

Enjoy—as will I!
Namaste,
Tandra

....

SEPTEMBER

Tandra at age fifty-one

TANDRA   Fantastic, huh? Fast, huh! Just like that!

D   Talk about co-creation.

TANDRA   I'm settling in to my new life just fine. I set up my website and have launched my private Reiki practice. It's all very exciting, but I'm still tight behind my left shoulder blade.

D   *I check in with Tandra's biological heart for a few minutes.* I *hear* "It's my cross to bear!" Quite literally! Its impression is marked diagonally across your back! I *hear* "Love and happiness are for everyone else—not me." Hmmm… Looks like some unwholesome beliefs are getting in your way.

TANDRA My right ear started ringing loudly when I lay down last night. Then a great pressure pushed my head down. Well, you know where you're going tomorrow, I thought.

D   *I place my hands on Tandra's ears for a few minutes.* I *hear* "Know your place and everything will be fine. Speak only when you are addressed. Be quiet. Don't rattle your cage."

TANDRA I want out of all of this.

D   It looks like a part of you still acquiesces to the old status quo. I *hear* "I have to do this. This is my life. This is my unhappy life. That's all it can be and will be." That sounds more like your mother. I *sense* that she passed down her beliefs and tried-and-true survival systems. And it looks like they were passed down from her mother and grandmother before that. You have internalized their beliefs and look at yourself through their lens.

TANDRA They were workers. They worked hard. That's all they knew.

D   This energy system reaches into your neck. Steel-like cables pull down your head. I *hear* "Know your place!"

TANDRA There were class issues in both St. Lucia and in England!

D   You take for granted that your options are limited. Your mother's, grandmother's, and great-grandmother's beliefs shut down your creative urges and any inspiration deemed inappropriate in their working-class ethos.

TANDRA Oh sure, don't get too big for your britches!

D   Unfortunately, it looks like this intergenerational powerlessness is potent.

TANDRA The primary objective in our household was survival. Learn how to survive and here's how to survive in this world! In their world, there was no art. There was no piano or music in our household. I don't remember playing games even. That survival mentality has been passed down from generation to generation!

D   And the sexual abuse from age six to thirteen reinforced that. The development of your poetic and creative thinking was also thwarted by your constant vigilance! By age six your energy bodies had already settled into fight–flight–freeze ecology. Ah good … The energy in your right brain stirs from its hibernating slumber. You are safe and you have permission to develop your imagination and creativity, Tandra.

TANDRA   Now that's a revolution. Art and purpose have always been for others, not me!

D   It's time to dream your life, Tandra. Dream and dream big.

TANDRA   Yes, more of *that,* please! I plan on starting right now, thank you very much.

D   You go, girl! Namaste.

TANDRA   Namaste.

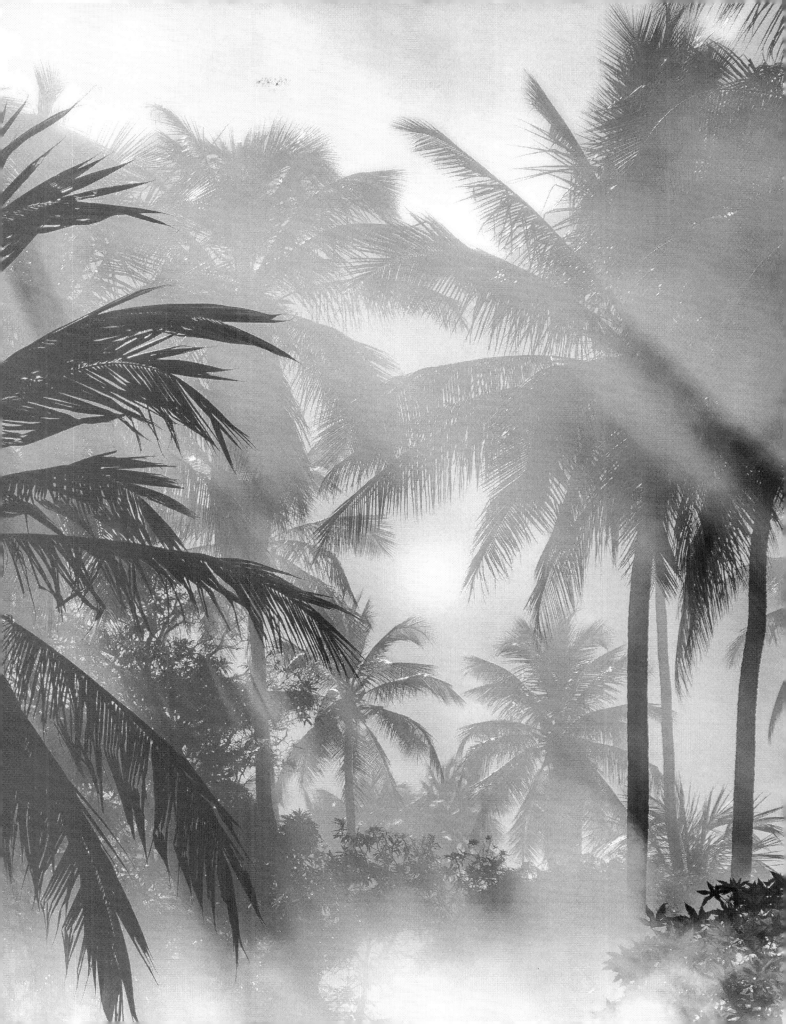

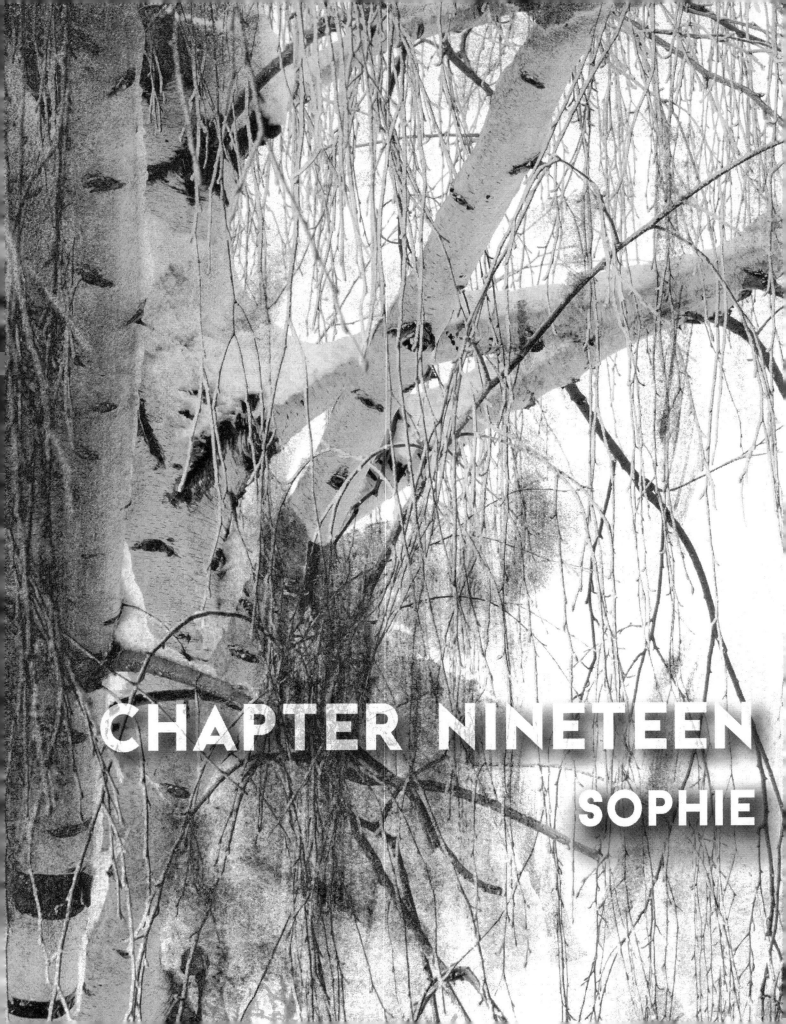

CHAPTER NINETEEN
SOPHIE

SEPTEMBER

Sophie at age sixty

SOPHIE   My craniosacral therapist recommended you. My feet hurt, my left heel especially. I have difficulty walking. It's been going on for months and getting worse rather than better. I'm starting to really worry. It makes me feel old. I mean, is this it? Am I going downhill from here? What do I need to do to shift this? What's this about? What's behind it? The pain in my feet is not shifting even though I am experiencing more mobility in other parts of my body. I'm an active woman and have been for years. I practise yoga, Tai Chi, and meditation several times a week and my diet is healthier than most. I've been on the organic bandwagon since the 1980s, way sooner than most. My craniosacral therapist suspects that an emotional blockage needs to be accessed in order to release the energy flow in my left leg. He thinks that I need to heal and integrate a submerged trauma.

D   Your timing speaks volumes about your readiness to shed. It's fall equinox, a most propitious time for a concerted effort at digging. *I rest my hands on Sophie's shins for a few minutes.* Hmmm … Your energy field is extremely compact and close to your body. Your aura is small. Thank the Goddess you practise yoga, Tai Chi, and meditation regularly; your well-being would be far more tenuous if you didn't. Also, your breath is surprisingly shallow considering your practices and diet. Hmmm …

A few minutes later:

I *see* you standing, arms by your sides, your heart burdened with sorrow and your eyes resolutely staring ahead. You are on a serious mission. You have held yourself together through thick and thin for years. I can feel that there was no choice, no other option.

SOPHIE   I'm a single mother! My two girls are in their twenties now.

D   One marriage?

SOPHIE   No, two. Both my marriages were super stressful and both ended because of massive betrayals.

D   *I shift my left hand to Sophie's left kidney while my right hand rests on her right thigh for a few minutes.* I *feel* that you bravely persisted through both divorces. *I slow down to drop deeper into the divorce file in Sophie's energy field for ten minutes.* I *see* your feet glued to the floor with your eyes wide open, blinded by shocking news. Your first husband has just declared that he is leaving you. Although you are heartbroken, terrified, and crushed, in a millisecond your mind shifted to your children and every cell in your being realigned.

SOPHIE   It sure did. What else was I supposed to do? I had to take care of my girls somehow.

D   Yes, I *hear* "I can do this! I can and must provide a safe and nurturing home for my children!" At that critical juncture in your life, you created a brave architect of survival. Every victim meets the energy of adversity with an architect of survival; they have to in order to survive. Your energy speaks of your resourcefulness and determination. However, under this courage, there's a frenetic and electric crackle. This static tells me that you are tormented by worry.

SOPHIE   Oh God, I'm always worried. Worry is my middle name!

D   Yes, and your encounter with fear predates your first divorce. Insecurity and anxiety were already chronic by then.

SOPHIE   I'm sure it was.

D   *I settle my right hand on Sophie's left thigh for a few minutes.* Your left leg reveals a bone-deep rigidity. I *sense* a much younger self emerging to present her story. *I pause to drop into the ethos of Sophie's childhood for five minutes.* We're here, little one … You are safe now … We're listening … Whatever you need … We love you. Hmmm … I *see* that you had a difficult father who abused you.

SOPHIE   Yeah, my husbands didn't have the copyright on that!

D   You are also triggered by adversity in the present. Your architect of survival is holding on for dear life. Your seat belt is on (this is a good thing), but you are moving through yet another fast curve on your roller coaster of a life. It's was all very scary, then and now!

SOPHIE   It always is somehow.

D   *I feel called to shift my left hand to Sophie's biological heart and glide my right hand to her left kidney. I settle in for a few minutes.* Hmmm … The energy in your biological heart is heavy and there's a dense ball of toxicity the size of a lime. I *sense* that betrayal is a theme in your life. Images of men's faces and upper torsos float above my right shoulder. Your father and husbands and …

SOPHIE   … and now I'm dealing with an administrator at the ashram!

D   Ah, this is the betrayal in your life now that has triggered your architect of survival into high alert. You are doing your best to keep it together, but you are white-knuckling it.

SOPHIE This latest disloyalty is throwing me for a loop! The ashram has been such a healing place for me! I despair whenever I think about it.

D Your sacred space has been violated. The ashram, your sanctuary, is now infected by betrayal. You are heartbroken again. There is a direct line from your biological heart, through the left kidney, and down into your left foot. I *hear* "I can't support you anymore. I'm tired. I can't do it, not without the ashram!" Your architect of survival is not sure she can pull it off this time, not without her safe refuge.

SOPHIE Well, where am I safe? Where do I belong?

D *Tears drop into Sophie's ears ... gentle Reiki tears. Love and compassion pools in her biological heart and once satiated her heart pours the healing energy into her kidney. Loud gurgles resonate through her torso and pelvis. The energy then travels down her left leg to her foot.*

Ten minutes later:

That's it, Sophie. Your connection to your guru is rekindled. You feel her support and wisdom and with her reconnect with Divine and sacred energy. This is only one layer. I suspect we'll be digging our way through several. We'll get there though.

SOPHIE Thanks. That was powerful. So much of what you expressed resonated with me.

NOVEMBER

SOPHIE I spent a month in England with my daughter and newborn grandson. It was great, but now I'm back, you know, that same old anxiety crept in almost the minute I walked into my apartment.

D *I place my hands on Sophie's shins.* Your energy is flowing beautifully. *Heat meets my hands almost immediately.* Your self-healing systems are up and running and your tight shield is thawing. There's clearly nothing like baby kisses and grandmother rapture to soften the edge of betrayal! Vibrant energy is still clearing stagnant energy from your biological heart, left kidney, and into your left foot.

SOPHIE The very warm and loving family experience in my daughter's home really touched me, you know.

D Indeed! Your grandmother love-fest was a restorative boost. Let's check in with your left leg. *I place my left hand on Sophie's thigh and my right on her shin for a few minutes.*

Hmmm, we're in a different time zone. I *hear* "I'm back here! I'm alone again in my barren home!" But you're not just speaking of your current home. I *sense* it's your childhood home, your crumbling home after your first baby and the home you live in now on your own.

SOPHIE   I'm alone again! *Sadness marks Sophie's facial features. Her body slumps heavily on the table.* I'm always getting the short end of the stick, in my family, my marriages, and now at the ashram!

D   I *see* you walking on barren land with little or no sustenance. Although on the verge of collapse, you are determined not to succumb. I *hear* "I'm OK. I don't need that much sustenance anyway. I'm brave and courageous! I will raise and educate my girls and create a beautiful home. I will thrive no matter what. I will grow and learn to live well. I will transcend my wounds and my ego. I will open my heart to love and compassion."

SOPHIE   I will.

D   I'm sure you will, but that's one hell of a list. Your architect of survival is on a serious mission to seek not only the essentials for survival but also a better life. It's a huge and beautiful undertaking sustained by courage! Bravery, though celebrated by most cultures and religions, is nonetheless a mechanism of survival rather than a life-affirming and nourishing expression of *being*. To be brave and courageous implies that you must move forward despite adversity every day.

SOPHIE   I was a single mother back in the 1980s! The support networks were not what they are today.

D   Add to this two divorces and a difficult father and you had serious challenges to contend with. Your bravery and courage are entrenched and so is your intrepid quest to create a good life for you and your children despite all odds. Is this a threat now though?

SOPHIE   No, not really. *Sophie's energy shifts. Gradually, she yields to peace and stillness.*

D   Your life force eases its drive to advance. Good, your courage campaign is on hold. Gentleness and serenity infuse your being.

SOPHIE   I'm safe!?! I am safe! What a change, huh?

D   Huge. Drink in this energy. Take your time.

Fifteen minutes later:

That's it Sophie! I *see* a smattering of angel dust penetrate and replenish your aura and energy body. Your torso shimmers with your angelic grandson's sweet love. Baby love, pure and so intensely generous, expands your heart chakra. You're now integrating your experience in your daughter's home. Your Sacred Tree is harmonizing with the earth and the source.

SOPHIE   That's a really big shift. I can't wait to see where that takes me.

EARLY DECEMBER

SOPHIE   My left foot is still sore! It's still hard for me to walk! It's so frustrating. I'm fit otherwise.

D   It's cramping your style, I *see* that. You like being active.

SOPHIE   I do.

D   *I place my hands on Sophie's shins for a few minutes.* A huge shift is occurring. There is nothing stagnant here. It's December after all; the winter solstice is right around the corner. You are decidedly on track and surrendering to the transformative impulse of this most potent portal. Your etheric field is very faint from waist to mid-thigh. Your cosmic underwear, as I call it, is torn and damaged. This weakness in your etheric field speaks of sexual trauma. Are you aware of any violation in your history?

SOPHIE   At age three, I ran away from the house one afternoon. An innocent escapade … an adventure … I don't know. I think my mother had fallen asleep on the couch. I was sexually assaulted by two teenage boys and found hours later lying on the ground, unconscious.

D   *I place my hands on Sophie's left thigh for a few minutes.* We're here, little one … We love you … It's all over … You are here with us now … *Teeny Sophie emerges from her fearful slumber. I reach out to her with love and much gentleness. She is extremely distressed and hurt. Within a few minutes we are connected and she receives our love.*

SOPHIE   Ouf …

D   Let me know if you get too uncomfortable. The shock is surfacing and yielding very quickly. Your yoga, Tai Chi, and meditation are facilitating this process.

A few minutes later:

Hmmm … I *see* that you tried to kick the boys off but did not succeed. Your left thigh reverberates with the brutal news flash: "I can't stop these boys! I'm helpless! Whatever horrible thing it is they are trying to do to me, I can't stop it. They're hurting me! I can't stop them. I can't!" *I feel called to reach for Sophie's left foot and hear* "I tried running away from the boys but failed."

SOPHIE   Ah geez … ouf … *Sobs shake Sophie's torso.*

D   *A few minutes later, I shift my left hand shifts to Sophie's left adrenal gland. A strident, high-pitched hum meets the heel of my hand.* Wait a minute here, something is missing … The helplessness and total powerlessness story does not fully express your experience. Teeny Sophie's radiant strength is not accounted for. You were found unconscious, right?

SOPHIE   Right.

D   You did not fail! Your "lifeless body" scared the boys away! They thought you were dead. Your possum strategy worked; it interrupted the assault! Your pre-emptive strategy was unsuccessful, but "playing possum," feigning death, totally worked!

SOPHIE   What do you mean I did not fail? I was raped, no?

D   Yes, but you saved yourself from greater harm. This is major news! It's very important to reframe the story so that it includes your cleverness and resourcefulness. As I witness it, the hum of your exhausted adrenal gland is yielding to a softer tone. You protected yourself! There are degrees of helplessness. You did something to help yourself and actually halted the attack! You weren't entirely powerless; even at three years old you had tricks up your sleeve.

SOPHIE   Really?

D   The awareness of this decisive fact is crucial to facilitate your healing and well-being. Witnessing that you were not able to run away, that it was impossible to kick off the boys, and that you were raped is momentous, yet honouring your possum strategy also has a great impact on your energy field because this was a determining event too. You did not have the power to prevent the attack, yet you stopped it. You totally did!

SOPHIE   I had no idea.

D   It's a massive shift in the story. That's it, as you acknowledge your resources, in this case the possum strategy, your personal power replenishes its stores in your second chakra, dantian, and your cosmic underwear is filling in. The holes and tears are healing as we speak.

Fifteen minutes later:

The fibres of your etheric body are now scintillating with blue light. *My hands comb Sophie's etheric field to amplify the shift.*

SOPHIE   Who knew?

D   You knew what to do to halt the attack! Namaste, it's an honour.

SOPHIE   Namaste.

LATE DECEMBER

SOPHIE   I was really tired after the last treatment. It took several days for me to feel I had enough energy to go out even.

D   I suspect we need to pick up where we left off. Are you OK with working through more of your trauma at age three?

SOPHIE   Yes. I really want to get better.

D   Ah good … Teeny Sophie is very present. *I rest my hands on Sophie's shins for a few minutes.* Hmmm … I now perceive a huge cowl of unwieldy, unbeneficial energy saturating your upper chakras and aura.

A few minutes later:

Hmmm … I *sense* culpability and self-blame. I *hear* "It's my fault. I ran out of the house and look what happened! Look what I did!" Oh dear, Teeny Sophie is taking full responsibility for the violent criminal offence perpetrated by two adolescent boys.

SOPHIE   I wonder how I got that idea.

D   *My hands settle on Sophie's ears for a few minutes. Loud untruths greet my palms. I settle into the energy for several minutes, inviting it to leak into my palms. I see* Teeny Sophie emerging from her unconscious state in the hospital. Ah … It's your mother's admonishments that haunt you still.

SOPHIE   What?

D   I *hear* your mother saying "Look what you did! Never do that again! You hear me?" In that instant, you perceived yourself as responsible for the assault. I *hear* even more loudly "Look what I did! It's my fault! I'm a bad girl."

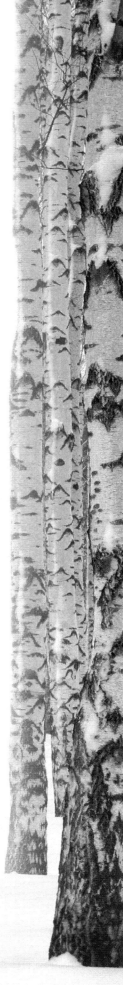

SOPHIE   Oh dear ... I had no idea.

D   Here you are, in a hospital after being raped, lucky to be alive, and your mother does not welcome you back to the land of the living with a huge hug and a kiss. She did not celebrate the fact that your life was spared or express love and relief. Instead of a hero's welcome, you woke up to your mother scolding you, blaming you for the harm you did to yourself and for the trouble and grief you are causing her. Over and over you *hear* "Look what you did! Never do that again!"

SOPHIE   Of course, I ended up thinking it was my fault and that I was a bad girl! She punished me!

D   Yeah, and that's not the full story. Your mother is a wreck.

A few minutes later:

I *hear* "Where was I when she slipped out of the house? What time was it? Was I sleeping? Was I awake? What was I doing?" It makes sense: to know that your daughter slipped from under your nose, ran out in the street, and roamed the neighbourhood for a long time only to encounter two young teenagers who rape her is unbearable. It looks like your mother unconsciously/consciously passed on her guilt to you. It's a Grimm tale indeed.

Once upon a time, there was a dear little girl who was loved by everyone who looked at her, but most of all by her grandmother, and there was nothing that she would not have given the child. Once, she gave her a little white nightgown, which suited her so well that she would never sleep wearing anything else. One afternoon the dear little girl got up out of bed, opened the door below, and crept outside. The sun shone brightly so she meandered through the village with ease and wonder. She gazed in merriment at all the windows that glittered in the lemon light. And just as she walked by the wood, two wolves met her. Teeny did not know what wicked creatures they were, and was not at all afraid of them.

"Good day! Good day!" said they.

"Thank you kindly!"

"Whither away today?" said they in unison.

288

"*To my grandmother's house.*"

"*Where does your grandmother live?*"

"*Just a little farther past the park; her house stands under the three large oak trees. The nut trees are just below; you surely must know it,*" replied Teeny.

The wolves thought to themselves: "*What a tender young creature! What a nice plump mouthful she will be. She's much better to eat than the old woman.*"

So they walked for a short time by Teeny's side and then they said, "*See, Teeny, how pretty the flowers are about here—why do you not look around? We believe too that you do not hear how sweetly the cardinal sings; you walk so gravely along, while everything in the wood is merry.*"

Teeny raised her eyes, and when she saw the sunbeams dancing here and there through the trees and pretty flowers growing everywhere, she thought: "*I suppose I can take Grandmother fresh flowers; that would please her.*" And so she ran from the path into the wood to look for the flowers. And wherever she picked one, she fancied she saw a still prettier one farther on, and ran after it, and so got deeper and deeper in the wood.

The wolves jumped on a rock. They intended on waiting for her, and then to steal after her and devour her. And scarcely had the wolves settled on the rock than with two bounds and a skirmish to reach for Teeny first, they were off the rock. The older and bigger wolf was ahead of his brother and swallowed Teeny up before he even had to share.

When the wolf had appeased his appetite, he lay down and fell asleep and began to snore loudly while his sulking brother lay about in a dejected heap. A policeman was just passing the rock. "*Do I find you here, you young sinners?*" said he. Startled but still light, the youngest wolf scampered off. "*I have long sought you!*" said the policeman to the big fat wolf. Then just as he was going to fire at the lumbering wolf, it occurred to him that he might have devoured Teeny, and that she might still be saved, so he did not fire. He took a pair of scissors and began to cut open the big round stomach of the big bad wolf. When he had made two snips, he saw Teeny, and then made two more snips, and the little girl sprang out, crying, "*Ah, how frightened I have been! How dark it was inside the wolf.*" Teeny quickly fetched great stones with which to fill the wolf's belly, and when the wolf awoke, he wanted to run away, but the stones were so heavy that he collapsed at once and fell dead.

Then both were delighted. The policeman drew off the wolf's skin and went to the station with it. And revived Teeny thought to herself, "*As long as I live, I will never by myself leave the house, to run into the wood, when my mother has forbidden me to do so.*"

JANUARY

SOPHIE I experienced anxiety for two days after the last treatment. It calmed down after. Since then though, I'm more aware of my constant anxiety. It's like a fluttery, worried energy.

D *After resting my hands on Sophie's shins for a few minutes, my left hand climbs to her right kidney and adrenal gland while my right hand rests on her right thigh.* Your right kidney pulsates. Panic experienced during traumatic events in your past are still buried in your kidney, and that tremor of fear attaches itself to events in your daily life now. There are many layers here.

A few minutes later:

The energy is malleable and set for a release. Are you ready to do what I call a hard-drive cleanse?

SOPHIE OK. Let's do it.

D I'll focus on the right kidney because it is calling me. But the kidneys work as a pair so you will have sensations and clearing in both.

A few minutes later:

Ah … I *sense* that the terror experienced while unconscious during your attack is recorded here. Although unconscious and playing possum, you lived through the horror of the attack, blow by blow. And Teeny Sophie who is unconscious is floating far far away from her Sacred Tree. She has no idea that this experience has ended and that you now thrive. We're here, little one. We love you.

SOPHIE I'm here, little sweetie. I'm here …

D That's it … Open your heart and arms. Embrace Teeny Sophie and celebrate your triumphant survival.

A few minutes later:

Offer her a peaceful, safe, and restorative home in your heart. Create the safest bedroom ever with the coziest bed ever. Slip her into little PJ bottoms and a top. Tuck Teeny in. Kiss her, hug her, and snuggle in with her. Rest together while watching a coloured light project dancing animals and swimming mammals on the walls.

A few minutes later:

That's it, Sophie. Surrender to sleep together.

SOPHIE   She's right here with me. I feel her so vividly.

D   You're doing great. She's softening.

A few minutes later:

Oh … Part 2 is presenting already.

SOPHIE   It's OK. We're OK.

D   I *sense* the flight–fight–freeze overload and the accompanying flash when the pain exceeded your threshold when you were penetrated.

SOPHIE   Ouf…

D   Yeah … Unfortunately, the level of pain you experienced altered and weakened the energetic map of your cells and molecules in your right kidney. It's like an oil change. Out with the lightning bolt of horror caused by the intense pain and in with the love.

A few minutes later:

Your left foot is probably totally numb by now, maybe both.

SOPHIE   They feel like wood. I can't move them. Ooow.

D   It's OK. That feeling is temporary. It means we are doing our work. The shock and trauma are leaving through your feet to the earth. And love and compassion are flowing in, filling in all the space the release is creating.

SOPHIE   Wow! This is powerful.

D   You have done a lot of work; that's why it's melting off you like butter. Keep up all your practices. I look forward to working with you in a month.

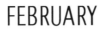

FEBRUARY

SOPHIE   The last session was intense. I feel better now, but I still feel really jumpy.

D   *I rest my hands on Sophie's shins for a minutes.* Hmmm … There is a lot of fear in your system. I *sense* that all the clearing we did in your right kidney has stirred up your adrenal glands. They want a hard-drive cleanse too.

SOPHIE   There's more?

D   Our adrenal glands and kidneys work in a team, so it makes sense that you can shift their vibration, especially now that your kidneys have shifted. *I rest my hands on Sophie's adrenal glands.* Hmmm … I *see* exhaustion in both adrenal glands. They're like tight little dried raisins with lightning bolts shooting out in all directions. They're not designed to produce flight–fight-freeze hormones every day, especially every time your daughters leave the house.

SOPHIE   Ah, I'm always afraid when people leave that they will never come back … that I'm seeing them for the last time … Not only my daughters—everyone! But especially my children! I always ask them to call me when they get home. I can't help it! They humour me and do it.

D   That's an intense way to live! I *sense* that you relive your mother's trauma every time someone leaves the house. You worry that your daughters will be attacked like you were. And that if they are, you will be buried in guilt and sorrow like your own mother was. It's a double trigger.

SOPHIE   My daughters are in their twenties!

D   Yep, that's fifty-seven years bearing the brunt of your trauma and twenty-five years of overlap with your mother's trauma. It's enough to make your knees buckle and more than enough to exhaust these poor little Napoleon hats on top of your kidneys. Hmmm … There's more.

A few minutes later:

I *see* a teenage Sophie frozen from head to toe, totally out-of-body, unable to express sexual desire and unwilling to engage with a suitor. It seems you had a hair-trigger fear response to sexuality when you were a teenager. Your fear totally thwarted your sexual awakening.

SOPHIE   I was terrified of sex! I still am!

D   Sexual energy can be a trigger for anyone who has been raped, but this is a double whammy. Your sexual awakening, such as it was, was thwarted, especially because you were surrounded by teenage boys. Your attackers were teenage boys. This unconscious link and trigger was extremely potent, and you couldn't get away from it unless you stayed as far away from the boys as possible.

SOPHIE   That's exactly what I did! I wanted nothing to do with it!

D   You were an adult when you opened up to the possibility of being sexually active, when men approached you rather than teenage boys?

SOPHIE   Ahhh, my ankles ache. My right leg is asleep! It hurts. It's completely numb!

D   *My hands glide down to Sophie's right leg and settle in for a few minutes.* We awakened the whole line. Something about what I just said. I *sense* you are out-of-body. Hmmm … You are in bed with your second husband.

SOPHIE   Oh, he was a possessive and controlling man!

D   You were out-of-body during sex with him.

SOPHIE   Probably.

D   Actually, I don't think you knew if you were coming or going in general. You were so fearful and stunned.

SOPHIE   He was a tricky personality. He was passive–aggressive and extremely manipulative.

D   In other words, he was toxic. He never did a day of therapy in his life and really should have for his sake and others around him.

SOPHIE   I feel so lucky I got out! *The energy release is sudden. The teenage boy and man file is fumigated. I open the window and Sophie sits up to get her bearings. A strong gust of wind wraps itself around her, sweeping the toxic debris out of the studio.* Good riddance!

We both glow with excitement. We hug in celebration of our complicity and to express gratitude to the earth and the sun. We are both blessed by their grace.

OCTOBER

SOPHIE   I'm a wreck. Everything hurts. I am so stiff! I'm getting old.

D   *I rest my hands on Sophie's shins.* Whoa … What's going on in your life?

SOPHIE   Huh?

D   Well I don't *sense* that this is really about aging—your wheels are not falling off—so has something happened?

SOPHIE   Really? … Well … ugh … My Tai Chi teacher inappropriately touched me. I'm deeply disappointed. It makes me so sad. I love Tai Chi, loved the class, and I really thought I had found a really good teacher. My neck is really sore.

D   Your energy is swirling in a tornado of doubt and fear. It's all the same familiar emotions, but the movement pattern is unusual. You are out-of-body, rattled, and confused. It looks like you haven't fully acknowledged the impact of your teacher's sexual harassment. Your narrative appears unclear, and some of your feelings are still suppressed.

SOPHIE   I respect my teachers! That's what it's all about, isn't it? That is what it is about in my tradition.

D   At this decisive juncture in your student–teacher relationship, you trust your teacher more than you trust yourself. Meanwhile, your body screams injury and violation. Your indecision is unfortunately absolving your teacher of his guilt. Oh dear … This is an old pattern. It goes deeper than that. I *sense* that you trust others more than you trust yourself because you think that others are more intelligent than you are.

SOPHIE   They know more, don't they?

D   No one knows more what is best for you than you. Trusting other people's judgment more than your own cuts you off from your intuition and inner wisdom.

SOPHIE   Well, I'm deeply sad and disappointed. He knows so much! I just don't understand how it could happen. *My hands shift to Sophie's stomach for a few minutes.* I really understand how it can happen to young women! But me, my belly hangs out and my arms flap! How can he want *that*? I'm not attractive anymore. I have grey hair!

D   I *hear* "I really thought I was invisible to men. I don't want to be involved with a man!" Hey, when did crones stop having sex? They're not necessarily celibate, you know. It's a choice you can make, but the choice is not made for you.

SOPHIE   Women are attractive until age fifty-five. I'm sixty!

D   Says who? Sexist men? Your internalization of the dominant sexist narrative about menopause and aging? You're in great shape! The soft flesh business is absolutely relative. You exercise, practise yoga, eat a plant-based diet, and on and on.

SOPHIE   I like to look nice. I like to dress well, that kind of thing! You seriously mean I need to go on guard again? I thought I was through with that.

D   Guard no, awareness yes. You are only now learning to trust and be open.

SOPHIE   I was open!

D   Open, not really, aware not really either. Unbeneficial beliefs about aging, specifically about aging in a woman's body, created an illusory security shield. You essentially felt secure in an armour of self-denigrating beliefs and low self-worth: I am unworthy of that kind of attention so I am finally free.

SOPHIE   I really think that, you know.

D   This supposed freedom comes at too great a price, Sophie. It robs you of your personal power and distinction. Your crone power is reduced to an illusory safety zone without men's attention, rather than a fuel for living an expansive and effervescent life, with a sexy relationship if you so choose. Your generation has the resources to transform our cultural misconceptions. But for that you need your voice! No wonder your neck is sore: you are silenced!

SOPHIE   Well, I haven't told anyone about it. I've been doing Reiki on myself to clear his energy off me.

D   Your practice is beneficial, but it can't stand on its own without action. It's essential that you welcome yourself back into your body. You can do so by honouring your experience and speaking up.

SOPHIE   He even offered me the class for free! He said, "You don't have to pay for this class." I felt like a prostitute. It was so confusing. I felt like I let it happen. I feel complicit. I should have said something sooner.

D   At three years old you couldn't speak up, but now you can. You can write him a letter, talk to other teachers at the school, alert other students, or choose to report him to the police.

SOPHIE   Can he charge me with slander?

D   Your truth is not slander.

SOPHIE   I was trying to forget. I can feel that now. My neck was full of knots and my body was protesting my concerted effort to put it behind me. I feel so much better. Phew! OK. I'm going home to think about what I am going to do.

D   You're a beautiful crone. Work with it! Take your power! Decide what is best for you. Speak up in whatever way feels right to you! You are doing this for you, not for him. You come first.

Namaste.

NOVEMBER

SOPHIE   I had a lovely trip visiting my grandchildren. I feel stiff and tired though. I'm frustrated with the amount of pain and discomfort I'm experiencing.

D   Did you follow through with your Tai Chi teacher?

SOPHIE   I wrote a letter to him before leaving. I opened my mailbox and email with some trepidation when I got home, but there was nothing. No response so far.

D   I'm delighted to hear you decided to write to him. *I rest my hands on Sophie's shins for a few minutes.*

SOPHIE   I felt so much better after I spelled out my take on the events that afternoon.

D   You are still coming down from it all. Your left kidney is hopping. You are still in flight–fight–freeze mode.

A few minutes later:

Hmmm… Your second husband's energy is surfacing.

SOPHIE   I thought of him just the other day. It doesn't happen often anymore.

D   I *sense* you were so bewildered back then. I *hear* "Why is he doing this to me? Why is he harassing me?"

SOPHIE   I was so overwhelmed.

D   Both these men violated you. I *sense* your second husband was a dangerous man. He was driven by urge to have power over you. Hmmm… Are you aware that you are traumatized by your sexual relationship with him?

SOPHIE   I was out-of-body the whole time.

D   Yes, for sure. That hurts in and of itself, you know.

SOPHIE   I didn't know what to do.

D   It doesn't look like you said no.

SOPHIE   I submitted, basically. I didn't feel I could say no. Is my first husband knocking around in there too?

D   WOW … Your left kidney is responding well. Your whole left body is now vital.

A few minutes later:

Whoa… You're jumping ahead! You are clearing the man file: first husband, second husband, Tai Chi teacher, whoever … Your self-healing mandate is on board with clearing the whole lot out of your life now!

SOPHIE   Well. I'm sixty… and I finally give myself permission to embrace freedom with or without a man.

D   Yes and the old "I am undesirable, men don't want me, and that's for the best" belief is morphing into a conscious decision to speak up and to stop looking for a man because you really need one to be complete.

SOPHIE   I have girlfriends who are still looking desperately for a man; for me, it's time to move on from that desperation. I'm so free now. And I love it! I can do whatever I want whenever I want. It's amazing!

D   Namaste.

SOPHIE   Namaste.

CHAPTER TWENTY
ORION

EARLY MAY

Orion at age thirty-four

ORION   I'm anxious and angry all the time. I'm not grounded. I'm confused about what to do next. I hate my job as an art administrator. My art is not really happening either. I feel so stuck.

D   *I rest Orion's head in my hands for a few minutes.* Woowee! Your left-brain hemisphere is cranked up on high alert. A fierce architect of survival greets me at the gate. She's a fast-talking, clever, and aggressive Little Orion at age … hmmm … nine.

ORION   Hahahah! Yeah, that's me all right.

D   Yeah, she's in control and she's making sure that I know. She's the official architect of survival on duty. She's alert and anxious and she has a most important mission. OK, wait a minute … Ah … She is the officious guardian of a secret.

ORION   Oh?

D   She's not the only one who is pumped up. Your body is buzzing. *I shift my hands to Orion's chest.* Do you smoke cigarettes?

ORION   I've been trying to quit for years.

D   Nicotine is definitely your stimulant of choice. *I move my left hand to Orion's pancreas.* But I suspect sugar runs a close second. Do you eat a lot of sweets?

ORION   Yes, that too.

D   Your pancreas is doing backflips to calibrate your blood sugar levels. *I shift my left hand to Orion's adrenal glands.* And you drink coffee … right?

ORION   Eeek … three strikes and I'm out!

D   Literally, that buzz perturbs you enough to significantly weaken your connection to your Sacred Tree and the nourishing energy of the earth and the sun. Nicotine, sugar, and caffeine are an integral part of this little one's survival strategy. I *sense* that at age nine, you deemed it absolutely necessary to keep a secret locked up, not only from others but also from yourself. Sugar, coffee, and nicotine keeps the withholding pattern alive and well.

ORION   I hate it. What am I still in denial about? I've done so much work!

D The good news is that despite all of that, you're more in your body and Sacred Tree than one would expect. It's clear that you've done a lot of emotional work and have healed many traumas already. I also *sense* that you have had many wise and supportive guides on your journey.

ORION Yeah, I really have. I've been blessed.

D You've been really working hard and it shows. And you are clearly on a mission right now. You really want to crack the nut and get to the other side.

ORION I'm really struggling. I need things to change … I really need to quit smoking.

D OK, let's see if it's the right time to tiptoe past your guard dog. *I pause. I hear a charged silence. I wait. Orion suddenly shifts on the table. Another Orion at age nine greets my interest and presence swiftly.* Ah! The traumatized astronaut who created the buzzy guardian of the secret is here. Hello, little one, we're here and we love you. We're honoured by your presence. We're listening.

ORION Whoa! … Wow! … I can feel that.

D Yes, there's a lot of energy moving. There's no resistance. You're all ready to be reunited.

ORION I'm so there.

D I *hear* "I *know* a lot." You sure do, and beyond your age for sure! I can *see* that you're a beautiful oracle.

ORION Nine was a really hard time for me.

D Very much so; you were keenly aware that you were living in an unsafe home. "I *know*. I know a lot." I *hear* again.

ORION We moved in with my stepfather then.

D Ah! He's a problem.

ORION Oh yeah, for damn sure he is.

D You don't trust him and he's hurting you. But there are other children too, right?

ORION I have two stepsisters.

D Hmmm … It looks like your little oracle really saw her new siblings. You perceived their anguish and suffering.

ORION They're both still really fucked up.

D   You were so young and yet I *sense* that your third eye was wide open; you saw the unfiltered truth. I *see* it with you. … You intuited that your stepfather was sexually abusing one or both of his two daughters, your stepsisters.

ORION   I KNEW IT! I've always suspected!

D   Yes, and your stepfather looms large and overhead while your little oracle crouches in fear.

ORION   I hate him!

D   You had to create a boundary somehow. The information and the threat were overwhelming.

ORION   It's so fucked up!

D   It sure was and he was on to you. He silenced you. He knew you were a threat. It's a double whammy. You couldn't handle really knowing, so you shut your intuitive perception down, and he terrorized you to make sure you kept your mouth shut. *Hard tears of helplessness and rage trickle down into Orion's ears and onto the pillow.*

ORION   Oh geez…

D   The secret was safe, yet everyone was in danger.

ORION   Totally! It still is!

D   You've done so much work. That's why both the nine-year-old architect of survival and the victimized astronaut showed up together today. Together, you are a potent force that will no longer be disempowered. Together, you can change the culture of silence in your Sacred Tree and eventually in your family too.

ORION   I sure want to… Ouf… quite the download!

D   Yeah, this was a big information-gathering session. Your day-to-day consciousness is going to reorient itself in a new configuration in relation to the truth and your sixth chakra. You might remember events and start seeing things from a completely different angle. Just give yourself the time to absorb and integrate your intuitive wisdom. Rest. You'll probably need more sleep than usual. You will most likely experience fatigue as you forego the family mythology and embrace the true narrative.

ORION   OK, I'll keep that in mind. Thank you.

D   Namaste. It's an honour.

LATE MAY

ORION   I'm still struggling. I'd love to quit smoking.

D   *I place my left hand on Orion's belly and my right on her right thigh for a few minutes.* Hmmm … Your abdomen is tied in knots. It speaks of chronic tension. *I then rest my left hand up to rest on Orion's liver for a few minutes.* Whoa, your liver is super-hot! It's like molten lava in there. Hmmm… Your liver and gallbladder are blistering with rage and hatred.

ORION   I hate him! I hate him!

D   You were all in danger, this is an old boundary. Hmmm … There's more to it though. Hmmm…

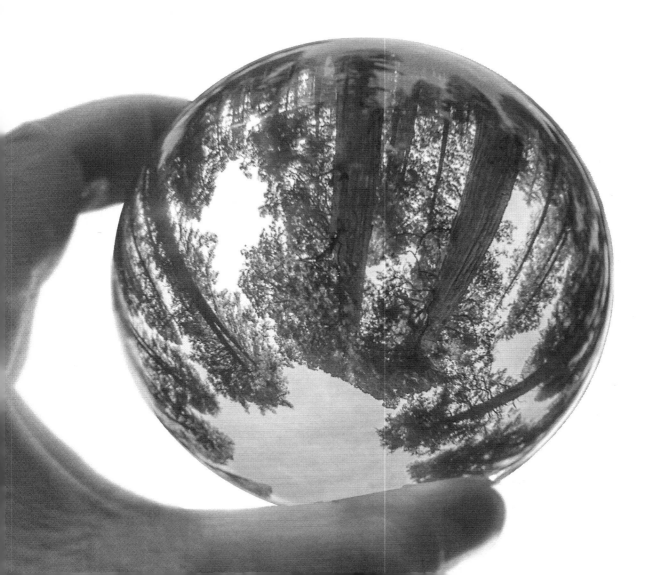

A few minutes later:

I *sense* that you hate yourself too! You hate yourself because your silence unintentionally made you an accomplice—being in on the secret enlisted you as his accomplice.

ORION   Aaagh!

D   It was terrifying and repulsive. Deep within, you are disgusted because your integrity feels contaminated. It's intense! You're haunted by guilt and self-hatred for unconsciously collaborating with their abuser and, most importantly, for not protecting your stepsisters.

ORION   That's so intense!

D   It's huge, you practically hate yourself for not stopping the violence. You were nine years old, Orion—how could you?

ORION   I get it! I was just a child, for crying out loud!

D   Exactly. And the information you perceived intuitively was so terrifying that you had to silence it within yourself to survive. The charge was too great. Sugar worked, right.

ORION   Oh yeah, I ate tons.

D   At age nine you did not have the resources to absorb and integrate the magnitude of your knowledge and its implications. Hmmm … The little oracle knows more.

A few minutes later:

Was there a break between your stepfather's two marriages when he lived alone with his daughters?

ORION   Yes.

D   He probably abused them in your collective home, but you *sensed* that they were in even more danger when they lived alone with him.

ORION   My mother basically married a pedophile!

D   Yes, and you intuitively knew that at age nine. You intuitively perceived that your mother was unsafe and she didn't know; your stepsisters were unsafe and you knew your mother didn't know; and you felt unsafe and you knew for sure that she didn't know that either.

ORION   It's such a mess!

D   Yes, and unfortunately your stepfather is not actually the biggest problem—at nine years old, you were keenly aware that your mother was no longer protecting you, your stepsisters, or herself. It was terrifying! You were abandoned and unsafe.

ORION   I was abandoned; that's just it. Once she married that guy, it was over!

D   Yeah, and you've worked on that already and transcended a huge percentage of this pain. But what lingers and is intolerable now is the denial of your intuitive perception. Although necessary at the time, keeping your third eye shut perpetuates the cycle of fear and isolation by cutting you off from your Sacred Tree, the earth, and the sun. You were not only cut off from your mother's love and protection; the dream team ends up cut off from the flow of unconditional love and compassion as well. It's a major ouch!

ORION   It's super intense. I get all the layers. I feel the block.

D   Yes, and add to that your self-hatred. You still pace to and fro between rooms banging doors.

ORION   Yep, that sums it up.

D   Let's compassionately witness your distress and terror at age nine. Try cuddling on the couch with both: your overwhelmed oracle and your architect of survival high on sugar. You have the resources now to end the cycle of violence by stepping in as their official caregiver. They are both safe with you. Embrace them. Compassionately witness their experience softly and tenderly. It's safe to be together, whole, and connected to your scared tree, the earth, and the sun.

Ten minutes later a brilliant green light suddenly gushes out of Orion's heart and fourth chakra. Wow! That's it! The vibration of unconditional self-love and compassion is now shifting your vibration.

ORION   Whoa, intense.

D   Yeah, intense and magnificent! It ain't a Bell commercial, that's for sure. Unconditional love is so beyond our sentimental definition of familial or romantic love. It's so vast and all-encompassing. It's so beautifully intense and powerful!

ORION   Amazing!

D   Haaahahahah! Good, eh?

ORION   Yeah … Hahahaaa.

D   Namaste!

MID-JUNE

D   Happy summer solstice! Intense, huh?

ORION It's huge this year for me.

D   Let's see what the solstice high tide is bringing in. *I slide my hands under Orion's head for a few minutes. I hear a quiet growl.* Hmmm … Your nine-year-old watchdog and secret-keeper is in high gear.

ORION I'm avoiding my stepsisters and they're avoiding me.

D   I *sense* that you avoid each other to avoid stirring your shared secret.

ORION It's still such a mess.

D   Yes, and for as long as you are separated the truth has less chance of surfacing. This dynamic will clear in time. Let's focus in on you and see what's creating the resistance. Hmmm … *Orion is overwhelmed with grief. My hands shift to her chest, focusing on her heart for a few minutes.* Your little nine-year-old oracle and traumatized astronaut is reaching out again.

ORION I'm still so upset by all of this.

D   We're here, little one. We love you. I *hear* "Everything's different … Everything has changed … Everything!" Hmmm … You feel abandoned, lost, and threatened in your mother's new marriage and home. You have lost her to him.

ORION Yeah, that was pretty much it after that. *Tears moisten Orion's cheeks.*

D   It's more than that too.

A few minutes later:

You feel disoriented and alone in your new school. You miss your supportive teachers and old friends. Everything familiar and comforting has vaporized.

ORION It was unbelievably awful.

D   Your isolation and helplessness was overwhelming.

ORION To say the least.

D   Let's conjure up a wave of unconditional love and compassion. Wow, your fourth chakra is beaming again. You clearly have cultivated this energy in your spiritual practices. Bring that awesome power to your traumatized astronaut at age nine, in that house and at school.

Ten minutes later:

That's it; let the wave swell, so much so that the cumulative force propels it toward your navel, down through your pelvis, out your perineum, and through your legs and feet. Allow any lightning bolts of trauma still trapped in your cerebrospinal fluid to soften out of your body and into the earth. Fantastic! Ah… wait a second, your heart meridian in your right arm is clogged!

ORION   Actually, my right arm is totally numb.

D   Something is blocking the energy in the heart meridian in your right arm. Something is preventing you from letting go. Hmmm … Let's see here. *I shift my hands to Orion's right arm and tune in to the resistance for a few minutes. I sense* that you are holding on to your mother and stepsisters. It looks like you want to save them too.

ORION   Of course I do!

D   You are aware that they are drowning.

ORION   Their lives are such a mess!

D   I *sense* that the pull is so strong that you are in danger of being pulled down by the undertow of their unacknowledged trauma. Orion, it's OK to be the first one in your family to reach the shore. Years of therapy later, you are within reach. You can let go of your stepsisters and mother for now.

ORION   Really?

D   Yes, you have the permission to embrace your own healing. Let it come to fruition now and trust that theirs will unfold in its own time. It's more than OK to be on your own healing schedule.

ORION   I hadn't thought about it that way before.

D   Survivor's guilt, that's what that is. The energy is still not moving. Oh Orion, you are not in the clear yet; you are holding on to your stepfather too—you want to make sure he doesn't get away with it.

ORION   Well, he's dangerous, isn't he?

D   Don't worry; he won't get away with it. You can make sure of that later, when you are thriving. For now, I recommend you try letting go. Let the nourishing nectar of unconditional love and compassion bloom and prosper in your heart. Unleash that powerful flow!

ORION   There it goes ... Wow!

D   Hahahaa! Your oracle and guardian of the secret are riding the wave! You guys have the right to divorce him, you know. You don't have to wait for your mother to do so. You can launch the process: file the papers, so to speak. Hahahaaa ... I *hear* "Did I hear divorce? YEAH! I hate him." Hahaha ... Your nine-year-old dream team sure likes that idea.

ORION   I'm so done with him.

D   Hatred was the only defence you had. It was your last-ditch effort to create a boundary with the guy. Give yourself permission to file the divorce papers. Make your healthy "no" loud and clear. That's it! Now, say "yes" to healing. Reach for the shore. You have the resources to create healthy boundaries now!

ORION   Holy shit. This is huge.

D   It's self-love in action. It's going to go a long way, Orion! It's heart-healing par excellence. Summer is the season of the heart, by the way. Congratulations for courageously embracing the heart-healing offered to you at this time!

ORION   Happy summer solstice, Dany!

D   Thank you. Happy summer solstice to you, Orion!

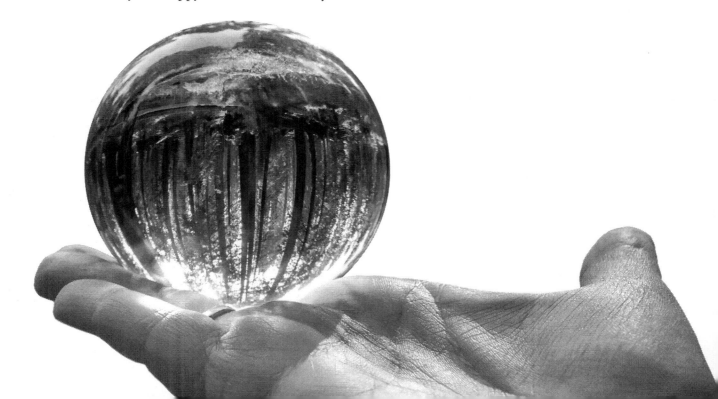

EARLY JULY

ORION   Same old, same old. I feel slightly crazed. The solstice was intense, wasn't it?

D   *I rest my hands on Orion's shins for a few minutes.* Yikes! Your adrenal glands are working overtime. Your nicotine–sugar–caffeine cocktail is raging.

ORION   It's totally out of control. I'm drinking coffee and eating cookies non-stop and smoking all the time. I'm basically chain-smoking at this point.

D   *I rest my left hand on her left kidney and with my forearm connect with her right kidney for a few minutes.* Your adrenals are hooked into fight–flight–freeze mode. You're still producing high levels of stress hormones. You even depend on the jolt to get up in the morning.

ORION   I feel like shit. I'm sleeping a lot and dragging myself to work and barely getting anything else done. I come home and crash on the couch.

D   Yeah, I can *see* that you have a hard time motivating yourself to do anything and if you do, you then have a hard time focusing.

ORION   I hate everything. The old shit, the new shit, whatever!

D   Despite your triple-stimulant cocktail, you have no energy to do what you love or to love what you do. Your adrenals are depleted.

ORION   That's what my naturopath said.

D   It's a widespread syndrome, and it often hits in the mid-thirties or forties. Those hormones are designed for high performance in moments of crisis. They are not designed for sustained effort and concentration or just plain waking up in the morning.

ORION   I can't get up in the morning without a coffee.

D   You're not alone in this. Coffee shops dispense caffeine and sugar at high profit margins on every corner. Our culture and market economy support and enable your addiction to your body's fear chemistry.

ORION   I'm so addicted! It's out of control.

D   Most of us are, and most people don't think about how these yummy treats generate fear either. Cranking up the fear program is no way to start the day. Yet it's a pandemic. The energy of life is unconditional love. Fear is the antithesis of love and trust.

ORION   I can totally see that.

D OK, that was the bad news. *My hands shift to Orion's biological heart and settle in for a few minutes.* Despite the adrenal mayhem, your heart is still clearing and healing. The wounds that surfaced in the past few treatments are nonetheless on the mend. You wholeheartedly embrace your nine-year-old dream team. You also acknowledge that you have the resources to be your own mother, teacher, and friend.

ORION That's such a relief to hear.

D OK, let's check your right arm. Hmmm … You're still holding on to your stepsisters' pain.

ORION I actually think about them all the time … and I keep thinking of the pain experienced by women and girls around the world. It's everywhere!

D While you're integrating your familial truth into your day-to-day consciousness, you're also compassionately witnessing the impact of unlove in all other victims of sexual abuse. The more you heal your heart, the less overwhelming it will be. In time, your compassion will express itself through meaningful action and transformation within yourself, your family, your community, and the global community.

ORION I so want that.

D You'll be part of the solution, Orion. *I feel drawn to Orion's ovaries and rest my hands on them for a few minutes.* Hmmm … Your left ovary also bears this outrage. Your tiny ovary, barely the size of a walnut, stores your thundering repulsion of not only your stepfather but of all perpetrators of sexual abuse.

ORION God … he makes me sick.

D Yes, and you were transplanted into a violent and sexually abusive home just as your body was beginning to change.

ORION I'm still hanging on to that old shit?

D That old shit is none other than sexism itself. At nine years old, you were at a turning point in your life. It's at this critical juncture that girls construct their gender identity. Your stepfather intensified the onslaught of sexist bigotry at that pivotal juncture in your life. It's no wonder that some of your disgust is stored in your reproductive system!

ORION Eeeweee!

D You and your dream team have the resources now to reject the sexist limitations imposed on you culturally, politically, and personally.

ORION Not a moment too soon!

D   Yeah … talk about fuelling your feminist engines … They were revved up before all of this. In time, you'll transcend the rage and connect with the healing power of your compassion.

ORION   Yes, I'm ready to move on to that, please.

D   Compassion is a way more sustainable energy than fight–flight–freeze hormones. See what you can do in terms of slowing down on the sugar–coffee–nicotine combo. These substances are feeding your fear ecology. They're obstructing your powerful heart energy.

ORION   Yeah … I can see that.

MID-SEPTEMBER

ORION   Waaa! There is a lot going on. I told my mother about him!!! I told her that he's a pedophile.

D   Wow, you let your oracle speak her truth! How did it go?

ORION   My mother can't hear it. She denies the whole thing!

D   She has a lot at stake. It might take her a while. She might never face it. One has to wonder what she is experiencing as his wife. It can't be pretty. To believe you and support you and your stepsisters, she would need to acknowledge that she is married to a pedophile. The implications are vast and probably extremely scary for her.

ORION   Yeah … I can see that.

D   Breaking the silence is a profoundly empowering act. It's yours regardless of how she reacts. You're still on your healing schedule and she on hers. You're not letting her slow you down.

ORION   This whole thing about staying on my own timing is really helpful.

D   It's liberating, isn't it?

ORION   Totally!

D   *I rest my hands on Orion's shins for a few minutes.* It's fall equinox. Let's see what else you're cookin'. *I slip my hands under Orion's head.* Oops … You've sprung a leak. Beneficial energy is streaming out of your fifth chakra! *I cup my hands above Orion's throat for a few minutes.* You're bursting with excitement!

ORION   Yeah, well there's so much happening. I've decided to shift away from the arts. I really love the energy healing course I'm taking.

D   All super good, but you're burning the beneficial energy off faster than you can generate it! Hmmm … Instead of building on your nascent clarity and soaking in the nourishing experiences, you're propelled into activities that drain your system. I *sense* that you're talking a lot.

ORION   It's so true, I'm on the phone for hours every day.

D   Bingo. You're talking so much that you are leaking your precious new resources before they have a chance to nourish you on a cellular level. Your sugar–caffeine–nicotine–infused verbal enthusiasm interferes with and limits the depth of your transformation.

ORION   I can see that. I get that. When I used to talk about my art projects too soon, the energy would sputter right out of them. It was lethal.

D   Exactly. When you talk about your ideas, you manifest the energy on the earth plane. So, why do the project then? On some level, it's already done; it's already out on the earth plane. You've basically just blown it off. The same principle applies to all your new endeavours.

ORION   I can feel that.

D   Healing your fifth chakra will also help you harmonize your habits and choices on the earth plane with your spiritual goals—with your purpose.

ORION   Now wouldn't that be a delightful change.

D   Yes, it would change everything! It's so hopeful, isn't it?

ORION   It is. I can feel things changing deep inside me. I do feel hopeful! It's such a breath of fresh air.

D   You do not have to be depleted, Orion. Abundance is your birthright. Let that beautiful nectar of hope, joy, and clarity pool in your heart. Let it accumulate.

A few minutes later:

That's it! Allow that energy to build so that your heart compass can steer the ship at this juncture. The fall equinox is around the corner.

ORION   Oh yeah… right!

D   Invite the nectar to replenish all your cells and energy bodies. The fall is the perfect time to learn how to conserve. Fall encourages you to store your harvest for the winter. It's also about moving inward, toward the yin and light within. Let your leaves fall and whatever habits are not in alignment with your essence. It's really good time for shedding whatever is not useful!

ORION   Nothing like timing, right?

D   You're in the flow, that's for sure. Namaste.

ORION   Namaste.

EARLY OCTOBER

ORION   I started a three-week cleanse. I'm taking a tincture to accelerate detoxification and I'm on a strict diet: no salt, no sugar, and mainly green vegetables and brown rice.

D   Yay! And your fifth chakra has stabilized. It's purring. This is a victory. Your choice to embrace a cleanse program is a definitive act of self-transformation. It's a sign that resistance is dissolving.

ORION   Woo hoo!

D   Wow! Both your feet are firmly planted and connected to your roots. You're in your Sacred Tree. Congratulations! You're not frantically running around it!

ORION   I feel so much better already.

D   I'm so sure, but be prepared though, this part of the process is marked by frequent exits from the Sacred Tree, falling out and landing on your butt.

ORION   Oh yes, there's still some of that, for sure.

D   Certainly, but your cleanse supports you. You're more likely to pause, breathe, reassess, and find your way back into your tree again.

ORION   I'm meditating more.

D   Even better! And the really good news is that the tinctures are supporting your liver. It's releasing some of that excess heat.

Five minutes later:

So good! Your days of having a hard time getting up in the morning and focusing on what you love are numbered. You will soon have the clarity and energy to execute whatever you need to do to transform.

ORION   I do feel a lot clearer.

D   The fact that you are not eating sugar is huge! Although sugar addiction is normalized in our culture, high levels of sugar in the body read like white noise from a TV that has no reception. At Burning Man one year, my gift to the playa was a Reiki treatment for all members of the village I was camping with. The one condition I imposed on the recipients is that they come for a treatment when they were high on their substance of choice (I was kind of doing my own research). After a week of doing Reiki on people who were high on everything from marijuana, hash, mushrooms, acid, ecstasy, or cocaine but who were not necessarily habitual users, I finally encountered the candidate who was more separated from his Sacred Tree than a sugar addict: he'd been high on acid for seven days straight. *Orion's eyes pop out of her head.*

ORION   Really?

D   Shocking, isn't it? That something so harmful can be purchased by anyone everywhere and almost everyone is on it! Something we can compare to acid for seven days straight!

ORION   Wow! OK. I'm pumped. I'm staying on the cleanse, that's for sure. By the way, my right arm has been hurting lately.

D   *I shift my hands to Orion's right arm for a few minutes.* This is another facet of the excess liver fire. Ah! You have been working on your liver energetically too! You're pushing this fire out. You are successfully disentangling this unbeneficial energy on your own.

ORION   I am? Oh good … I'm not sure what do to with it now though.

D   You're hanging on to your sword. You're a formidable warrior on a mission to break the cycle of violence in your family. You want to fight for your stepsisters too. It's quite the agenda.

ORION   Makes sense.

D   You got this far. Throw in more loving kindness and compassion.

Ten minutes later:

Whoa! You got it! This inner strength doesn't need to be fuelled by rage anymore. Honour the high vibrations of love, compassion, kindness, patience, and generosity imprinted in your liver and gallbladder.

ORION   In my liver?

D   Yes, love and compassion are the high-vibration imprints in your liver. The wood energy in your liver fuels the regenerative cycle of your Sacred Tree and evolution. You'll see! Your outrage will simmer down and you will honour your peaceful and loving intention to heal your wounds, help your stepsisters heal theirs, and now help others too as a light worker. Let your peaceful warrior emerge!

ORION   Wow!

D   Wow is right. You are doing amazing work. It's exciting!

ORION   It feels so good to be witnessed.

D   You are your first client, you know. You're doing it. You are embracing your new practice and healing yourself.

ORION   Wow!

D   No need for words. Enjoy and celebrate! Make sure you mark this moment in some way in the next few days. It's important to honour your birth days, not just the day you were born physically but all the many other initiatory births!

ORION   Namaste.

MID-OCTOBER

ORION   I'm almost done Level One of the course. I'm on track with my cleanse. I'm still totally off sugar!

D   Woohoo! Let's check in with your pancreas. *My left hand settles in for a few minutes.* Oh goodie, it's softening. Hmmm … Let me settle in here. Ah … An architect of survival high on sugar something fierce is presenting herself! You're about fourteen, I think.

ORION   Oh, that's me then, for sure. I went on Skippy peanut butter binges. I gained twenty pounds in a few weeks once.

D   She's holding on! Let's listen in. I *hear* "If I lose my armour, who will take care of me?" Hmmm … I wonder how excess weight protects you. I *hear* "If I'm fat, I'm less attractive, so then he rejects me."

ORION   Shit!

D   Yeah, you gained weight to prevent your stepfather from sexually abusing you.

ORION   It makes so much sense!

D   Wait a minute, the energy is moving fast. Your cleanse is really moving a lot of energy. I just got a whiff of potent toxins. Ah… You're also shedding shame! I *hear* "I'm disgusting."

ORION   I am!

D   Oh Orion, you made it through with the resources you had! So what if you ate sugar, drank coffee, and smoked cigarettes. All these substances performed a service. Survival is a messy business. Have you ever seen the runt of a litter? They don't look so good, do they? What are you going to do about it? Shame them? Blame them? No, you're going to scoop them up and love them back to life!

ORION   I'm knee-deep in shit! I feel so humiliated!

D   Take care of your architects of survival as you would the runt of a litter. Pick off the fleas, offer delicious food, provide a safe shelter, and smother its soft belly with kisses. It's sometimes hard to love the little girl who is abandoned by her mother, the little oracle who hides in terror, the "fat" teenager who binges on Skippy, or the chain-smoking adult. Yet witness them with compassion and curiosity. They survived with the resources they had. Fifteen minutes later:

Orion's heart energy bursts with powerful self-love again. You're doing great! Keep going…

Five minutes later:

Okay, now shed that leftover self-disgust and shame while you're at it. That's your stepfather's energy that's still clinging to you. FedEx the lot to him COD right now! His actions can lie with him, whether he embarks on a healing journey or assumes his accountability or not. It is his karmic load to carry.

ORION   Aaagh!

D   You are not the perpetrator; he is! And you didn't abandon yourself; your mother did.

A few minutes later:

Okay, now dump your mother's self-loathing too, while you're at it. Bathe all your cells in the healing light of your unconditional love. That's it! You're doing great. Quite the load, huh?

ORION   Woo, I think we need to open the window.

D   We sure do! Hahahaaa ...

FEBRUARY

Orion attends my one-day Reiki Level One workshop with one of her stepsisters. Her first practice session is with her stepsister. The first perpetrator energy she had the honour of encountering and clearing is none other than that of her stepfather! The house shook and the reverberations of that healing still echo in my healing studio to this day.

Thank you, Reiki.

Thank you, Orion.

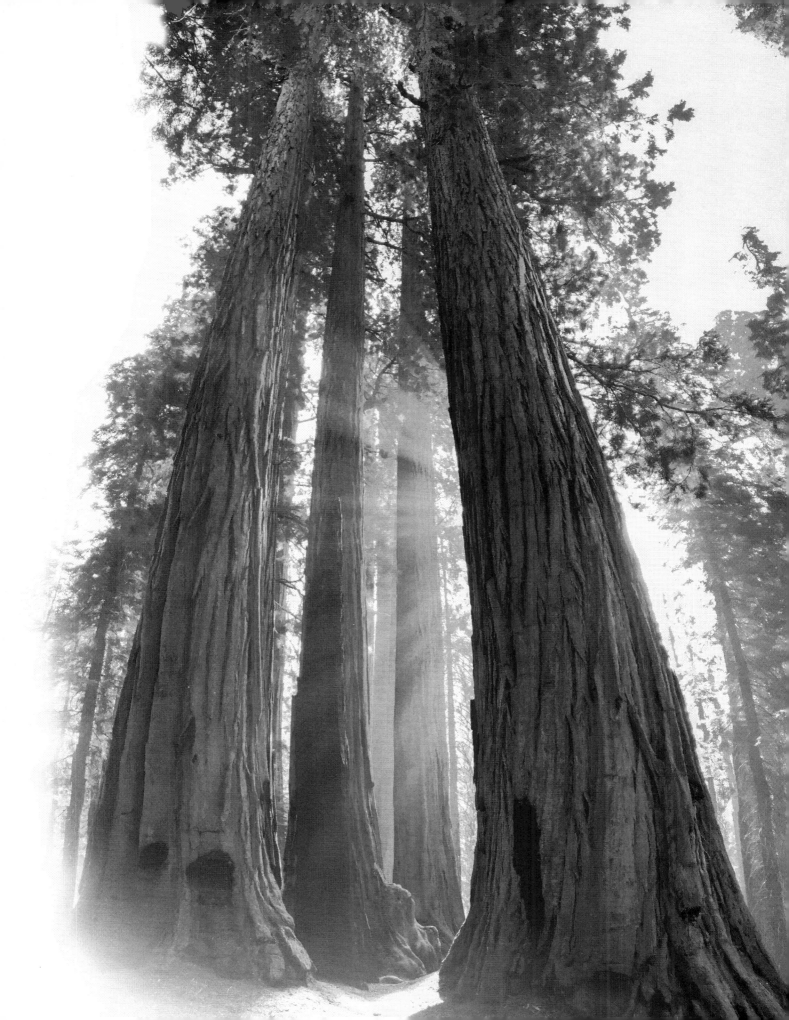

CHAPTER TWENTY-ONE
RAEL

EARLY MARCH

Rael at age thirty-eight

RAEL   I was raped at seven years old by my father. I've done years of talk therapy. I really wish I felt better. I can't say I do. I'm a productive artist, a single parent, a teacher, and an activist, but I still feel stuck somehow. I'm still anxious a lot of the time.

D   *I slip my hands under Rael's head for a few minutes.* I *sense* dissonant chords throughout your body. Do you feel everything sharply?

RAEL   I do!

D   These intrusive sensations express your history of abuse. I *sense* that pain, discomfort, shame, sadness, and rage often invade the present and overwhelm your consciousness.

RAEL   I'm tired of living like this. I know it's not my whole life—that it's my past … but something about it is not shaking off.

D   Exactly. I *sense* that your mental energy body is burdened with an old belief. I *hear* "I'm powerless. I'm powerless"… nothing more … nothing less … just that: "I'm powerless!" Over and over again. And you're a super competent and engaged artist, teacher, and parent! *Rael slips into a deep meditative state almost immediately; her years of therapy and processing provide us with a solid base to go deep fast. After a five minutes a young Rael reaches out from under her oppressor's energy.*

RAEL   I feel like I'm stuck under him for life!

D   You have been stuck under him—that's a good way of putting it. No wonder you get angry, sad, and overwhelmed sometimes.

A few minutes later:

I also *see* that his attack damaged the etheric fabric from waist to mid-thigh. I refer to this portion of your field as your cosmic underwear. Yours is gone, unfortunately, vaporized by violence. You have no filter or protection to assure you that you are secure. It's no way to live!

RAEL   *Young Rael speaks up through the din of the present.* I can't get him off me!

D   *I shift my hands to Rael's pelvis for a few minutes.* It's OK, little one, we witness your distress. Life without cosmic underwear is a dubious affair, to say the least.

A few minutes later:

Women around the world in all eras could weave a cloth that covers the entire planet with the light fibres that were torn off their bodies. The good news is that we can energetically weave light filaments together again to restore this imbalance immediately.

Ten minutes later:

RAEL   Oh my God … That feels so much better!

D   Doesn't it now. Cosmic underwear is the best thing going! No wonder the lingerie industry is thriving. I think we're all seeking to restore and celebrate this fundamental aspect of ourselves.

MID-MARCH

RAEL   I feel much better. This is so different from talk therapy. I do feel more space between myself and my father, more so than ever before. It's such a relief. But even though I'm productive, I still often feel quite anxious and upset.

D   *I slip my hands under Rael's head for a few minutes.* Hmmm … I *sense* that your father's attack was so violent that he caused a neck injury.

RAEL   He hurt my neck for sure. I wore a neck brace for a month.

D   My sense is that the pressure on your neck was potent enough to injure it very seriously. I feel your life was in danger.

RAEL   Yes, my rage and fear remind me all the time.

D   This is partially why you have been plagued by powerlessness—not just as a feeling in your emotional body but as a deeply entrenched belief in your mental body. We only cleared part of it in the last session. Not only were you raped; your life was in danger. That's a whole other level of abuse and trauma.

RAEL   Ugh.

D   You're doing great, Rael; the shock and trauma are surfacing and ready to release. The intensity concentrated in your neck, marking your bones and tissues, is softening.

Fifteen minutes later:

That's it, Rael, you can release that trapped lightning bolt. The glacial terror you experienced can stream though your spine, out your tailbone, and out through your feet on its way to the earth. She gladly receives your pain.

RAEL   *Little Rael speaks up.* Ooow! I feel like my neck is going to break! I'm so scared.

D   You're OK, little one. Your heart and soul spun under the assault on all your senses. We're here.

A few minutes later:

You're not alone, little one. And we know you made it through. We love you. We're here to get you out from under his weight and thrusting. You're not alone anymore. It's over. You can climb into Rael's heart now. You're safe.

RAEL   I still feel really scared. It's so intense.

D   You don't have to die to be free from this trauma. That's an old belief. You thought that this was imprinted for life.

A few minutes later:

RAEL   Oh … I do feel the imprint leaving my body. What a relief!

D   You are releasing an intense layer of shock and trauma. It's a lot. So many organs are burdened by this level of trauma it takes a while for your subtle body to release it all. Besides, your liver is involved. That's how I know you were scared for your life. The liver stores the most intense emotions, including terror and fear of death.

Ten minutes later:

There you go—you're doing great—I can feel your energy softening—that traumatized astronaut trapped in that specific moment is now returning from its out-of-body journey. Little one, we're here. You are alive and we welcome you here, now. We love you.

RAEL   I really feel her.

D   I do too and I *see* your heroic resourcefulness. You harnessed your strength and courage to torque yourself out from under your father's life-threatening grip, weight, and pressure. You saved your life! We celebrate your vigour and the blessed gift of your presence and essence.

RAEL   I can really feel her!

D   Hold her in your arms. Embrace her. Let her know how proud you are of what she did and how happy you are that she is alive. Celebrate her strength and determination to live.

RAEL   Ouf...

D   Hmmm ... Something else is coming up. I *hear* "I should have died! I should have died!" I *sense* that your father's assault on your life taught Little Rael that her life had no value. This belief was planted in your seventh chakra, your Sacred Tree's gateway to the sun. The transgression is his, little one. He could have killed his daughter. Your life is not the misdeed. His violence is. Your tapestry of karmic energy reaches far beyond this moment under him. Your wisdom and potential are so much greater, richer, fuller, more beautiful, and infinite. He owns that moment and you own your life.

RAEL   Intense.

D   OK, we are not out of the woods yet; more images are coming. *I rest my left hand on Rael's abdomen and my right on her right thigh.* I *see* Little Rael taking a bath after being raped. You were desperately trying to scrape yourself clean.

RAEL   *Little Rael blurts out her horror.* I hate that little girl. I hate her vulnerability.

D   Let's give all of that to your father. Let him have it, all that hatred and loathing. He's a vile criminal. Little Rael was hurt; she's not disgusting. She's beautiful and hurt.

     A few minutes later, Rael's energy does an about-turn. Let's love that little girl to bits, take care of her, soothe her, and bathe her tenderly. Climb into the tub with your Little Rael. Embrace her lovingly. Help her in whatever way you deem necessary. Do whatever she needs.

     A few minutes later:

     There you go; unconditional love and compassion are flowing from your heart. The warm water transforms into a million bubbles of light, reflecting the seven healing colours of the rainbow. Infinite love penetrates your pores and bathes all your cells and molecules. Your heart resonates with calm, stillness, and joy.

RAEL   I so look forward to bathing when I get home!

D   It's going to be a long, delicious bath. Place your hands on your heart to keep your unconditional love flowing. Receive.

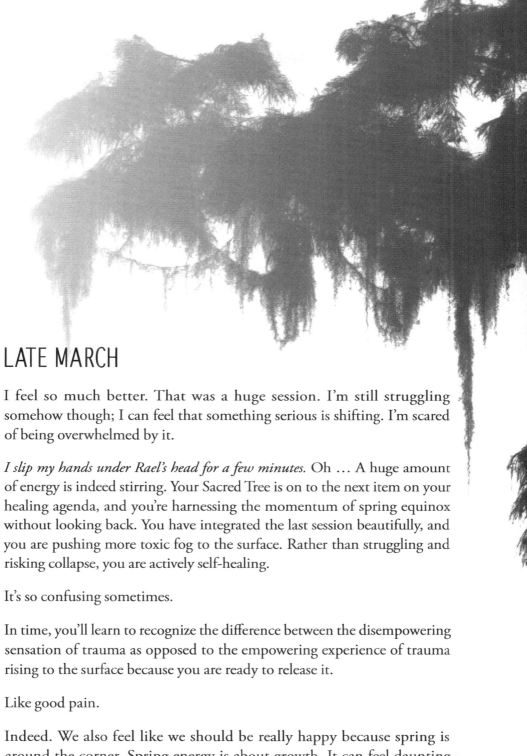

LATE MARCH

RAEL   I feel so much better. That was a huge session. I'm still struggling somehow though; I can feel that something serious is shifting. I'm scared of being overwhelmed by it.

D   *I slip my hands under Rael's head for a few minutes.* Oh … A huge amount of energy is indeed stirring. Your Sacred Tree is on to the next item on your healing agenda, and you're harnessing the momentum of spring equinox without looking back. You have integrated the last session beautifully, and you are pushing more toxic fog to the surface. Rather than struggling and risking collapse, you are actively self-healing.

RAEL   It's so confusing sometimes.

D   In time, you'll learn to recognize the difference between the disempowering sensation of trauma as opposed to the empowering experience of trauma rising to the surface because you are ready to release it.

RAEL   Like good pain.

D   Indeed. We also feel like we should be really happy because spring is around the corner. Spring energy is about growth. It can feel daunting sometimes. OK—let's see what this is all about. The energy is most dense over your eyes and ears. *I cup my right hand on her right ear and my left hand hovers above her eyes for a few minutes.* Hmmm … I *sense* that you were force-fed adult pornography by your father. Were you about nine?

RAEL   Yes. I sat on the edge of my parents' bed just a few feet away from the TV. *Little Rael immediately reaches out for help.*

D   The explicit copulation images damaged the etheric field over your eyes and the groans and grunts pierced the etheric field over your ears. It's all the same energy field as your cosmic underwear. We can clear the charge of the toxicity and weave new filaments of light.

RAEL   *Little Rael is plunged into the experience.* It's so gross!

D   And really scary. You're not alone, little one.

        A few minutes later:

        I *hear* "He wants me to do what these women are doing!" You're frozen. I *see* you sitting motionless, utterly trapped in your father's gaze as he transposes you onto the synthetic copulation. Your child ears, eyes, and consciousness are raped by your father's desire and the porn industry's caricature of sex. Your skin prickles under his foul gaze.

RAEL   *Rael bolts up, sitting on the edge of the table, her back rigid as a plank.*

D   *My left hand settles on her back at heart level and my right hand rests on her right shoulder.* Your flesh is imprinted by your intense feelings of degradation and humiliation. Your spine arches rigidly, expressing your fear and resistance. Your breath stands still as his penis erupts onto your back.

RAEL   *Little Rael's cry pierces the air.* Get him off me—get him off me—get him off me! *Rael's back now arches in horror and protest.*

D   Now and forever! Every trace of the physical, emotional, mental, and spiritual violation attached to this memory can be released now.

        A few minutes later:

        You can get Little Rael out of that room now! Go get her and burn the room down. Incinerate the reeking atmosphere: the bed, sheets, lowered blinds, murky daylight, semen, and the Fuck-TV. Reach out to trapped Rael with love and compassion. The criminal activities in the room reek, not her!

        A few minutes later:

        Do whatever works for you. Do whatever your imagination is telling you to do. You have the resources to do it all now. You have the personal power, clarity, courage, and strength to get her out of there. Little Rael will never again be trapped by your father's distortion and contamination of parental love.

Ten minutes later:

That's it, Rael! Little Rael comes out smelling like roses! And he sure as hell doesn't.

RAEL The room is burnt to the fucking ground!

D Woohoo! Now your spine can soften. Yield to the life force and feel its rejuvenating pulse and embrace.

A few minutes later:

That's it—your whole back is cleansed. You own it again. Embrace all your bones, muscles, flesh, and tissues. Every molecule is yours, and all cells dance with the earth and the sun. You are free. Your self-healing capacity mends all holes, rips, and tears in your etheric body. Your back is secure, your eyes are clear, and your ears are purged. Witness your field as it lights up, singing its brightest blue. Replenish your cosmic underwear while you're at it. Taste the vitality in your spine. Savour beauty with your eyes. Relish a sweet song in your ears. Receive.

RAEL Oh my God, that was intense. I thought I would never get through it. Look, I can turn my head. I can look back. And I'm OK with you behind me. I've always hated the feeling of having someone behind me. But now it's OK. I normally hate to be touched on the back. Wow!

D Yeah, you can be 3-D again. You own and control your whole body and all the space around you.

RAEL I feel so much better. Thank you so much. It feels so validating. And now I'm not alone with it. It's so amazing to hear your voice and feel your respect. You're right there with me. It's so amazing to be in it with you.

D Yes, and the horrid humiliation and terror are history. Both of you are here now and can feel love and compassion and so much gentleness.

RAEL Look—I can move my back. I've always been so stiff!

D Hahahahaha … Enjoy!

APRIL

RAEL   I've been thinking about my mother a lot. I mean, where was she? Why didn't she protect me? I know she was abused by her father, but still.

D   You were raped by your father, but more importantly you were abandoned by both of them. Your mother's neglect is a core wound. Sexual abuse trauma actually piggy-backs on top of abandonment trauma and not the other way around. To feel unloved and unprotected is even scarier than being raped.

RAEL   I really feel the extent of it these days. It's so huge.

D   It definitely is. *I slide my left hand on her abdomen and my right on her thigh for a few minutes.* Hmmm … Silt is stirring in the dark recesses of your reproductive organs. I *sense* that beyond abandoning you, your mother colonized you. While your father's attacks taught you what it's like to be a girl—ambushed, objectified, violated, and powerless—your mother taught you that patriarchy, and its systemic hierarchy of violence, is the way of the world. She taught you that there was no way out.

RAEL   I remember her telling me, "That's how it is! They do *that* to us."

D   That's full-on colonization. Your mother's internalized sexism was a virulent force.

RAEL   It sure was. It's brutal.

D   You were a biological prisoner in a war against women. Pinned down by both their patriarchal thumbs, I *sense* that you perceived your persecuted girl body as the enemy. Your reproductive organs still bear the brunt of your rejection.

RAEL   I'm a feminist and an activist, I know this! I should have been on this!

D   We often know it inside-out intellectually, but it's hard to get at all the layers in our heart and subtle bodies, especially the mental body. I haven't worked on a woman yet who does not have some internalized sexism still lurking somewhere. Little Rael did what most of us do when we are trapped in an ethos that is presented to us as an unavoidable oppression: we reject the part of ourselves that we perceive is binding us to the corrupt contract.

RAEL   It runs so deep!

D   It really does. And let's not forget that we are digging ourselves out from under the weight of countless generations of oppression. You are a feminist and have been for years, yet we are now reaching a much younger you still stuck in confusion and fear. That young Rael is an architect of survival just doing what she can with the resources she has to survive. It is her you are healing now, not the victim. Architects of survival are die-hards—thank the Goddess for that. But when it comes to integrating them and releasing ourselves from their grip, it's a different process from healing the victimized self.

RAEL   It does feel different. I see—I have to find all aspects of me that are still trapped in that survival mode.

D   Yes, and it just takes time. Even though many years later you mobilized your rage and became an activist and have railed with thousands of other women against the misogynist contract that normalizes atrocious acts of violence, this self-rejecting architect of survival is still active. For as long as she is hooked in, the victim aspect of you is not fully released from the negative charge of sexism. First, we heal the victims, then we release the strategies of survival. And by the way, I can *see* the extent to which you transformed your helplessness into defiance. "Fuck you and the horse you rode in on! Fuck you all!"

RAEL   Yup. That's me.

D   Exactly, and that Little Rael was another part of you. Hmmm ... All of this talk is pushing another fog bank out of your body. *I rest my left hand on Rael's right shoulder and my right on her right thigh for a few minutes.* There is more abuse on its way out of your field. It looks like your father's eyes insinuated themselves into your tissues.

RAEL   Ach ... I remember him staring at me.

D   I sense that he caught every glimpse he could get.

RAEL   Ach ... in the hallway between the bathroom and my room.

D   His fantasies plundered your Sacred Tree. His desire alone violated the sacred parent–child contract. This, too, is sexual abuse.

RAEL   It was awful. I couldn't go anywhere without him undressing me with his eyes.

A few minutes later:

D   The energy is clearing rapidly. It's very liberating to release an invasive gaze.

RAEL   Yeah, the relief is palpable.

D   You're doing so great.

A few minutes later:

You are rejecting your father's power over you in all your subtle energy bodies. It's fantastic. You are truly getting out from under your parents' thumbs. You have worked hard for this. Your personal power is growing exponentially. I recommend you try to rest in the next few weeks while you integrate this huge energetic shift.

RAEL   I feel so much lighter. Thank you.

MARCH

18 months later

Rael at age forty

RAEL   I feel it took me all this time to integrate the work we did a year or so ago. I eat better. I feel great at forty. I don't know—I just felt like I emerged suddenly on the day of my fortieth birthday. A huge weight dropped off—like a big sigh of relief. I feel more me.

I'm off-track though. I stopped exercising in December. I think the looming breakup with my girlfriend was weighing on me. I didn't quite keep it all together. We broke it off a few weeks ago. It's a good thing, but I need to get back on track.

D   *I rest my hands on Rael's shins for a few minutes.* You are in your body and in your Sacred Tree! This is fantastic, considering the breakup and all. Your right hip is congested though. *I rest my hands on her abdomen and hips for ten minutes.* Your right sacroiliac joint is not fluid.

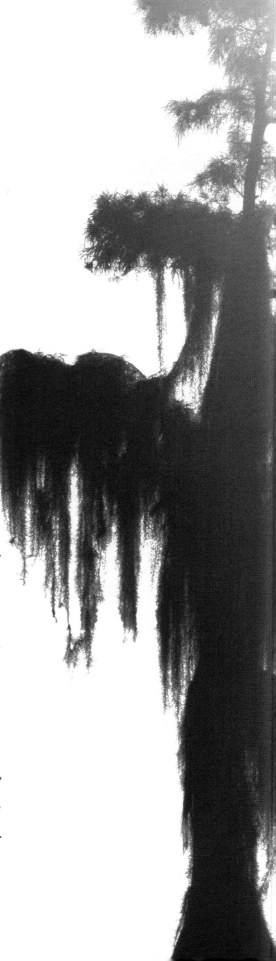

Let's work through this. Hmmm ... Your right ovary is dense and prickly. Is your menstrual cycle regular?

RAEL   Ha ... It hasn't been for years. It's also very painful.

D   Does your period often start after openings?

RAEL   It does!

A few minutes later:

D   Basically you get your period once your show opens. You get so caught up with your art that your menstrual cycle has quit the moon cycle and now adheres to your professional schedule.

RAEL   That's a little much!

D   Yeah, the moon is powerful enough to govern the oceans, but your singular focus is stronger still. It's only when your work is done that your body can soften into its biological and hormonal functioning.

RAEL   It's unrelenting!

D   Yeah, it can't just be about the work though—your stress levels are through the roof. *I place one hand on each kidney and adrenal gland for a few minutes.* Hmmm ... I *sense* that if your work is well received, you are proud of yourself. If it's not, you descend in a spiral of self-loathing and self-doubt.

RAEL   Oh yes, that old thing. It's a nightmare.

D   To be trapped in a conditional love relationship with yourself is a nightmare. Hmmm... You love yourself when your work is loved and appreciated; otherwise, you hate yourself. These are stark and high-pressure conditions to create in and, for that matter, to live in.

RAEL   It's awful.

D   It's a sure way to live on the edge when your artistic expression and self-worth are prey to the art critics' fickle tastes and politics! It's no surprise that the chronic threat of rejection and self-rejection causes strain in your kidneys and adrenal glands.

A few minutes later:

Do you have a lot of daunting deadlines coming up?

RAEL   Yes.

D   Well, you're actually right on schedule!

RAEL   I am? I'm so behind!

D   Spring is around the corner. It's an optimal time to cleanse your liver and gallbladder. Self-hatred and self-loathing are imbalances stored in the liver and gallbladder energetic orb. In other words, your Sacred Tree is right on schedule! It's harnessing the energy of spring to push out those low vibrations. They're in the way and you're ready to release them.

RAEL   Yeah, makes sense. It's time to implement a little more balance.

D   It's more than that. You're already self-healing. It's time to support that seasonal and dynamic opportunity to grow and evolve. It's not all about the work, remember?

RAEL   Ah! Something good is already happening and I didn't recognize it.

D   Exactly. Rest. You're really tired. Give yourself more "me time" to help soften the transition after your breakup. Your creativity will then have energy to draw from. First things first: spring cleanse, replenish, evolve, then produce.

RAEL   I'm on it! Thank you so much!

APRIL

RAEL   I finished a ten-day cleanse a week ago. I feel so much better. I'm not going to eat dairy or wheat anymore. It's so clear that I function better without them in my system.

D   *I settle my hands on Rael's shins for a few minutes.* The cleanse is really stirring things up in a good way. Hmmm … You're out-of-body though—a ten-year-old Little Rael is awakened by the drastic shift.

RAEL   My ten-year-old? I never think of her. That's the time in between the abusive events. I really never think of that time.

D   She has burst into the present and she has a story to tell. Your spring cleanse has diluted the glue that kept her shut out.

RAEL   Hmmm …

        A few minutes later:

D   I *hear* "I'm sad. I feel confused. I'm so tired. I'm tired all the time. I don't sleep well. I feel unsafe. I hate my bed."

RAEL   Whoa …

D   That's not all, she has more intensity brewing. *My left hand shifts to Rael's left thigh for a few minutes.* I *hear* "I so wanted to be loved. I let it happen. I'm ashamed." *My left hand shifts to Rael's left knee and I settle in for a few minutes.* Wait, there's more—I *hear* "I am scared. I'm scared all the time."

RAEL   I'm still fearful!

        I settle my hand to Rael's left calf for a few minutes. I *hear* "I feel so much rage it strangles me. I did not sign up for this. I'm really worried about what is going to happen to me. I'm scared. I don't want any of it. I want to die."

RAEL   Ouf …

D   Ouf is right. This is quite the download from your cleansing liver. You had a hard go of it when you were seven years old, but it sure sounds like the years after that were just as tough. Your little ten-year-old is uprooted and her roots are stiffened and parched.

RAEL   Ha! I repotted all my house plants last weekend. I got bigger pots and bought the right soil. I untangled all their roots. I really got into it. Now I'm watching them grow every day.

D   Lovingly soften Little Rael's roots and nestle them in the most soft, comforting, and nourishing earth on the planet. Oh—she's loving this and responding very quickly. She welcomes your soothing touch and she's now drinking the earth's energy and looking up to the sun.

RAEL   It's so good to get in touch with this part of me. I had no idea. It's so easy to get stuck on the obvious headlines.

D   Exactly, the process of healing from sexual abuse often tends to overshadow the pain of abandonment and other wounds—including the level of despair and suffering that creates

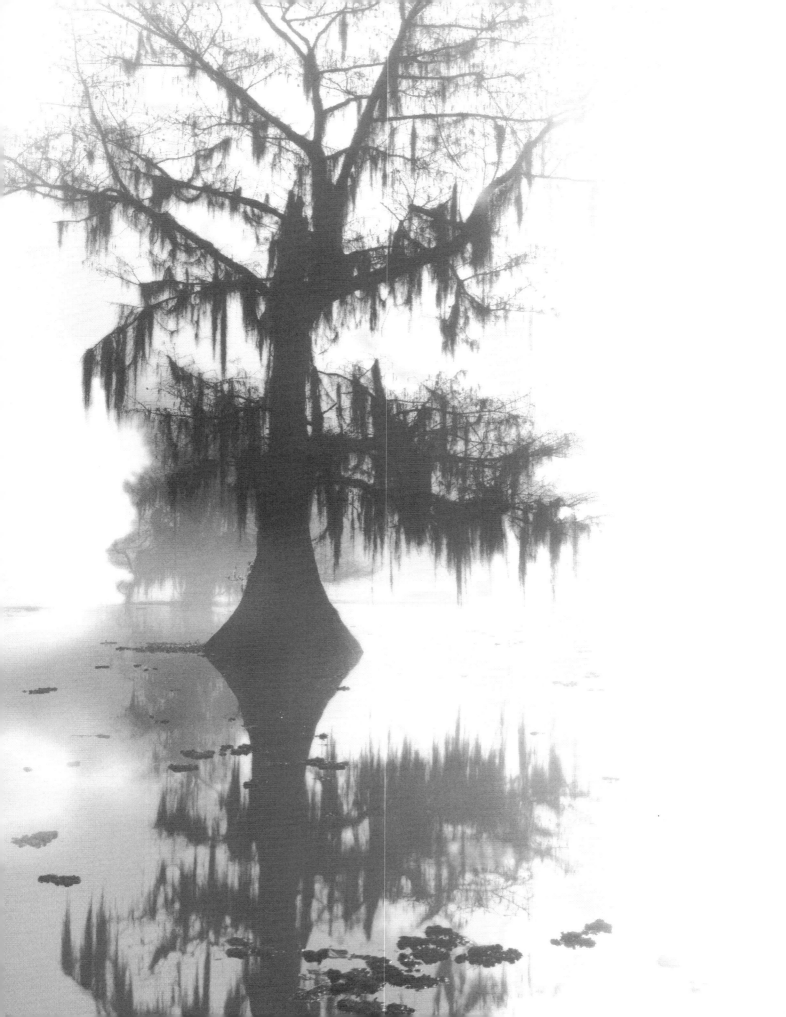

an architect of survival who will consider and sometimes embrace the need to get out with as drastic a measure as death.

RAEL   It's so intense.

D   Yeah, wanting to die is a survival tactic. If I die, I will be free. If you are trapped and feel powerless, then it's a conceivable and enticing strategy. Unfortunately, I don't think it works all that well. I encounter so many distressed souls who have committed suicide who are still attached to family members, friends, or sometimes strangers. For all their desire to get out, they remain trapped in the vortex of their suffering on the earth plane and do not find the path into the force field of unconditional love.

RAEL   I think that all my talk therapy really focused on the victims. It's a whole different approach to consider my strategists. They're not victims—they're actually really resourceful.

D   Exactly. In every war and battle there is a brilliant strategist, and for every victim there is an architect of survival. It's quite the crew. Besides, how else are we supposed to win the day?

RAEL   Yeah, I can totally see that.

D   Unfortunately, for as long as we remain hooked into these strategies, even beyond the grave it seems, we remain hooked into the adversity that created the unbeneficial and painful charge in the first place.

RAEL   We really need to do the work, don't we?

D   Yeah … and find the earth, the sun, and the Sacred Tree—that's the only way I know of getting out of fear and into the flow of love and compassion here and beyond.

RAEL   I get that.

D   Besides, if we do the work, then we get to savour our magnificence.

RAEL   It's totally win–win.

D   It sure is. Namaste.

MAY

RAEL   I'm fine, but I've been thinking about my father a lot—something's up.

D   *I settle my hands on Rael's shins for a few minutes.* You are more grounded than usual, yet you're still very anxious. Well, at least you're grounded and anxious. That's a change in the right direction.

RAEL   I feel shaky. Something is coming up. I'm not sure what it is.

D   I *sense* that you're living in both a new and old script simultaneously. Your conscious self has not caught up with your spirit yet. I *sense* that part of you still assumes that you are alone and disconnected from love and compassion and will always be. Now that's an old belief rearing its ugly head.

RAEL   It's true. Somewhere inside I always feel alone and afraid. I get so stressed out about everything.

D   My sense is that though you are artistically productive, you need to find other activities that help you connect with the spirit living inside this body. Oh dear … you're all cooped up. You need fresh air and some exercise. That's the first step. The weather is stunning and the gardens are already in full bloom, yet you're still huddling inside trying to survive the winter blues. Waves of old anxiety and fear are swallowing you up and dragging you down in their chilly undertow.

RAEL   You're right—I haven't spent time outside at all.

D   It's time to shake it off. Your old skin is flaky and dry and barely has a hold on you. Some wind, some sun, some exercise, and you can rattle that heavy mantle off your Sacred Tree. It's old and weak; you're not. You can climb out of the old and into your clear, strong, and empowered Sacred Tree.

RAEL   I got an asymmetrical haircut and it was all too much. I had to adjust it. It was making me crazy.

D   Why? Was it too much fun? I'm joking … OK, there's more to it—we're going to settle in here for a while. I'll check your upper neck and skull. Hmmm … Your sphenoid bone is out of alignment. It's not just the haircut. The sphenoid is the foundation stone of the whole skeletal structure. It's shaped like a butterfly and its body houses the third eye and the sixth chakra.

RAEL   Ugh …

D   You've got that right. AHA—here it is—a nasty belief is surfacing from your sixth chakra. I *hear* "Life's a bitch!" Now that's a phrase you heard a lot.

RAEL   YES!

D   My *sense* is that you internalized your parents' cynical gaze at a really young age. Your parents' view of the world has been blocking you from perceiving the world with your own most-sacred third eye. It's cutting you off from your inner wisdom and intuition.

RAEL   For Pete's sake, I don't really identify as cynical … but I do catch myself thinking that life sucks pretty often.

D   It's a thought that carries an intensely non-beneficial energy. Nothing kills your connection to your Sacred Tree like cynicism. It's the enemy of the third eye. Cynicism is a cold and bitter isolated island, all rock and no trees. It's no place to live, that's for sure. It's even more gruesome than despair because it propels despair forward, casting a net far and wide into the future. It chokes all potential for new growth, enthusiasm, curiosity, joy, trust, and faith.

RAEL   I can see that.

D   That, plus the fact that your life actually was a bitch the whole time you lived with them, so there was not much evidence to the contrary. It's quite the bumper sticker for a couple of perpetrators to endorse: "Life's a bitch, not us."

RAEL   Isn't it now?

D   Yes, it's rather useful for them that you go on thinking that life is the bitch while they remain unaccountable for their actions. Totally noxious. You can let it go.

RAEL   Oh my God … I feel so much better.

D   Shedding unbeneficial beliefs and clearing your mental body is like a power wash. You'll feel even better when you start enjoying some Nature time. It's really important that you do.

RAEL   I will. Thank you so much.

JUNE

RAEL   I'm experiencing joy even in the simple day-to-day events, like feeling the breeze on my skin. I feel more sensitive and open. I laugh more. And I'm really excited about my projects!

D *I settle my hands on Rael's shins for a few minutes.* It's an exciting change indeed, but, woowee, your right adrenal gland is on overtime! It's bouncing around like a ping-pong ball at a professional tournament. You are pumped. I *sense* that when you're happy, you become so excited that you zap your system with a mega-dose of stress hormones.

RAEL I'm always in flight–fight–freeze!

D Yeah, at first, the stress hormones tickle your nose and the buzz is good, but it soon swirls into an uncontrollable frenzy. The next thing you know you're having some insanely sweet snack.

RAEL That's exactly what I do. What the hell? The next thing I know I'm stuffing my face with some ridiculous cupcake.

D And then it's uphill from there. Your accelerated heart rate and frenetic pace race ahead of you until you crash.

RAEL … right back in the old shit again.

D It takes practice, this happy thing.

RAEL That's so true. The next thing I know I feel totally stressed-out again. It's like the old anxiety never leaves … it lurks underneath everything … even when I'm happy!

D Oy vey, your right kidney is dense too. Hmmm … Let's drop in here for a while. *I rest my hands on Rael's kidneys for five minutes.* Oh … A tiny Rael is still stewing in her parents' toxic brew. Oh … She's been left behind! She is an infant and still trapped in that house. She is a living, breathing, and miserable Little Rael from the time before your official start date for the abuse in your narrative. Rael, would there really be a time without abuse in that house?

RAEL Huh?

D Really? With everything that went down after age seven, can you really assume that your childhood home was safe before that? Knowing what you know about your parents now, in terms of all your conscious memories since age seven, can you imagine them truly loving and caring for you?

RAEL God no.

D I know this is horrible to sit with. This is a core trauma. Your parents hurt you long before your father raped you and your mother failed to protect you. The sexual abuse is an add-on—it's not the core of your pain.

RAEL   Ugh … I always feel sad when I look at my baby pictures and, weirdly, almost like I look … gross.

D   My sense is that you see that you were neglected. Let's scoop Teeny Rael out of that toxic stew forever. Love yourself to bits and nestle Teeny Rael in your heart. You are her primary caregiver now.

Now in a deep meditative state, Rael softens into her Sacred Tree. She rests in this peaceful ease for ten minutes. You're doing great. Your heart is opening. What you see in yourself in those pictures is your most painful traumatic experience, the foundation under everything that comes later. Beautiful baby, you weren't gross. You were grotesquely mistreated.

RAEL   It's so HUGE.

D   You have the right to separate yourself from your biological tribe. You have the power to create the space in your heart to unconditionally welcome and love all your younger selves. Unconditionally create a loving, safe, calm, and happy home for all Raels at all ages.

RAEL   I feel awful.

D   I *sense* that. Something is blocking your love from flowing. Hmmm … I'm getting a whiff of nasty criticism in your third chakra. *I shift my left hand to Rael's solar plexus for a few minutes.* It seems to be the home of an internalized censor who viciously judges your art before it's produced.

RAEL   Ah, of course—I'm applying for a grant.

D   This harsh internal judge weasels its way in every time you cast your work into the public arena, even before you have actually manifested it. This grant jury becomes an internalized and magnified savage. It knows no bounds. It will even pounce on your first thought.

RAEL   We've been here before!

D   We have. Open your heart to your creative and expansive self too, not just the victims. Love all of you!

A few minutes later:

I also *sense* that you have been on the art world roller coaster without a break for too long. You have been *on*, producing non-stop for more than a decade. I *sense* that it's time to press the pause button, sit back, observe, ingest, digest, and then launch into Part 2 later. And you need time outside. It's summer! It's time to smell the flowers! Go to the Toronto Islands for the day, whatever. Get your ass in Nature. You need to refuel and reconnect.

RAEL   Oh that's such a good idea.

D   And take time off over the summer!

RAEL   I so need it. It's so hard to do.

D   It's a necessity, especially for artists and freelancers. You have to trust that if you need a break, you can take a break and stop worrying that you will lose ground. The most efficient way to lose ground is to run on empty and risk burnout. And more importantly, you need to feed yourself in order to have something new and relevant to say. My *sense* is that you are at the end of Part 1; you launched your artist voice and ran with it. What is your Part 2 all about?

RAEL   I have no idea.

D   Perfect. It's the right time to take the time to figure it out.

RAEL   That sounds so good. I need to rethink my summer in a major way.

D   Plan on hanging out with your neglected Raels, enjoy summer, the season of the heart, together. And spend time outside! Take the time to rekindle your connection to the earth and the sun. You will *all* feel better. Guaranteed.

RAEL   You know, I still haven't even really been outside yet. OK. I need to go for a walk and look at the gardens in my neighbourhood and come up with another plan.

MID-SEPTEMBER

RAEL   I just got back from a week of camping at a woman's festival in a retreat centre in South Carolina. I just flew in at midnight last night! It was amazing! I'd heard about it for so long.

I never thought it would be like this! Wow! It was so profound! I put up my tent and set everything up on my own! No butch around to help me, haha. It was so amazing. I spent a lot of time just standing and breathing and looking at the stars. I've never felt so safe in my entire life! I even felt safe walking in the desert at night.

D   Talk about taking back the night! And throw in a major dose of Nature. Alleluia! This kind of space really exists! And it's not just at retreat centres and festivals, but everywhere and every day. *I rest my hands on Rael's shins for a few minutes.* Your first chakra is going through a paradigm shift. It's a realization that sits in high contrast with your previous perception of yourself on the earth plane. Your cells and molecules are still soaking in the desert's unconditional love balm.

RAEL   The space is created by artists and activists. All of it is beautiful, joyful, zesty, and cathartic! I participated in a sweat lodge ceremony. My first time ever. It was dedicated to women survivors of sexual abuse. I thought I would release and purge; instead, I felt strong, beautiful, and healed. It was a celebration! I don't feel like a victim anymore! I realized that I could feel safe in the world. I really thought I would never experience that. I didn't think it was possible. I'm safe. It's really over!

A few minutes later:

Ouch, my chest is hurting!

D   A crust is cracking. Your little eight-year-old Rael loved the festival! She does not want to leave that exquisite and enchanting world.

RAEL   OMG! I saw eight-year-old children, like me, yet so unlike me then: unrestrained, exuberant, joyful, and safe. Wow! *Tears flow.*

D   The strain and effort of your healing journey rumbles in your chest.

A few minutes later:

A profound realization is pouring out of your heart. I *hear* "It's over—It's over." It really is over. You have made it out of the tunnel. You are safe and free.

RAEL   I did the work because I had no choice. Really, what else could I do? I felt so awful. WOW! I've really emerged on the other side!

D   It was definitely a win–win week. Your third eye is gloriously open. That's one hell of a festival! I *sense* that you listened to your intuition throughout the week.

RAEL   I totally knew where to be and what to do. I just floated and listened.

D   You were on a different program: you knew what you needed to enjoy yourself and savour life. Rather than painstakingly monitoring everything and searching for what you needed to be safe, you perceived the opportunities for love and compassion. No fearful detours; just a non-stop train to joyful fulfillment.

RAEL   WOW! That's new! Really, really, new.

LATE SEPTEMBER

RAEL   I've been feeling upset … lots of sorrow surfacing. It's such a surprise and a drag after my amazing time at the festival.

D   *I rest my hands on Rael's shins for a few minutes.* It is fall equinox and you were blessed with an intravenous hit of unconditional love and high vibrations at the festival. It's turning your world right side up. The feeling of safety you experienced in the desert still churns in your veins; this feeling is so different that it's taking you a while to acclimatize.

RAEL   Yeah, it has been surprisingly tough. As if the desert wind cleaned some stuff off so I can see I still have all this gunk stuck to me—all this shame.

       A few minutes later, Little Rael tries to push the sticky mess away from her neck and head. I want it off me—I don't know how! I keep having memories of my father raping me. *Her throat tightens. She turns her head to the right and left, her lower back arches, her breath accelerates, and her face reddens. Little Rael whimpers as a shiver crawls up her spine. The memory of her distress climbs into the here and now.* I feel stuck. My neck is twisted at a wicked angle. I can barely breathe. It feels like it's about to snap! I'm so scared it's going to break! Oh my God, I don't know if I can do this!

D   You have the personal power now to transcend this moment of powerlessness. You have the strength to set yourself free.

RAEL   *Little Rael spits her rage.* I feel like my life was hanging on a thread! I almost died! My father could have killed me!

D   Yes, he almost did. We've been here before—there is more to it though—what other Rael lies in the darkness unloved?

A few minutes later:

Hmmm … Were you taken to a hospital?

RAEL   Yes, my mother took me the next day.

D   And your mother, of course, did not reveal the true cause of your injury. She concocted a story in which you were to blame for the "accident."

RAEL   Of course she blamed me.

D   You heard the blasphemous story loud and clear. The whole thing was your fault: you did something stupid and you got yourself hurt. And the hospital staff did not investigate. You were seven years old. You could answer questions after all. You must have been visibly in shock. You were brutally attacked less than twenty-four hours ago; surely, on some level, it was possible to see you were traumatized. One can only hope that things have improved since then.

RAEL   Yes, we can only hope.

D   That's a whole other level of neglect. After X-rays, physical examinations, much prodding, and none of the compassion, perceptive analysis, tender care, concern, or time that you needed … What happened?

RAEL   I was sent home with a huge neck brace for a month. It was so tall that I could barely open my mouth!

D   Rather convenient one might say: you literally could not divulge the secret.

RAEL   Yeah … For a whole month my jaw was painfully clamped shut. It was awful.

A few minutes later:

D   Ouch—it was excruciating. Your neck stiffened and you really ground your teeth under the pressure.

A few minutes later:

Hmmm … I *sense* that, emotionally, you were taken through the wringer as well.

RAEL   Yes, my father, mother, sister, and friends mercilessly teased me.

D   I especially *hear* your mother. "Look what's happened to you now! Haha!" As if this is one more calamity you brought on yourself. She unabashedly blamed you. You were publicly humiliated for one night and thirty days and thirty years and she blamed you.

RAEL   Shit!

D   Let's just sit here for a while. Your vertebrae moved once and you almost died, so rightfully so, they are determined to never move again. It's deemed too risky.

RAEL   I can't stand being touched on the neck. It feels argh … ugh! *Rael shudders at the thought.*

A few minutes later:

D   Your distress was frozen and locked in place by the month in a stiffening restraint. You can allow your vertebrae to move now. You can allow them to align now. You are strong enough now. You are safe now.

Ten minutes later:

Woowee … The joints between your cervical spine are expanding. *Rael hangs on for the ride, bravely clutching at the blankets, trusting yet drenched in her old fear. Blood flushes in. The tissues become viscous. A gentle wave of unconditional love rinses the cells and molecules. As Rael reconnects with her inner wisdom, the vertebrae glide into alignment.*

RAEL   BLAME? He's to blame, not me! I thought it was shame! Blame! I can whack that right back at them. That's way more cut-and-dry. Shame is sticky … and somehow more about me. I'm lovable; that's clear. I'm not taking that blame for one more second! Wow! I feel as though I'm finally clambering over the edge of the cliff and back onto the rock.

D   Yes, you're back on the sacred land where you felt utterly happy to be alive!

RAEL   Yes, not just safe, but happy and free too.

D   You didn't just take back the night, you took back your life.

RAEL   I'm so grateful to be alive. Wow!

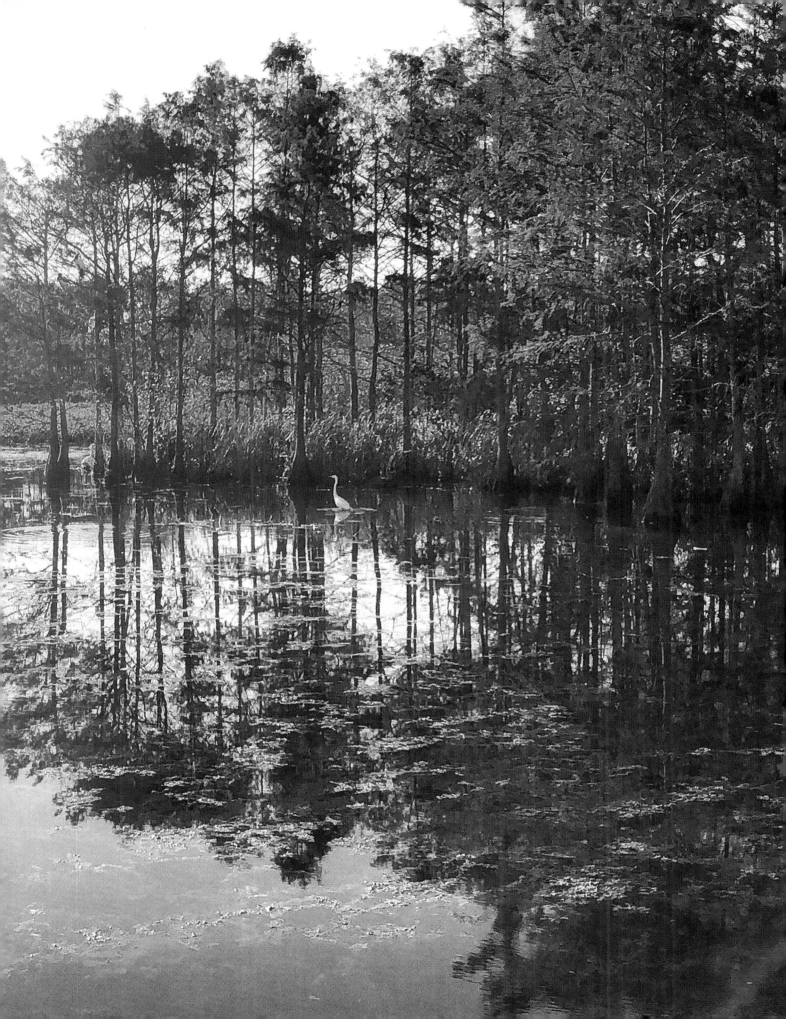

CHAPTER TWENTY-TWO
MASUMI

EARLY APRIL

Masumi at age twenty-seven

MASUMI   I have been in therapy for years dealing with issues linked to my sexist, authoritarian Japanese father. I still struggle with depression. It seems worse right now.

D   *I rest my hands on Masumi's shins for a few minutes.* I *sense* that you're in your first Saturn return. How old are you?

MASUMI   Twenty-seven.

D   Well, you're right on schedule. Saturn is in the same place it was as the day you were born. Let's say that the riverbed over which your life force flows is this wide. During your Saturn returns, at ages twenty-eight and fifty-six, the river goes to one-eighth of its width. The flow is so compressed that the current increases tremendously and with it your life force. You are in one of the two mega-portals gifted to you in this lifetime.

MASUMI   The level of intensity has taken me by surprise.

D   It's like being in a pressure cooker. Saturn returns are bound to feel intense, but they present initiatory opportunities to grow and evolve. When we harness their momentum, we are propelled into a higher frequency.

MASUMI   It feels low to me at this point!

D   *I rest my left hand under Masumi's abdomen and rest my right on her thigh for a few minutes.* Growth hurts because it entails change. Most of us resist change even if it's for the better. This gateway is a sacred call to transformation. It's intense because a very big light is shining on every aspect of your life that is holding you back. Although colossal, this force is buoying you.

MASUMI   It sure as hell doesn't feel like it is.

D   If you're on board, the energy feels encouraging and supportive, but if you're hanging on to the shore and resisting, it tears you to shreds, or it feels like it. Welcome to your first Saturn return! That explains a few things, doesn't it?

MASUMI   It sure does. I couldn't understand why in this particular moment I feel so utterly disassembled, like I'm revisiting everything. I thought I had cleared out all this stuff. I haven't been this challenged in a long time. I had hoped that I would never feel like this again. I thought I had done the work.

D   The work is never-ending. You know the old analogy of peeling the onion. Your Saturn return has just peeled off a layer. You're invited to look again.

A few minutes later:

Hmmm … You're out of your Sacred Tree. Despite the therapy and work, you're still unplugged from the earth and the sun.

MASUMI   I don't feel grounded, if that's what you mean.

D   Yes, that's part of it. But it's also about being out-of-body, having been dissociated to some extent since early childhood. It looks like the sting of your upbringing in a Japanese patriarchal family oppresses you still; you're right about that. You're a disheartened and weary warrior.

MASUMI   It's so intense right now.

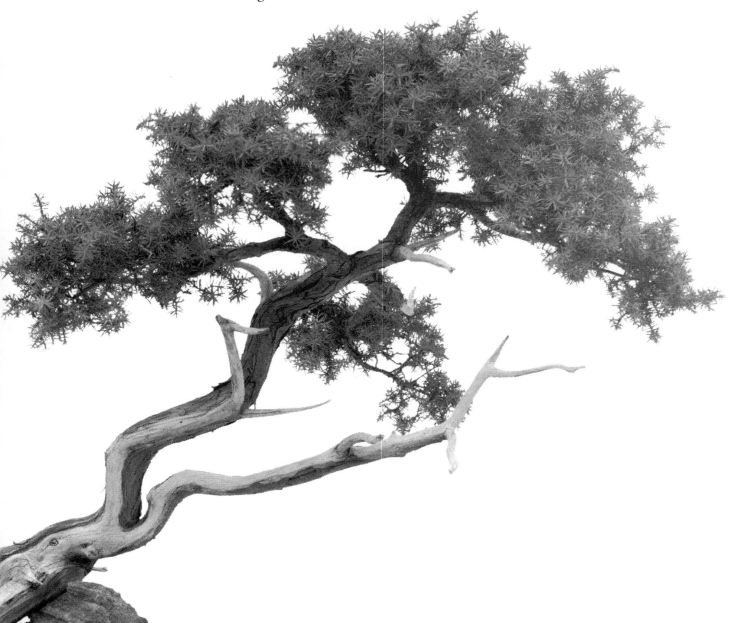

A few minutes later:

D   You're still colonized energetically—that's the bad news. You're unfortunately still living and breathing within the confines of your father's sexist energy. That's why you feel like shit. The good news is that you feel like shit; if you were numbing this pain out, you would miss your Saturn return's initiatory opportunity. Your Sacred Tree is not letting you miss your appointment with transformation.

MASUMI   I thought I was falling apart.

D   You're not falling apart, the status quo maintaining the colonizing straitjacket is. *I slide my hands under Masumi's head for a few minutes.* A battle is raging. Your father terrorized you and enshrined himself as a God-like authoritarian ruler, not only in the household but in your energy body. Your seventh chakra is invaded by his autocratic power and absolutism.

MASUMI   What the hell?

D   Yeah, his overbearing energy is blocking your portal to the sun. Hmmm… It's blocking your sixth chakra as well. This interferes with your intuition. He taught you to listen to him, not yourself. As a result, you are plagued by self-doubt, confusion, and apathy.

MASUMI   I am!

D   We are clearing his invasive and domineering energy out of your sixth and seventh chakras now.

A few minutes later:

This is your scared space. No one should be in here but you, especially not a dictator! This energy blocks your access to the sun. How can your Sacred Tree grow if you cannot reach for the sun?

MASUMI   I can really feel that.

D   Are you going home now?

MASUMI   Yes.

D   Good. Take it easy for the rest of the day. Soften into the energy of the sun now tickling your branches. Try to sit in silence too, no TV or computer. Create space for your intuition to speak. Give yourself the opportunity to hear yourself think.

MASUMI   OK. It's a really different way to look at things. I'll try. Thanks.

LATE APRIL

MASUMI   That was intense. I had to lie in bed all day after that session.

D   You cleared out your father from your upper chakras and spiritual centres. It doesn't get much bigger than that. Your Sacred Tree was robbed of its branches! Let's see how you integrated this shift. *I slide my hands under Masumi's head for a few minutes.* Hmmm … Your mouth is also sealed. I see your father's hand hovering over your lips. He silenced you then, and still does now.

MASUMI   That's so ironic. I have to talk all the time at work. That's what I do all day.

D   Ah … but I *sense* that your true voice has not emerged yet.

MASUMI   Sadly, no.

D   *My hands rest on Masumi's chest for a few minutes.* I *sense* that your heart is bleeding. Your father's imperious and cold arrogance wounded you. His attention was empty of love and care. It looks like every interaction reinforced his power over you and his ownership of you, nothing more. He ruled and you obeyed. That's one hell of a dry contract. Not exactly what you need out of a caregiver.

MASUMI   Ugh.

D   *I rest my right hand below Masumi's right breast. Within a few minutes a sizzling lightning rod surfaces.* An energetic rod pierces through your breast tissue down through to your liver. Rage and despair are literally shooting through you. Hmmm … A Little Masumi is surfacing. You're four years old. Hmmm … It's late at night … You're crumpled in the backseat of the car …

MASUMI   Oh … yes … we were driving home after a party. My father was drunk and driving recklessly. I remember my parents yelling at each other. My brother and I huddled together in the backseat.

D   And your father hit your mother?

MASUMI   Yes, he did!

D   Your mother's screech reverberated in the car. Then, crying and screaming, she threatened to leave the car. *My right hand glides to Masumi's solar plexus and I settle in for a few minutes.* Your father stopped the car and your mother clambered out … The argument continued. *Masumi's solar plexus rips as the threat of being separated from her mother tears into her.*

MASUMI   I was so scared. I thought I would never see her again.

D You were abandoned by your father already; the threat of being separated from your mother created a terrifying chasm of unlove and danger. You feared that no one would be there to love you and care for you. *Masumi shifts her body. Little Masumi's distress is palpable.*

Let's scoop Little Masumi out of that car and into your heart. It's OK, little one, you're not alone. Masumi loves you and will take care of you.

A few minutes later:

That's it, console Little Masumi, cuddle her and reassure her. Let her know that she will never be alone or helpless or at the mercy of your enraged and inebriated father again. Let her know that you are her primary caregiver now.

A few minutes later:

You're a dynamic duo with the power to reject your father's authority and aggression. Ouf... Stay with her, the horrendous fear of losing your mother is releasing. The traumatic charge of that event, the lightning bolts trapped in your tissues all this time, are releasing through your spine, legs, and feet and into the earth. That's it! You're doing it!

MASUMI Ugh!

A few minutes later:

D Hmmm... I also *see* your mother getting back into the car. The storm eventually abated.

MASUMI Yes, it did, fortunately.

D There's more to that story, but in terms of that specific moment, the energy has cleared. The earth is composting it as we speak. Acknowledge all the space created in your body today. Invite love and compassion to fill this newfound space. Allow all your cells and molecules to bathe in the healing energy of love and compassion. Receive and give yourself some time to rest over the next few weeks.

MASUMI I need to catch my breath.

D As you mentioned, you've worked on a lot of these traumas before. That's why the energy releases very rapidly. However, you're now learning how to release the lightning bolts of trauma stored in your organs and tissues. Create time and space to encourage the release to continue. Take long baths or lie in bed or on your yoga mat so you can learn to trust the throbbing wave of release. You have the power to do this on your own too. I'm not the one doing it, you are.

MASUMI OK, I'll try. Thanks.

MAY

MASUMI   I'm feeling better, but I'm still frustrated at work. I even had a few panic attacks.

D   *I slip my hands under Masumi's head for a few minutes.* I *hear* an exquisitely beautiful female voice. *I cup my hands over Masumi's ears.* Your mother's soothing voice hovers in your right ear.

MASUMI   My mother was an opera singer! I loved listening to her sing.

D   Her beautiful voice reached your spirit! It inspired and cultivated your creative impulse. Within the cocoon of her sound, your passion for art and artistic expression blossomed. Yet this joyous energy hangs on the outskirts of your energy bodies. Your connection with your creative voice is ambiguous.

MASUMI   That's unfortunately true.

D   While your creativity was nurtured by your mother, it was thwarted by your father. A thick fog clogs your right-brain hemisphere. Your creative centre is depleted.

    A few minutes later:

    Hmmm … Your father's sexist disdain crushed your connection to your genius and life purpose.

MASUMI   Makes sense.

D   Thank God for your mother's gift! Although she didn't have the power to protect you from your father, her nectar fed your spirit nonetheless. Your gift could not blossom then, but it can now.

MASUMI   I so yearn for that.

D   Let's water that little sapling now. Lots and lots of love, please! *Masumi's body visibly softens into the surface of the massage table. She slips into deep meditation for ten minutes.* Let's see here, your sixth chakra is still congested. We have more work to do here. I *sense* that your father expected outright obedience all the time. Unfortunately, your obligation to submit to his authority barred your sacred connection to your intuition and imagination. Please serve an eviction notice now. This is your sacred space!

    A few minutes later:

    Hmmm … There's more to it. I'm drawn to an aggressive thumping energy in your right cheek. *My left hand hovers over Masumi's cheek. It's still storing the charge of her father's offence.* Did your father slap you across the face?

MASUMI Yes, he did!

D Often?

MASUMI Yes.

D His strikes were an affront to your Sacred Tree. In doing so, he violated your dignity and eroded your self-worth … and your connection to your beautiful, expressive, and capable Sacred Tree. *Tears stream down Masumi's cheeks. My right hand slips down to Masumi's jaw and I settle in for a few minutes.* Your jaw is clenched shut. You were silenced.

MASUMI I was not allowed to respond to my father.

D Yes, you were muzzled and so was your love of art and your creativity. Defeat and humiliation are formidable foes. *I'm drawn down to Masumi's right shoulder and arm and settle in for a few minutes.* Your arm is numb. It's like concrete it's so heavy.

MASUMI I wasn't allowed to defend myself or my mother. When I was slapped across the face, I had to stand still.

D Your energy shudders in the wake of your statement. The sting of your father's violence still reverberates through your being. Let's liberate your arm from your father's debilitating shackle. You're allowed to hit back now. If that's what you need to do, let him have it. Pummel him to the ground. You have the strength and enough rage to fuel a mega-rampage. *Masumi embraces her personal power and lets her imagination run with it.*

Ten minutes later:

That's it, your father's invasive energy is detaching. You're clearly winning! Free yourself from his tyranny! That's it, the helplessness and despair in your liver are also dispersing.

A few minutes later:

Great! Your heart chakra is now opening. Ooh… The soft tones of your mother's voice reach your creative spirit. Oh good, the creative energy in your mother's voice is penetrating your field and stirring your creative fire in your right-brain hemisphere. The energy in your sixth and seventh chakras is also stirring. Receive, dear Masumi!

MASUMI Ouf … I feel dizzy!

D Tectonic plates are shifting. It will take a few days for all your energy bodies to settle into their newfound freedom. It's disorienting at first when the door of the cage is flung open.

MASUMI   You're not kidding.

D   Take your time. And go straight home to rest. Eat light. Take it easy tonight.

MASUMI   I don't even try to go back to work anymore. Thank you.

NOVEMBER

Masumi at age twenty-eight

MASUMI   I've had a breakthrough! I've been working diligently with my therapist for the past few months to access my inner strength and clarity. I intuited that my father had been having affairs since I was a child. I asked my mother if this was true, and my mother was honest and willing to talk. It all makes so much more sense now.

D   *I rest my hands on Masumi's shins for a few minutes.* Your energy is swirling in all directions as you reshuffle the deck. It feels like a lot of new information to integrate in your day-to-day consciousness. This one realization sprawls over many years of lived experience in your parental home. It's like the light feels too bright all of a sudden.

MASUMI   Well, it changes everything!

D   Let's see if we can lower the wattage a bit … because nothing has really changed … Little Masumi knew … in your bones you knew that your father was unfaithful and deceitful. *I rest my hands on Masumi's kidneys for a few minutes.* You have already lived through the truth; it's only your conscious mind that is catching up with the program.

MASUMI   I knew … you're right. I did know.

Fifteen minutes later:

D   That's it, your energy is settling down as you connect with your intuitive knowledge. You're starting to feel strong and solid again. Your tree is bending, but it's not breaking.

A few minutes later:

Good! Your heart is opening. *I slide my left hand to Masumi's chest and my left on her right thigh and settle in for a few minutes.* Welcome all the traumatized astronauts into your heart—all of you, at all ages, who experienced your father's lies intuitively. That's it—you're doing great!

MASUMI   I so knew … *Tears stream down Masumi's cheeks.*

D   And you've been working hard, Masumi. Compassionately witness your journey and tireless dedication to your healing.

MASUMI   It's been relentless lately.

D   Yes, and drink in your growth and learning. Invite all your cells and molecules to absorb unconditional self-love, the earth, and the sun. That's it, there's a big beautiful world beyond your father's betrayal and lies. Wholeheartedly align with the vibrations of honesty, respect, integrity, and trust. Encourage these vibrations to imprint in your cells. Yes! That's the world you now live in, Masumi.

MASUMI   What a breath of fresh air. I feel so much better.

EARLY MARCH

MASUMI   I felt suicidal on Sunday. I have not felt that deeply depressed in six years. How can I be here again after six years of therapy? I can't do it! I can't go there again! I was so scared. I was pinned down on my bed for most of the day. I couldn't move. At times, I could hardly breathe.

D   *I rest my left hand on Masumi's solar plexus while my right remains on her right thigh for a few minutes.* Hmmm, I faintly see a little nine-year-old Masumi. She's sitting alone in an enclosed space. I feel it's daytime, yet she sits in murky darkness. She's extremely frightened. Where is she?

MASUMI   I'm in the basement! My mother used to lock me down there! I was so scared when I was down there.

D   On Sunday this Little Masumi crawled out of the basement and into bed with you. She is surfacing and reaching out to you. What's her story? What's happening? It's OK, little one, we're here. You're not alone anymore. What is scaring you?

MASUMI   It's so intense!

D   *I shift my left hand to Masumi's right adrenal gland for a few minutes.* Little Masumi feels isolated, but an emotion more strident than fear is surfacing. Hmmm … You feel more alone than ever, you feel betrayed. Ouch! Who's hurting you? Hmmm … Your brother, now about twelve years old, has turned on you.

MASUMI   AH! I started writing about my brother in the creative writing course I'm taking. I had no idea. I've done so much therapy around my father. My brother has never come up. It's so intense. I really didn't expect this.

D   Hmmm … Father and son are now allies! Your brother was learning the ropes, and the sexist hierarchy was beginning to structure your youngsters' world.

MASUMI   Of course, I just hadn't thought about it before.

D   Yeah, the two of you were not united against him anymore.

A few minutes later:

Your brother, now a little man, was assuming his new position in the household. He's not just a kid anymore. At age twelve, he's stepping into his sanctioned patriarchal role as eldest son. He is now more powerful than his mother and little sister.

MASUMI   Of course he is!

D   Little Masumi then had two male perpetrators to contend with. Once your ally, your brother was now a traitor!

A few minutes later:

He bullied you. The little man is making you do things you do not want to do.

MASUMI   It's devastating!

D   Betrayal is brutal. I *hear* "My brother? He loved me! We were so close! Now, he threatens me and scares me! He humiliates me! I'm alone against my father! The house is a really scary place now."

MASUMI   It really was.

D   Yes, and I *sense* you run to the basement to seek refuge. Once a jail, now it's your sanctuary. You sit alone in the dark and space out. Your traumas recede into your dark unconscious. The basement becomes your temple of survival. It's a place you go to when you need to forget.

MASUMI   Oh dear …

D   The pain and panic you experienced on the weekend is a testament to your strength and the power of your writing. You accessed your heartbroken and terrified traumatized astronaut and the numbed architect of survival in the basement.

MASUMI   I really did not make the connection.

D   Yet you listened and with compassion wrote her story. The emotions overwhelmed you for a few days, but now that the connection is conscious and the betrayal has been named, you can integrate your Little Masumis and welcome them into your heart.

A few minutes later:

They no longer have to be alone and frightened in the dark basement. They are both a part of a dynamic team, you at your age now, your Sacred Tree, the earth, and the sun.

A few minutes later:

They are not abandoned at the bottom of the hierarchy anymore. They are reunited with your powerful creative spirit!

MASUMI   We have a lot to write together.

D   You sure do. It's exciting. Keep going. Keep writing!

LATE MARCH

MASUMI   I'm feeling much better. I started a liver and kidney support program yesterday. My naturopath recommends Unda 1 and 2 as well as nettle leaf tea and lemon in my water. She also recommended vitamin D, more protein in my diet, regular exercise, and some high-EPA fish oil.

D   Right on schedule. The vernal equinox is the most optimal time of year to cleanse. *I rest my hands on Masumi's shins for a few minutes.* Hmmm ... You're not grounded, and your sacrum is out of alignment. *I slide my left hand to her abdomen and right hand on her thigh and settle for a few minutes.* Your sacroiliac joints are extremely stiff, especially on your left side. They feel locked in a fearful and rigid stance.

Ten minutes later, Masumi's right hip suddenly releases. She wheezes. Her breath becomes shallow as fear takes hold of her. She feels weak, helpless, and powerless. Little Masumi's experience at age nine overwhelms the present. It's OK, Masumi, little nine-year-old Masumi is here with us. We love you. You're not alone. We're here to help. I can feel that your connection to the earth and the sun is faint. You feel like this feeling is bigger than you. You're terrified. It's OK, little one. We're holding you. We're here. You can trust us. We're here to get you out of there.

MASUMI   It's so huge.

D   You can release this terror. You think you can't survive this sensation, but you can. It's huge, but you're even huger. You don't have to live with this vibration in your bones and tissues any longer.

Ten minutes later, the nine-year-old traumatized astronaut and architect of survival feel Masumi's strength in the now. They both yield to the feeling of safety and love. Love and compassion slowly seep into your consciousness and a new level of awareness is emerging. Oh good, they both feel your strength and agency.

A few minutes later:

Ah, your third eye is opening. You're dropping into your Sacred Tree. *Masumi sighs.*

MASUMI   Mmm ... I really feel it. It's so different!

D   Yes, and you can now *see* that you are in the middle of a very long journey. You are now aware that this lifetime is only one among many. Your mother is only one of the many biological mothers you have had, and the same applies to your father. From this vantage point in your Sacred Tree, you acknowledge that you are strong enough to end the multigenerational cycle of sexist violence.

A few minutes later:

MASUMI   Whoa, what's that?

D   You feel your strength and wisdom in your bones. You're connecting with the beautiful matriarchs who sit around a fire in the centre of the earth. Acknowledge the great-grand-mothers' love and wisdom clearing the path with you. They have heard and seen it all, your story and every person's story. They hold the stories for us. Let them hold you.

MASUMI   I've never felt anything like this.

D   You're not alone, Masumi. Let the matriarchs' wisdom penetrate your cells.

A few minutes later:

The unbeneficial energy in your left hip is also stirring now. Good! Let's release it. It's ready.

A few minutes later:

Your descending colon is welded to your left ilium. The fascia is rigid, and the soft tissue of the colon is attached to the surface of the hipbone. *I slide my hand to Masumi's left hip. Her tissues respond almost immediately.* That's it, Masumi, breathe. Clarity is emerging. You were joined at the hip with your brother until age nine. Your sibling bond was amplified by your solidarity against your common enemy, your father. Then, one day your brother became a little man. He abandoned the sinking female vessel.

A few minutes later:

That's it, release the pain and panic you experienced when your brother betrayed you and bullied you. The matriarchs witness your pain. Let them burn it in their sacred fire. Your brother does not have control over you anymore. Invite the smoke to cleanse your pores and molecules. You're doing great!

Fifteen minutes later:

Now in a deep meditative state, Masumi's entire left body vibrates at a higher frequency. Your energy rises out of the mire of that sexist hierarchy and out of the patriarchal Japanese cultural tradition. You are keenly aware of your mother's and grandmother's powerlessness, along with the centuries-old repression of women in Japan. The weight of this disharmony at the heart of your family and culture is lifting off. You are ending the cycle of violence for three generations of Japanese women: yourself, your mother, and your maternal grandmother, as well as countless more. You are the first in your family to release yourself from the cruel hierarchy of sexism. Receive.

MASUMI   It's big.

D   You're big. And you are setting yourself and so many others free. Namaste. It's an honour.

MASUMI   Namaste.

APRIL

MASUMI   After the last session, I had the worst stomach flu ever. I threw up for hours and retched late into the night. It seemed like it would never stop. Part of me wonders if it was a huge detox. I felt much better the next day.

D   *I slip my hands under Masumi's head for a few minutes.* You are shifting to a higher frequency. It was a most efficient detoxification, for sure. I do need to focus the energy on the bones in your skull though. Excellent, it's like butter. You're already releasing stuckness in your skull. Your dural membrane is softening and your third eye and seventh chakra are also clearing.

Ten minutes later:

Woowee … The energy is surging down into your neck. Let it flow, Masumi. This is what you have been working toward. There goes your fourth cervical vertebra! She's rushing on back into alignment right now. No point waiting. She's on a mission.

A few minutes later:

Bingo! *The current pushes through so suddenly that Masumi loses her breath for a moment.* Wow! Your fifth chakra just burst open. This is fantastic. Your throat chakra is the bridge to your upper chakras. You are strengthening your spiritual awareness and ability to manifest your spirit on the earth.

A few minutes later:

OK, the flow is now streaming down to your heart, stomach, and pelvis and down to your sacrum at the base of your spine.

MASUMI It's like filling and emptying at the same time!

D All your chakras are recalibrating! After six years of therapy your energy body is now shifting to a much higher frequency. You will now taste the fruit of your six-year self-love apprenticeship. *Masumi stretches her arms out and stretches her legs and feet.*

Ten minutes later:

Hmmm … Your left ovary is releasing sorrow and angst. It's linked to your brother's betrayal. This ties in with the work we did on your left hip and colon in the last session. You're harmonizing your energy with the sacred feminine, freeing your reproductive organs from sexist restraints. But … hmmm … something that feels like torment, something really potent, is gurgling to the surface.

MASUMI Both my legs are totally numb.

D *I rest my hands on Masumi's thighs for a few minutes.* Hmmm … Both legs are encased in an old belief: "It's sad to be Masumi." Well, let's just say that it was sad until now. It was sad to be Masumi while trapped and colonized. It's sad to have experienced abuse and misogyny. You are no longer constrained by any of that though.

MASUMI Huh?

D You are more than what has happened to you to date in this lifetime. That was a whole lot of bad weather, but it's not who you are. It's not sad to actually be you, your true self and Sacred Tree. Feel those chakras humming!

MASUMI That sadness is not me? I've always been sad!

D No, it's only a feeling you experienced a lot and now identify with. Feel your energy fields soaring up and beyond the onslaught of sexist weather! Soften into the joy and power of being connected to your Sacred Tree, the earth, and the sun. Invite all your cells to harmonize with this liberated frequency of all your chakras.

A few minutes later:

Kaplunk! That's great, Masumi. The old belief just came crashing down. Hahahaaa … Receive.

MASUMI Wild!

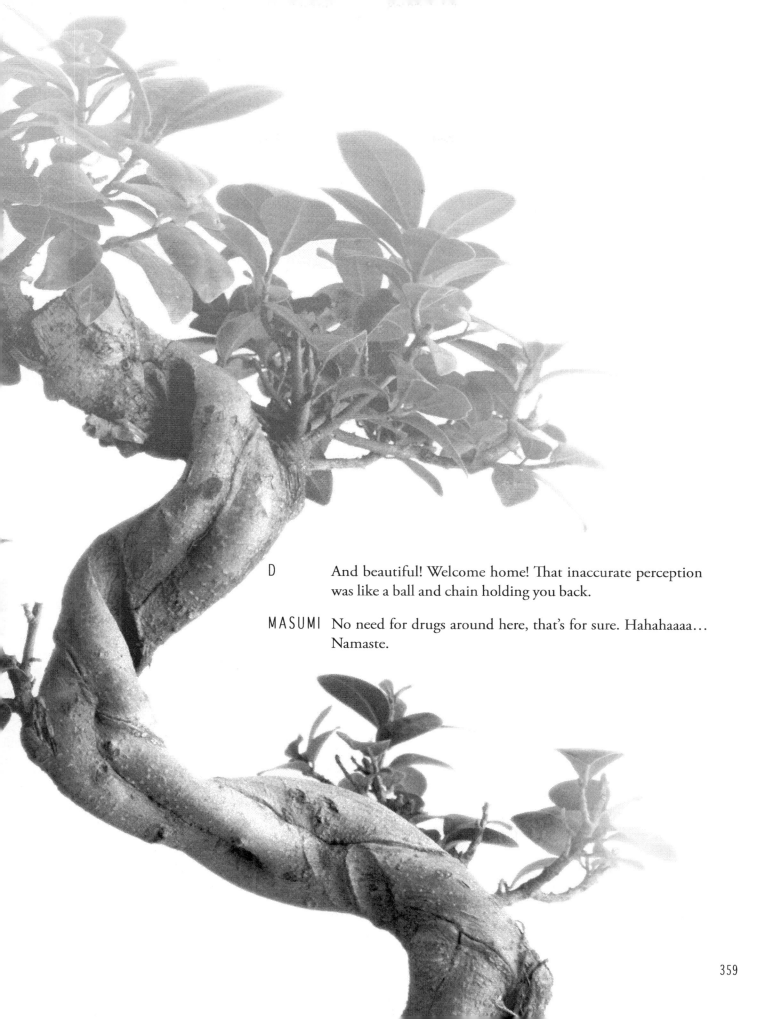

D   And beautiful! Welcome home! That inaccurate perception was like a ball and chain holding you back.

MASUMI   No need for drugs around here, that's for sure. Hahahaaaa… Namaste.

EARLY MAY

MASUMI   I still feel depressed and slightly restless. I don't feel settled.

D   *I rest my hands on Masumi's shins for a few minutes.* I *sense* that you're walking on eggshells. You don't believe that you have the power to set yourself free. You're stunned, and physically you're too static. Like a snake that rubs against a rock to shed its old skin, you need to move your body to fully inhabit the well-being available to you right now. The fumes of your sorrow, despair, and helplessness linger in your aura.

MASUMI   I'm all cooped up. I haven't been outside yet this spring.

D   The old skin is loose and flimsy. You can step into your newfound freedom by dancing, doing yoga, and engaging in outdoor activities. You need to breathe yourself free. You need to shake it all off, literally!

A few minutes later:

Hmmm … The energy in your right kidney just surged. *I shift my hands to Masumi's kidneys for a few minutes.* A glacial panic squashes your entire field. Hmmm … Who's here? *I settle in for five minutes to drop in to this vibration.* Ah, a tiny Masumi is surfacing. She is still in utero.

MASUMI   You can feel that?

D   You're already you. You're already living this lifetime. It just takes patience and silence within to tap into this level of life experience. Anything pre-verbal takes more time and stillness to tune in to. Hmmm … Tiny Masumi is overwhelmed by fear. Oh … I see—your mother is in shock. A canyon has just appeared under your mother's feet. She sobs violently and her distress rattles every pore of your tiny floating body. Her turmoil and uncertainty engulf you. I *hear* your father yelling too.

A couple of minutes later:

Ah, your father is having an affair!

MASUMI   It makes so much sense.

D   Yes, I *sense* that it is the first time he is unfaithful. The betrayal rips your mother's heart open, shaking the foundation of their union and the paradigm that makes her life make sense.

A few minutes later:

Your mother's spirit is tumbling in a heap of despair and submission. You experience your mother's acquiescence and desolation first-hand, front and centre, in the best seat in the house, so to speak.

MASUMI   Whoa … intense … No wonder I've been living this pain so viscerally.

A few minutes later:

D   You are in it; the experience permeates your entire body.

MASUMI   It really makes so much sense.

D   At six months in utero, you are living through an experience your mother in her late twenties did not think she could survive. In utero, you already know your mother's shattered trust, devastated heart, and powerlessness. You also know your father's power to devastate and master. The misogynist stage is already set.

MASUMI   Oh God.

D   Yeah … not exactly the welcome committee one hopes for.

MASUMI   Sure isn't. Even then, I was in it.

D   That's why it's so intense and has taken the time it has to clear the imprint. You've known nothing else. Get outside, move, and let your energy bodies reconfigure to a new vibration without sexism and powerlessness in to your cells.

MASUMI   That might take a while.

D   Not necessarily. Let yourself change. The stage is set.

LATE MAY

MASUMI   I want to write! My day job has run its course. I have decided to apply to creative writing graduate programs across the country. I have a mentor encouraging me to follow my dream, to honour my desire and unleash my voice. He believes in me! I now have the courage to speak of my writing publicly. I want to launch my new plan.

D   *I rest my hands on Masumi's right leg for a few minutes.* Fantastic news. Hmmm … Your enthusiasm and clarity are potent, yet a part of you is still disconnected from the well-being and personal power you have access to now. You are out of the menacing woods, no doubt. Yet you still trudge on a path day and night in a forest with trees so tall that the sun never reaches the forest floor. Your body still soaks in your father's stench and shadow. Which part of you has not joined the party yet? Who still feels trapped and powerless?

MASUMI   I'm really not sure.

D *My hands focus on Masumi's right shin for a few minutes.* I *hear* "I feel dead." Well—young Masumi in her twenties sure opens the conversation up lightly! I *hear* "I want to die. I think of killing myself all the time. And I don't do it! I don't have the courage. I'm a failure."

MASUMI Ah, yes. I always felt like a failure for not actually going out and doing it! Even when it came to killing myself, I failed.

D I *hear* "The world is not worth living for! I don't want any of it! I'm not signing that contract. NO! I want nothing to do with it! I don't want to be here!" You are accustomed to young Masumi's despair. The shadow of your powerlessness trails behind, snaking its long tail around your ankles. Your death mantra drowns your inspirational call to creativity and self-assured action. Your protest was fundamentally important, for sure. Saying no to sexism was vital. Saying no to subservience was crucial. But to say no to your own right to live is a whole other matter.

MASUMI You're not kidding.

D This is all very intense but … hmmm … there's a whole part to the story that's missing. I *sense* that you were a rather busy camper in your twenties.

MASUMI Huh?

A few minutes later:

D I *sense* a strong energy streaming through this young woman's bones. It looks like the industriousness of your young adult life lies buried. Your dauntless "no" to life does not reflect the entire narrative of your young adult life. Something is missing. A dynamic drive abounds. What *were* you doing in your twenties?

MASUMI Oh? I worked in a very competitive milieu.

D What else? There's more.

MASUMI I completed my undergraduate degree with honours.

D There's more still. What else?

MASUMI Hmmm … Oh yeah, I trained for half-marathons and ran four of them.

D OK, I think that about summarizes it.

MASUMI What? I haven't remembered any of this for years! I had no idea. I never talk about that job, or my undergrad, or my experiences as a half-marathon runner. Where has all of this been? I don't see myself like that at that age! I just remember wanting to die.

D   I'm honoured to introduce the two of you. This young woman is your maverick architect of survival. She was working tirelessly, setting the stage for you to live an empowered life, even while young Masumi's misery and trauma threatened to swallow her up each day. Even though your traumatized astronaut's despair clouded your perception, your maverick was on the job.

MASUMI   The split is potent.

D   Yeah, the one feels like she is drowning; and the other, your architect of survival, swims, or rather runs, like hell—half-marathons, no less.

A few minutes later:

They're the two sides of the same coin. Yet, in this case, the traumatized astronaut's pain suppressed the memory of your valiant effort and action. When walking on the edge of a cliff, does one really remember the colour and texture of the earth or does one recall the vertiginous abyss that lies inches away from one's feet? The haunting menace of the chasm organized your perception. Young Masumi's ethos is the victim's pain and sorrow, but your maverick impulse is your spirit's quest for freedom, accomplishment, and spiritual nourishment. Let the twain meet. Yummy! Receive!

JUNE

Summer solstice

MASUMI   My maverick has been visiting me a lot, sporting her different clothes and uniforms. The process of integration was really challenging for two days. It was humbling. I realized that I have never been fully present for myself or for others.

D   *I rest my hands on Masumi's shins for a few minutes.* Hmmm ... My *sense* is that you are remembering the crushing fog of dissociation. Although the pain of victimization is more tangible, the pain suffered when living in a dissociative state is also very intense.

MASUMI   It feels awful.

D   It sure does. Numbness actually really hurts, and it's a beautiful day when one becomes aware of this. *I shift my hands to Masumi's kidneys, and as usual Masumi's energetic field responds dramatically.* Fear leaches out of your right kidney. That's it—breathe. You're doing great! That young architect of survival is softening into your love-filled heart and releasing herself from her old and no longer useful strategy of dissociation. She is soothed by your body's substantiality, emotional vitality, and spiritual alertness. That's it! You are releasing your attachment to the dissociative response. Love and compassion are flooding in. Receive.

MASUMI   Oh! What's that?

D   Your energy is responding very quickly. Your upper chakras churn to the resonant chant of loving kindness. You celebrate your maverick's fortitude and accomplishments. The ordeal of disconnection from your Sacred Tree, the earth and the sun, from lovers, friends, and colleagues wanes as the full Technicolor spectrum of your lived experience blossoms. Your vitality flourishes in your brain hemispheres, third eye, and heart.

MASUMI   Wow!

D   Amazing. This is so great. But … hmmm … there's still some resistance in your right leg. *I shift my hands back to Masumi's right leg. I focus on Masumi's right shin for a few minutes.* Ah … I *sense* that your creative voice is exhausted! But the journey has just begun! What's going on?

MASUMI   I don't know.

D   I *hear* "I don't know if I can take another step! I feel fearful, despairing, and pessimistic." Hey you, what are you doing down there in the right shin along with the young Masumi who would rather be dead?

A few minutes later:

Oh dear, your artistic spirit is hooked into that era of your victimization. Your maverick, as potent as she was, is exhausted and has far less resources than you do now. She toiled despite all odds to embody power and success. You can give her a much-deserved break. You, at your age now, can embrace your creativity with all the resources you have now.

MASUMI   But I write about my experiences in my family and about what I endured! I draw my inspiration from my past. If I heal, I'm afraid of not having the impulse to write. I'm afraid of not having anything to write about.

D   When your energy is aligned, you have more stamina, clarity, excitement, passion, and joy to feed and sustain your artistic process. How can helplessness support your productive creative venture? How can misery and sadness support a demanding daily schedule? Anguish and torment are exhausting and unsustainable. You know, you've been living it. Who needs to be unhappy to do what they love? No one, artists included. To heal is to liberate yourself from subjugation. How can agency and personal power negatively interfere with your artistic process? Healing involves understanding your abuse. How can wisdom negatively impact your output as an artist? How can breaking your silence dry your ink? Not, not, not.

Align with your resources now. Align with your dreams and desires now. Align with your life's purpose now.

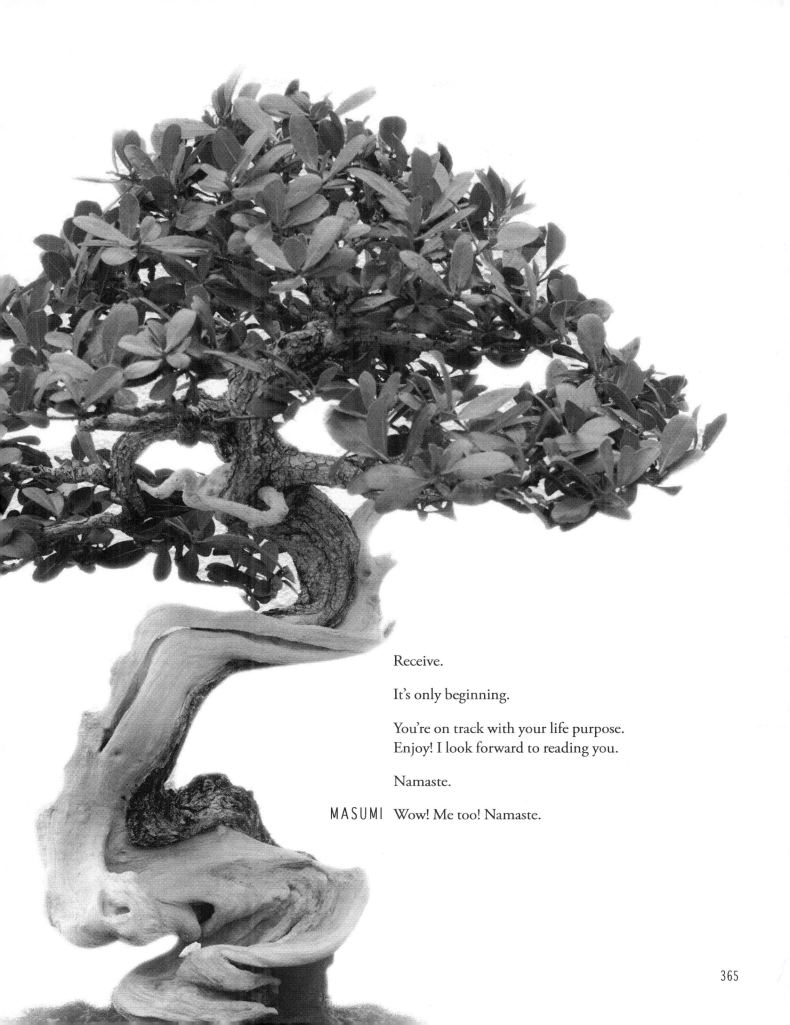

Receive.

It's only beginning.

You're on track with your life purpose.
Enjoy! I look forward to reading you.

Namaste.

MASUMI Wow! Me too! Namaste.

CHAPTER TWENTY-THREE

ANJU
PART TWO

EARLY AUGUST

Anju at age forty-three, a year and a half later

ANJU It's so good to see you. I've been experiencing intense soreness in both my breasts! I went for a mammogram. An alarmist nurse prescribed an immediate biopsy. It's scheduled for later this month! I'm nervous, but I woke up two mornings in a row with the thought: "I'm healthy—I am healthy—I'm well."

Oh, and my little five-year-old awakened in my Kundalini yoga class. You know the one who was distraught on the night of the phone call when my mother's brother committed suicide? She came and sat with me—in lotus—on my legs in lotus. I asked her what she needed me to do and she said, "Eat well and do yoga!" Last night, I had the biggest release ever: one hour of non-stop sobbing. I was mourning the loss of my loving ama that night at age five while simultaneously feeling embraced by Kali and the Divine Mother. I felt intense sorrow, yet I was aware that I was only mourning this particular mother in this lifetime while a divine mothering energy embraced me!

D *I rest my hands on Anju's chest above her breasts for a few minutes.* Hmmm … You have embraced your position as a matriarch. This is a fantastic positive shift. Your parents now trust you to make decisions.

ANJU I feel so much more energetic and clear. Something has really shifted in terms of my mother. I feel huge around her. She is getting smaller physically, but it's more than that. She is down there in the roots, caught in the mire of her painful past and her endless regrets. I've broken through the ground, so it's from that perspective that I see her now. I feel for her, but I am not caught up in the same way. I pray for her … you know … I'm really not sure she is going to break through.

D Praying is also compassion in action.

ANJU It so is. And my old thought patterns don't have the same grip on me as before; neither does my fear. Even though I feel intense pain exactly where they will do the biopsy on my left breast, and my right breast is still sore, I keep reciting my mantra and meditating every morning. It's really quieting my mind.

D *My right hand rests on Anju's chest above her left breast and my left sits immediately below for five minutes.* Hmmm … It's important to acknowledge that you live in a relatively new physical body. Our cells regenerate all the time. So your brother never actually touched *this* left breast. None of these cells were likely there during your adolescence.

ANJU   Oh … I never thought of it that way! It's so liberating to even consider this. It changes everything.

D   It sure does! What's stuck in your breast is an energy signature. It's totally fluid. Your physical body is the physical expression of the unbeneficial or beneficial energies in your subtle bodies. When the energy signatures in the energy bodies change, your physical body releases the old imprint and transforms.

ANJU   That's quite an empowering way to look at it!

D   It is. Most of us go through life feeling trapped in a body that controls us, rather than acknowledging our innate ability to self-heal.

ANJU   OK … This is quite disorienting.

D   It's confusing to your rational mind, especially if allopathic medicine has been the dominant framework. Regardless, your spirit knows that your body, all of it, is an expression of your spirit. This is where it gets even more confusing, because in this moment, it may not be wellness that best serves your spirit. Sometimes, we need adversity or illness to get with it, listen, and grow.

ANJU   Hmmm ….

D   Adversity and dis-ease is an initiatory process that helps you move you closer to your Sacred Tree and purpose. For instance, you may not like this whole biopsy mayhem, yet it is prompting you to focus on cells that need healing. You are called into action and have the opportunity to release the belief that your breast tissues are marked or scarred by your sexual abuse history. *Anju enters a deep meditative state for fifteen minutes.* That's it, Anju, clear it out, your brother's touch, whatever. Clear it all out! Your breasts have never been touched by him.

        A few minutes later:

        Allow love and compassion to flow through the denser tissue around your left nipple and through the area that is sore.

ANJU   Oooh …

D   Now invite your left breast tissue to meld into your chest; it does not need to be separate from you anymore. Feel your breast as an extension of your ribs, intercostal muscles, left lung, and biological heart.

A few minutes later:

Now feel your heart chakra and your breasts as one.

A few minutes later:

Surrender to the unconditional love in your spiritual heart. Feel it expand and fill all your energy bodies.

ANJU   Oooo … It's quite something!

D   Ha hahahaha … It sure is. It's so good. Keep going; you're gloriously on track.

ANJU   Thanks for that. Namaste.

D   Namaste.

MID-AUGUST

ANJU   I had my biopsy yesterday! I felt clear and grounded throughout. I even soothed a very scared patient in the waiting room! And you won't believe this … they come at me with this thing actually labelled and referred to as the biopsy gun!

D   Oh for Pete's sake.

ANJU   I know. Why does everything to do with women's breasts have to be linked with violence and aggression? Are the doctors and nurses really that ignorant of the symbolic significance of such language? They didn't even react when I pointed out the irony to them. Anyway, I remained clear and calm. I recited my mantra and gave them permission to do the procedure.

D   *I place my hands on Anju's chest above her breasts. She softens into a meditative state for fifteen minutes.* Your entire chest is vibrating with the frequency of unconditional love. Your etheric field was not pierced by the incision or the infamous biopsy gun. Your conscious authorization of the procedure protected you from their invasive and unconscious approach.

A few minutes later:

This is so great! You have taken ownership of your breasts. You claim your chest and fill your flesh with love and light.

ANJU   As I wait for the results, I remain clear that I am healthy and strong. I even decided to go to my Kundalini yoga class last night anyway. I had a huge emotional release. My left breast was a bit sore, but not today.

D   *I check in with Anju's kidneys for a few minutes.* Your kidneys are emitting some fear though. It's interesting. Foreboding and concern still activate some alarm, but the charge has nowhere to go. Your loving, centred, and focused approach cuts the wires that spread and transmit fear from the kidneys to the rest of your body. The cables are lying there dangling. This is so wonderful!

ANJU   It's over! I'm so grateful and relieved. *Tears of relief pour down Anju's face, pooling in her ears on their way to the pillow. Anju feels unconditional love flood her entire body. She softens in its embrace for twenty minutes.* Oh my God, this is so great! Ouuuhhh! *Anju and I hug. Joy wraps its sweet arms around us.*

D   Namaste.

SEPTEMBER

ANJU   I had a second biopsy in my left breast. I can't believe I had to go through it again! I'm way more nervous than after the first one. I find it harder to hold on to my peace of mind. Ugh, I finally went to a yoga class. I realize how out of shape I am. My physical body really is the final frontier! I so thought this whole process would be the other way around. I don't feel good. *Anju's hands hover over her thighs.* I feel stuck in my body.

D   *I rest my hands on Anju's shins for a few minutes.* You're bang on. Your whole right body is clogged. I *sense* that you not only resist exercise, you hate it.

ANJU   I do.

D   It's more than that though. I *hear* "Women who exercise are chained to sexist beauty ideals. They are disempowered slaves to the male gaze."

ANJU   I do think that! Of course I do.

D   While there is a lot truth in this statement, your belief does not include women embracing their physical well-being, alignment, and strength. Physical disharmony and imbalance are real barriers, not only physically but emotionally, mentally, and spiritually. This belief needs an upgrade to include the old maxim: sound of body and sound of mind. *I rest my hands on Anju's belly for ten minutes.* There's even more to it. I *see* you at twenty-nine years old. You're withdrawn, not sexual, and miles away from the brazen early twenties, sexy, shit-kicking activist in cowboy boots we met before.

ANJU   Oh … I was coming out of my über-performer phase. That's after I finished my graduate degree with honours and had lived and worked in India for a year. When I came back, I got a job that paid really well. I rented a semi-detached townhouse with two bedrooms and two bathrooms!

D   You were supposedly on top of the world, yet I *sense* you're stunned, dejected, and numbed out with nicotine and alcohol. Plus an angry "Fuck you all!" reverberates everywhere.

ANJU   I really thought I had made it. *Anju's eyes shift. Sorrow streaks her face.* I was knocking around that huge house a-l-o-n-e. All my friends were dropping out of my life like flies. They were all straight and white and all got married and had children around this time. They didn't have time for me anymore. *Anju's eyes widen as another layer of her isolation reveals itself.* The townhouse was in a very white neighbourhood in the suburbs of Calgary.

D   Ouch … That's intense. *I rest my hands to Anju's heart for fifteen minutes.*

ANJU   What the hell was I doing there? I was completely isolated culturally and geographically. Oh my God! I was so far from everything and anyone that might relate to me. *Anju's eyes search in the bleak landscape for a shard of hope.*

D   It seems that your twenty-nine-year-old prizewinner has arrived at rock bottom.

ANJU   Thank you for saying that. I'm a social worker. I thought I knew exactly what rock bottom looked like.

D   You didn't think it could look like this.

ANJU   I was so miserable. I watched mindless TV and I ate all the time. I overate, actually. All kinds of food; junk food mostly. I often felt stuffed and nauseated.

D   Yet empty. You felt heavy, yet you were not grounded at all. You were exhausted and despairing. You feel as though a beast had chewed on you and spit you out. I *sense* that at twenty-nine your depression and anguish were thicker than at any other time in your life.

ANJU   Oh and my relationship also ended around then … And then no one showed any interest for a few years. I really felt rejected, ugly, and absolutely undesirable. It was awful.

D   Undesirable because of your brown skin! Ouch. You feel trapped, encased, and sealed in. *Tears gush forth.* Your nascent self-love and the work we have done to date haven't reached your skin yet, the largest organ in your body! Internalized racism still festers in your pores.

ANJU   Oh! It feels like pins and needles.

D   The energy is rushing in, creating new pathways, rinsing the cells and molecules in your skin, welcoming its brown pigment and its rightness and its beauty!

ANJU   You know, I was looking at pictures of myself at that age just the other day. I looked so good at that time, so beautiful and strong. It's so ironic. Ugh … I feel tingling behind my left shoulder blade! Oh … AH! … Ha ha ha ha … OH … Ha ha ha aha ha … *Anju laughs herself silly as unconditional love fills and opens her heart.* Ha haaahahaha. Oh, that feels sooo much better!"

NOVEMBER

ANJU   I got the test results for my second biopsy. The calcifications in my left breast are benign. No C-word, thank the Goddess. I am well! I knew it. Even while I was waiting, I felt it deep in my bones. I kept telling myself: "I'm fine, I'm fine."

D   You do not have cancer and this is cause to celebrate, but you are nonetheless ungrounded. What's going on?

ANJU   I'm not sure. I feel off.

D   Your pelvis is numb again. It looks like your despairing twenty-nine-year-old is here with us again. *I hear* "I'm alone and unloved. All my relationships have hit the skids. No one wants me." *I intuitively reach for Anju's left shoulder. I settle in for a few minutes.*

ANJU   OUCH! That's so intense.

D   It's like a nest of angry bees in there.

A few minutes later:

Ah … The bustling density reaches down to your biological heart, that spot directly under the calcifications in your left breast we worked on last time.

ANJU   I felt so lost.

D   There's more to this story to tell.

ANJU   You know, I've been thinking, so much happened in that house. Once, I found my father unconscious. He was visiting me in Calgary and I had gone to work. I came home and couldn't get in. The chain was on the door and my father was not responding. I rang the doorbell and knocked loudly, but he didn't answer. I called 911 and they cut the chain and got in. He was out cold. It's then that I realized that my father was an alcoholic!

Another time, my brother and mother were visiting me. They both cuddled and hung on to each other at the table and then at one point they just laughed at me. This is useless, I thought. These people are useless. I have no family.

And I'd gone to India the year before, the older family members there constantly pestered me about men and marriage. Older people there think they have a right to criticize you—how you look—anything really. They do it openly. It's sanctioned behaviour. I was so disillusioned by my family there too. It was not the haven I was hoping for. I came back thinking: "Fuck you all!"

D   Really. "FUCK YOU ALL" in a major way. Here you are, at twenty-nine years old, on top of nothing, feeling estranged in a white neighbourhood and from your family in Canada and in India!

ANJU   You know, my family in India was not the panacea I thought it would be. I was not welcomed with open arms. It wasn't that simple. *Anju swallows loudly. Her throat feels constricted.*

D   Have you ever thought about how you would kill yourself? Have you ever thought about what you would do?

ANJU   *Anju utters without skipping a beat.* Pills! *Anju surprises herself. She is shocked by the clarity of this thought. Her eyes stare into mine.*

D   Did you have pills you thought might work?

ANJU   I had a bottle of Tylenol 2.

D   Reaching for that bottle in your medicine cabinet is imprinted in your energetic field. Your hand reached up and the plastic welcomed you. Its promise of relief soothed you. The familiar snap of the lid, the welcoming rattle of the pills, the capsules in your hand, your flesh against your mouth as you tossed those pills in … and then that sensation when they stick in your throat.

ANJU   I remember drinking wine from a mug!

D   Yes, you downed a few Tylenol 2s with red wine and your pain vanished. N-U-M-B, you fly. Free of your brown skin, of Calgary, of India, of your family, friends, ex-boyfriend, and everyone. Your legal and instant cocktail knocks you out cold, predictably, every time. Each time a little taste of death … dreamless sleep… a vast expanse of painlessness.

ANJU   I was on skid row in my own townhouse in my white suburban neighbourhood! It's the same thing. I was doing the same thing!

D   And you knew that if you added a few more pills to your beloved magic cocktail, you could slip into your death … your big death … and not have to wake up and go to work the next day.

ANJU   Oh … it was awful … How I would wake up and have to face life … And go to work … With all those people! Oh my God. I had no idea. I have never thought of this. I didn't remember this. I didn't remember. With all the liver stuff, it all makes so much sense. How is this possible? I knew I had forgotten parts of my childhood and adolescence, but something like this in adult life! It's shocking to me. I was so unhappy!

D   And so full of self-loathing.

ANJU   *Anju weeps as this new piece of her narrative fills in and fleshes itself out in her day-to-day consciousness*

D   The big-*C* scare has really galvanized your spirit, Anju. Despite the threat of the big *C*, you chose life. Now all of you can choose life, even your twenty-nine-year-old.

ANJU   Yes, yes, that's so true. We both do.

        A few minutes later:

        It's going to take me a while to integrate all of this. It's huge. It's quite the new piece of information. I feel quite out of it actually … WOW! I made it out, even then, I made it through—that's when I suddenly picked up and moved to Toronto. You know, it came to me almost overnight. The decision was made by the time I thought of it. I suddenly moved to Toronto. I just left and moved here. No wonder it was so sudden. It was do or die. WOW!

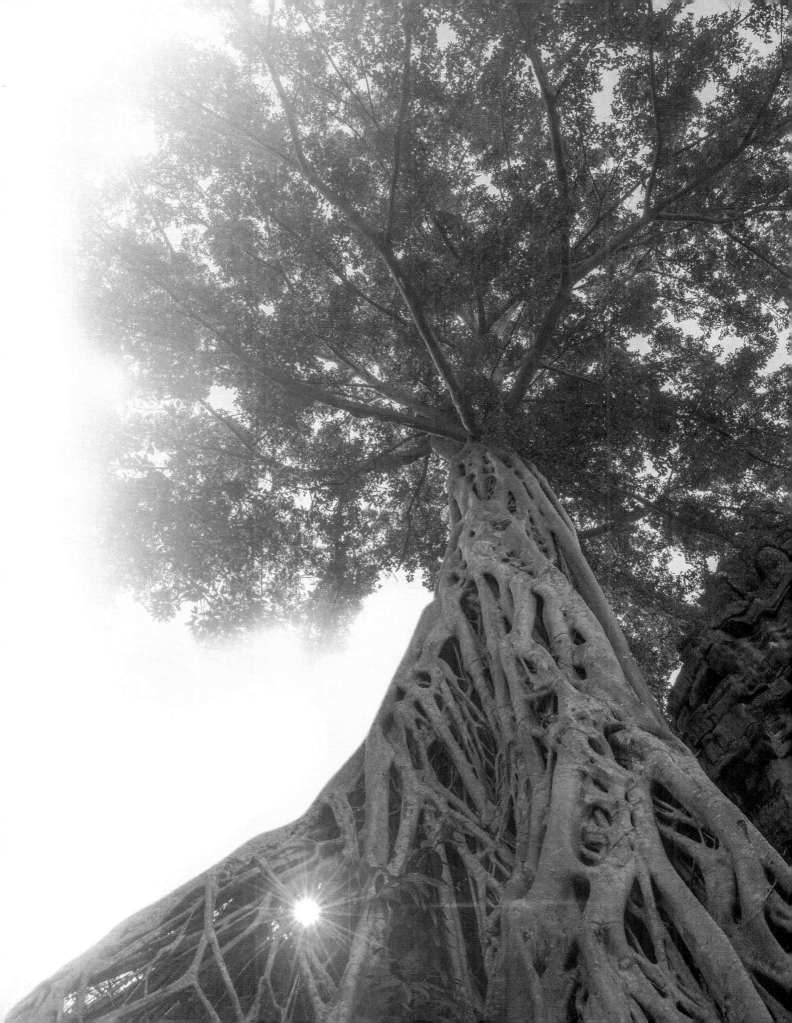

CHAPTER TWENTY-FOUR
FIONA

Dear Reader,

When I was young, I lived in a dysfunctional house where everyone smoked. I hated it and was always sick. I had a destructive and hateful relationship with my mother, who was verbally abusive, and a brother who was abusive in all ways. I came to feel that I was less than these people I despised because their needs were always put before my own.

In my adult life, I unfortunately reproduced the pattern over and over again. I entered into and stayed in horrible relationships, usually with very controlling people; not out of the fear of being alone, but most consistently out of the fear of being thought of as unwanted and unworthy. Sadly, those feelings of unworthiness were why I was in abusive relationships in the first place. I endured, and I suppose even sought out bad friendships, abusive partners, and thankless jobs because I felt I deserved nothing more.

What I got from all of this was a body that was twisted with dysfunction. Although I had done a lot of emotional work, I was still always sick and weak. I first came to Dany with torn fascia in my thighs. I have since come to understand that the fascia is a representative of the etheric body and that my fascia was both calcified to the point of fragility and therefore susceptible to being torn. I had let it grow too delicate to protect me, and with it I had let the world fray my cosmic underwear.

Fiona

....

FEBRUARY

Fiona at age forty-six

FIONA   My right thigh is extremely sore. Not only that—I'm a mess. My life's a mess. I feel totally fucked up.

D   *I settle my hands on Fiona's shins for a few minutes. I sense that you're not in your body or Sacred Tree and not connected to the energy of the earth and the sun. That can't possibly feel good.*

A few minutes later:

Hmmm ... Your mother's energy is overwhelmingly present. Well ... we know one thing for sure: your mother wasn't in her Sacred Tree either. She's stewing in quite a brew.

FIONA	Oh she's a piece of work all right.
D	And I *sense* that you have been overly subjected to your mother's misery and convictions. It feels as though you grew up soaking in her mess.
FIONA	Drowning is more like it.

A few minutes later:

D	I *hear* your mother's bitter voice: "I'm miserable. Life is miserable." Oh, and "I'm unhappy. So no one can be happy. Life is a goddamned miserably long mess."
FIONA	Yeah, her life was a mess and life with her was a mess all right.
D	Ah … I *see* that these beliefs are implanted in your first, sixth, and seventh chakras. As a result, your fundamental connection to the earth and the sun is precarious. You're on a bad line, so to speak.
FIONA	Figures …
D	Hmmm … Your mother was unplugged big-time, and unfortunately you're unplugged too at this point. She was not living from within her Sacred Tree—and neither are you because you learned this energetic pattern from her. So what we've got here is your Sacred Tree, uprooted and lying on the ground with its roots dried out and dangling in the air. For sure, that doesn't feel good.
FIONA	You got that right.
D	Beyond the obvious impact of your own adversity, you basically absorbed your mother's traumatized astronauts and architects of survival and sadly mimicked her chakras and energy bodies. Most of the damage was done before the age of seven and a lot of it happened in utero. This intergenerational trauma and stealthy explosives are creating havoc in your physical, emotional, mental, and spiritual energy fields and Sacred Tree.
FIONA	That makes sense to me.
D	OK … Let's see here. *I slide my right hand on Fiona's thigh and settle my left on her abdomen for ten minutes.* I *see* that your etheric body is extremely thin from your waist to mid-thigh—I call this section of the field your cosmic underwear. The threads are weakened, the glow is faint, and the weave is all loose and stretched out of shape. I *sense* unbeneficial energy from a variety of sexual partners.
FIONA	Oh yeah.
D	I also *sense* sadness, despair, shame, and self-loathing trapped in your second and third chakras. It looks like you've had a really hard go of it in terms of relationships.

FIONA   Yeah, I was fucked over a few too many times.

D   The deterioration of your field and cosmic underwear also speaks of your mother's story too. I *sense* that you're carrying your mother's wounds. Was she abused?

FIONA   Yes.

D   Unfortunately the cycle of violence is alive and well. You're caught in that mire as well.

A few minutes later: I *hear* your mother's voice: "This is it! It's really it! Expect nothing more. This is my lot and it's yours too. Don't you go thinking you can expect more. Trust me, I know."

FIONA   Yeah right, she knows nothing.

D   *I now rest my right hand on Fiona's abdomen and slide my left hand up to her liver for a few minutes.* I *see* that your liver is burdened with toxins. Actually, your organs in general are burdened with accumulated physical, emotional, mental, and spiritual debris. There's work to do here, but we need to work on your third chakra first.

   A few minutes later:

   Hmmm … Your will centre is depleted. *I glide my left hand to Fiona's solar plexus and settle in for a few minutes.* Your will is your "starter" energy. When this energy centre is clogged, it is virtually impossible to develop self-discipline or galvanize motivation. Sluggishness takes over, making it an uphill battle to focus on meaningful action.

FIONA   I'm not surprised.

D   On top of your will, your mother's unresolved baggage also eroded your self-worth, which is also mobilized by the third chakra. My concern is that it's a nasty combination with the sixth and seventh chakra depletion. I *sense* that your birthright alignment with your life's purpose is in jeopardy. The onslaught of your mother's intense history has interfered with your ability to trust your inner authority and listen to your own wisdom.

FIONA   What wisdom?

D   *I rest my hands on Fiona's right thigh for ten minutes.* I *sense* that your relationship with your critical, unconscious, and toxic mother was really adversarial. No surprise, really. Ouch … She spread her misery like Nutella on toast—thick and lots of it. I *see* that you fought tooth and nail, every day and all day, for your right to be and your right to be free. You fought bravely, that's for sure. You also fought desperately. Well, you fought—that's what you did.

FIONA   What else was I supposed to do?

D   That's all you could do. Your mother was a train wreck waiting to happen every hour on the hour.

FIONA   I left home at nineteen, and at twenty-three I walked away from it all. I had no choice. There was nothing else to do. I fucking cut the cord.

D   Partially … Your energy fields are still burdened with her energy. Well there's less of it now, but still, it's to be continued.

FIONA   I thought I was done with her.

D   Not quite yet; some of her energy still invades your cells. We cleared a lot of her energy out today. Besides, you have done so much emotional work already that the unhelpful energy is malleable rather than fossilized. You'll feel like you dropped twenty pounds after a few sessions.

EARLY MARCH

FIONA   I'm a nervous wreck. I'm tired of living like this.

D   *I rest my hands of Fiona's shins for a few minutes.* I *see* the energy in your head as a dizzying swirl of activity. Unfortunately your life-and-death battle with your mother rages on. I *sense* that you're on high alert 24/7. You are ready to defend and protect yourself at the drop of a hat. You created a fantastic architect of survival, Fiona, a vigilant freedom fighter who guided you and ultimately got you out of that house. Your heart and soul were at stake, so it was serious business. You needed that. *I rest Fiona's head in my hands for a few minutes.* Your Freedom Fighter's central command office is in your left-brain hemisphere. It's here that you plot your strategies of survival. Does your life now still warrant this level of alertness?

FIONA   Probably not. I'm exhausted by it all.

D   That's my sense.

Ten minutes later:

Hmmm … The right side of your face is burdened with shame. I *hear* "I'm ugly … and I'm aggressive." I *sense* that this is your mother's voice rather than your truth. It seems that you have internalized her perception. You see yourself as an ugly, aggressive, selfish cunt (your mother's words, not yours or mine by the way). In fact, if we listen to your mother, you deserved her every attack.

FIONA   Oh right, of course.

D   I *sense* that the field of shame spreads down to your right breast and lung. *I place my right hand above Fiona's right breast and my left below for a few minutes.* Hmmm … This is where you are storing some of your mother's shame linked to her own unhealed sexual abuse. Oooh … Your mother's power over you as a child and young teenager reeks of her own perpetrator's fumes. These emotional toxins have penetrated your flesh. Your breasts—the primary sexual ornaments and signifiers of your gender in our culture—are marked with the wounds of sexism, namely, disempowerment and abuse. Your mother had her share and so have you.

FIONA   Oh yeah.

D   *I feel called to Fiona's right shoulder. I shift my hands up closer to Fiona's shoulder and settle in for a few minutes. I hear* "I hit her! I hit my mother!" Ah … This is a different kettle of shame. I *sense* that you feel ashamed of the moment your Amazonian Freedom Fighter was born (thank the Goddess for her—we like her). One day you were trapped in yet another onslaught of verbal abuse. *Fiona drops into a deep meditative state and drinks in the energy for ten minutes.* It was just another attack, and yet a new set of resources emerged that day. You hit her back! The key word is *back*. You were a teenager by then and at that particular moment you tapped into a new resource: you realized you had the physical strength to fight back. I *hear* a loud and defiant. "Back the fuck off!" Good for you, Fiona! She had it coming. No shame in that.

FIONA   Whoa …

D   Yeah … You judge yourself harshly. You feel guilty and ugly because you responded violently. Your shame buries the dignity of your battle and the beauty of your will to survive. After years of abuse you defended yourself and set a much-needed boundary.

A few minutes later:

I *sense* that you blame yourself, Fiona, for the ugliness, abuse, violence, and harshness in that home. Let your mother carry it for a change. She created the environment. You responded. Survival is usually a very messy business. No shame there. It's her shame to carry. These are some nasty fumes to clear. Ouf … Clear, clear, clear. Good riddance, I say. Out, out, out. Are you OK?

FIONA   Yeah …

D   You're almost through it. You're doing great. It's melting like butter.

A few minutes later:

All the emotional work you've already done is really paying off. Let's liberate you and your architect of survival. It's best if you recognize your Freedom Fighter's heroic mission and celebrate the birth of her newfound strength and power. Celebrate her determination to protect you and your blossoming clarity, self-love, and self-respect. Thank the Goddess for all of it. You made it through because of it, despite your excruciating circumstances. Now let's see if we can convince her to luxuriate in a well-deserved day at the spa. It's working, Fiona, just settle in to this delicious respite.

FIONA   Whoa … I feel different.

D   Yeah, you can let your hair down finally. Your Freedom Fighter can rest and so can you. Savour the potential for rebirth into a life of thriving rather than surviving. The vernal equinox is around the corner. You're on cue for a big shift.

FIONA   At least there's that.

LATE MARCH

FIONA   My right thigh is still really sore.

D   OK … Let's see what the vernal equinox is shaking up in your liver and gallbladder. *I settle both a hand on Fiona's liver and the other on her thigh for a few minutes.* Hmmm … I *sense* that life at twenty-one was too much to bear.

FIONA   Oh that was a really hard time for me.

D   Yes, so much so that you wished to end your life.

FIONA   It was really dire.

D   Yeah … Your liver was totally swamped by despair. You felt you had nothing left and nothing to live for. You basically thought that you were nothing and that your life amounted to nothing.

FIONA   It was really rough.

D   Yet, it seems you gathered your last drop of energy to hobble away … raging … despairing … I see you dragging yourself down a long dusty road to somewhere, something, anywhere … to anything … You're limping away, as far away as humanly possible. You're so beautiful in your determination and will to survive. Wow, your liver and thigh also show us the strength you harnessed to get out of there!

FIONA   I did pull myself out, barely. It took almost everything I had.

D   Both your traumatized astronaut and your architect of survival in your liver and thigh are softening into your Sacred Tree. OK … Gradually, the ki energy is flowing through the mass; the texture is now sponge-like rather than rock-like. You're doing great.

Ten minutes later:

While this continues to unwind, let's see what else is up. Hmmm … I sense that there is more of your mother's energy around your head. I sit behind Fiona to cup her ears for a few minutes. Both your ears still ring with your mother's invectives. I sense that the verbal abuse climaxed when you were sixteen years old. Does that sound about right?

FIONA   Yes.

D   I *hear* "Who gives a fuck what I do, no matter what I do, it's the same thing. She just keeps yelling and screaming her head off!" Yeah—I know the feeling—the crack of dawn, six, nine, noon, three, five, seven, ten, midnight, two, three, five; no matter, nothing stops her. It was non-stop yelling around the clock. Anything and everything could trigger her.

FIONA   Literally anything.

D   Ouch … she's loud.

A few minutes later:

Oooh … she has a foul mouth too! I *hear* "You fucking ugly cunt. You whore! You're trash! You're nothing! You're less than nothing! You're just a selfish little cunt!" Talk about dumping. She is projectile-vomiting her shame and self-loathing onto you.

FIONA   She was totally out of control.

D   You know this now. The problem is, back then you didn't. Sixteen-year-old Fiona is still drowning in it. You were so utterly flattened and humiliated. Who wouldn't be? Your mother lashed out at you with all the vehemence and intensity her abusers dumped onto her. She was utterly trapped by the cycle of violence and became a perpetrator. She smeared her unresolved wounds, self-loathing, and humiliation on every aspect of her life, especially you. The fact that you're a girl makes such a huge difference.

FIONA   Yeah … I had to go down with her ship.

D   She knew of no other ship. No matter how much you glared, screeched, or clawed to gain some ground, she imposed her shame and humiliation on you. Humiliation is the most painful human emotion. It's the bottom of the barrel. Let's scrub the humiliation from the kitchen floor with fresh water and wash it out of your body, mind, and soul.

A few minutes later:

Let your mother carry the weight. Cast the whole lot off your shoulders and dump it where it belongs. With respect and love, celebrate your newfound freedom and personal power. Step out from under her distorted hierarchy enforced through fear and degradation. You have nothing to be ashamed of, Fiona. Nothing.

FIONA   It was such a hellhole.

D   You're not kidding. Oooh … Your fifth chakra is spewing. And it's not just what you had to yell back to hold your ground; your throat chakra is festering with negative self-talk. You had good training after all! *I cup my hands above Fiona's throat for a few minutes.* I'm *hearing* some the negative mantras you took in: "My life is mess—it is a total mess—a total fucking mess!" Not only are you focusing on what isn't working and what's missing, you're pissing on the whole parade. We just got a whiff of what your mother yelled at you. Can you imagine what went through her head? It's enough fucking bullshit to grind a whole generation to a halt. It certainly has been enough to paralyze you.

FIONA   Fucking hell!

D   That's it, Fiona, your fifth, sixth, and seventh chakras are spewing. *I rest Fiona's head in my hands for fifteen minutes.* Toxic beliefs are pouring out, untangling themselves and tripping over each other on the way out: "My life is awful. I'm a victim. I'll always be a victim. I'm suffering. I'll suffer for the rest of my life. I'm stuck. I'm trapped. I have no choice. I'm scared. I'm weak. This is what it's like to be a woman. It's our lot. It's reality." It's all coming out, Fiona. Internalized sexism and enforced powerlessness are truly vile. Just let it pour out. You've been carrying this toxic waste for long enough! Most women have this kind of soul-threatening patriarchal garbage tucked in the deep recesses of their psyches. It's centuries of oppression, generation after generation, great-great-grandmothers and so forth. This is the energy that is most damaged in our world: yin, the sacred feminine, the capital-*M* mother, Durga, Kali, call it what you will, but taste her strength and shit-kicking transformative power now.

That's it, Fiona, turn the wheel to end the cycle of violence inside and out. Dream, pray, chant, or scream your personal power into being. Visualize and focus on your potential and who you really are.

FIONA   It's totally rock and roll.

D   It's Patti Smith plus plus—that and the intense growth of the wood element in the spring. Delicious, isn't it? Your tree's wood is thickening and strengthening by the second. Hmmm … There's still some unbeneficial energy lurking. Ah … Your seventh chakra still holds on to some of your mother's bitterness and resentment. Let's open all your upper chakras and create a huge opening for the energy from the sun to penetrate and replenish your being. You need a mega dose of light. Receive. Ah … that's it … now you're clearing it all.

FIONA   Not a moment too soon. Whoa … I feel a bit dizzy.

D   That was an upper chakra power wash. Lie still for a few minutes. Take your time. Let yourself adjust to the new sensations. Your Sacred Tree is upright now. Block off some quiet and meditative time over the next while so you can practise drawing in energy from the earth and the sun as well as the high vibrations of love and compassion now accessible to you.

MID-MAY

FIONA   I'm frustrated. I'm still eating like shit and not taking care of myself.

D   *I rest my hands on Fiona's shins for a few minutes.* Your third chakra is still depleted. Your mother's screeching is like bucket-loads of swampy water dousing the fire in your will centre. *I join my hands on her solar plexus to nourish and tonify the chakra for a few minutes. I hear* "You're a loser. You can't accomplish anything. You're nothing. You're garbage." Well, how's that for a description of your mother? I bet you think she's rather accurate.

FIONA   Yep.

D   Your third chakra speaks of your relationship to yourself. What the hell is she doing in there? She's cutting you off from your inner strength.

FIONA   I am so tired of this.

D   Well, it stands to reason; how are you supposed to align with your life's purpose with gusto if a perpetrator pissed on your parade for years? Let's get her out of here pronto. This is your sacred space. No one should be in your chakra but you.

Hmmm … We still have work to do around your head. *I sit behind Fiona and hold her head in my hands for fifteen minutes.* Your seventh chakra is presenting more blocks. It's clearer after the last session's dump, but your mother's authority and power to terrorize you still interferes with your connection to the sun's energy. I *sense* that you do not have permission to even plug in. Your mother's dictatorial and abusive power usurped your birthright to connect to the sun.

FIONA   Whoa …

D   Yeah … Your mother wanted control of your whole life and being. She embodied a God-like, all-encompassing, omniscient presence of corrupt power and terror. She literally stood between you and the sun. This is the most monumental act of violence against a human being. This is what cult leaders and dictators do, by the way: they interfere on a soul level with your sacred connection with the life force. Her drive to overpower you disrupted this birthright alliance. Your mother drowned her own child's access to the transcendent dimension of life with her desperate addiction to external power: the junk food for her victimized self and the twisted lessons of patriarchal oppression.

FIONA   She is so out of there.

A few minutes later:

D   Hmmm … Your facial pores still ooze disgust. It's a monsoon of self-loathing. You feel ugly. There's more to this ugly business. Let's see here … Another incapacitating belief is coming out: "I am unlovable." *Fiona's arms and feet fidget. A shiver squirms its way through her entire skeletal structure. She jolts.*

FIONA   Oh fucking Christ, I hate the fact that I look like my mother.

D   Bingo. Thanks, Fiona. The repugnant and revolting energy is releasing. You'd internalized your repulsion for your mother. A cloud of toxic fumes is emanating from your face. Love and respect pour into your cells and molecules. *Fiona's face relaxes.* Claim your face … your bones … your earth.

FIONA   I'm so over it.

D   You can truly end the relationship now. You can choose to no longer be "daughter." You can choose to divorce your mother. Rather than be a daughter without a mother, you can liberate yourself and soften out of being her daughter. Reclaim your connection to the big-*M* mother. You can reclaim it all. You can really walk away this time … no hobbling … no dragging … no limping. You can walk your sacred walk with your feet firmly rooted in the earth's beautiful energy, your head high, touching the sky and your heart full with unconditional love.

FIONA   I am not her daughter, not for the rest of my life!

LATE MAY

FIONA   I feel much better.

D   *I check in with Fiona's solar plexus for a few minutes.* Wow! Your third chakra is on fire, as it should be. A beautiful steady flame burns. Your heart centre is opening up too. *My left hand glides up to Fiona's chest and rests there for five minutes.* You are shedding your mother's misery and your own. Ha! Your twenty-one-year-old who wanted to end her life is emerging from the deep well. Together, you embrace your freedom. Joy is gurgling to the surface. You have ended your relationship with your mother rather than your life, and that's a mighty good thing. Woohoo!

FIONA   This is so exciting!

D   It sure is. Let's see what else is cooking. I *sense* that your fifth chakra and throat are also opening. Fiona the activist and social agitator is emerging. You're seeing the big picture. The sexist social and cultural constructs that mutilated you and your mother are coming into greater focus. Your victimization is now your teacher. The violent language that once contaminated your throat is now perceived accurately as the voice of survival. You compassionately witness your right to use this weapon to defend yourself. With joy and gratefulness you embrace Freedom Fighter's valiant battle for survival. You're so on it, you can now see how courageously you fought! You didn't take your mother's shit sitting down, and that's a mighty good thing.

My hands rest on Fiona's chest for fifteen more minutes. Whoa … Another channel is coming through. Yikes! Mega second-hand smoke is exploding out of your lungs.

FIONA   We argued about her fucking smoking all the time!

D   *Pungent fumes attack our senses now.* Your mother was a chain-smoker. Her exhaust fumigated the house and invaded your body. *Fiona squirms under the memory of the attack.* Ouf!

FIONA   Whoooaaah! *The disgusting smell invades the healing room and for a moment threatens to swallow all inner peace and stillness.*

D   *With one hand still on Fiona chest, I sweep away the malodorous and injurious toxins. The intensity of the invasive assault softens.* Reclaim your lungs, invite all your cells and molecules to reject and spill out any remnants of nicotine toxicity on all levels: physical, emotional, mental, and spiritual.

FIONA   This is a huge pill to swallow.

D   Yeah, it's been swallowed, breathed in, and absorbed, and some of that waste is still in your system. *Fiona is walloped by this confirmation and affirmation.*

FIONA   I feel like it's the invasion of the 2000-something remake of the 1978 remake of the 1956 film based on the 1955 science fiction novel by Jack Finney: *The Body Snatchers.*

D   Yeah, it's your mother's body snatchers, literally!

FIONA   Fucking hell!

D   It's gushing out. Soften into the release, Fiona.

Ten minutes later:

You're going to taste freedom. It's coming. You're doing such great work. You are in an excellent place to embrace the full spectrum of energy available to you on summer solstice. Hold on to your hat: you are in for some big, fabulous changes.

AUGUST

FIONA   There has been a nasty breakup. It's just so FUCKED UP!

D   I thought of you on summer solstice. It was a big one for all of us. OK—here we are: your sexual relationships—your man file! We had to get here somehow. Your seventh chakra is presenting more fumes. Oooh … You're off-kilter and barely hanging on. You're unplugged again!

FIONA   Fucked over is more like it.

D   *My hands shift to Fiona's third chakra for a few minutes.* Hmmm … The breakup presents itself to me as a violent punch in the stomach.

FIONA   That's exactly how it felt.

D   The energy in your solar plexus and third chakra is literally caved in. The impact of your ex's attack took your breath away. Your flame is almost out cold again. You initiated the breakup though … right?

FIONA   Yeah. So you'd think I would feel otherwise.

D   Yes, but he sure didn't mince his words. I *hear* him lashing back with a virulent verbal attack. His violent words triggered you and smothered your self-esteem. Wait a minute … It's not just what he said; it's what you said too. You hate yourself and what you said. So many awful memories of your mother's abuse were conjured up: "You're nothing … fucking nothing … just a fucking selfish cunt." How much more to the point can a trigger be?

FIONA   Shit.

D   It's all there—clear it now—all of it. Soften into the release, Fiona.

Fifteen minutes later:

Celebrate your Freedom Fighter's right to defend you. It's OK. You did what you could with the resources you had last month. It can be different in the future when you have different resources. *I shift my hands to Fiona's pelvis.* Hmmm … Your second chakra is also burdened with your ex's toxic energy. Just what you needed, more of the very special President's Choice Memories of Ex—all of them, in fact— all the fuckers.

FIONA   Well, why the hell not at this point?

D   *Rage spews in all directions. My left hand shifts to Fiona's liver while my right rests on her right thigh.* Your poor liver! It is congested with your whole stinking man file—fuming at high temperatures. Hmmm … Have you been consuming more?

FIONA   Alcohol? I've been drinking my face off and gorging on greasy, fried summer party food.

D   Well sure—the trigger has you running for the hills. You're desperately trying to escape your painful emotions.

FIONA I am so done … so fucking done!

D   Yes, done, fucked up, fucked over, and fucking fed up. Agreed. But you're not so done feeling, processing, clearing, and healing your frustration, anger, and despair. Your right kidney, your liver's best colleague, is also contracted. This organ's vitality is severely compromised. The two most important filters in your body are speaking loud and clear.

FIONA Fucking hell.

D   Its OK, Fiona; it's nothing lots of water, low-fat foods, lots of vegetables, and some exercise and yoga can't fix. It will be much easier to drop into this protocol now that your ex's energy is cleared.

FIONA Yes … yes … yes, I'm on it.

OCTOBER

D   So what is the fall equinox brewing this year? You look radiant.

FIONA I am going on my own to India for six weeks after Christmas. This is a big dream for me.

D   *My hands rest on Fiona's shins for a few minutes.* You're landing on your feet despite your free-fall after the breakup. The impact of the conflict still marks your energy in your legs, but you are nonetheless aligning with your personal power. Your internal sense of direction is awakening, and your inner wisdom and intuition assuredly lead you to India.

FIONA I have been dreaming of it for years.

A few minutes later:

D   I *sense* that it is an auspicious time to make this dream a reality. Both your first and second chakras are welcoming the earth's and the sun's healing frequency. That's new. It's is a huge shift. It's a great time to realign with the high vibrations you're set to encounter in India.

FIONA I am so stoked.

D   Yes, and blocks in your third chakra are disintegrating as well. Withered self-hatred and bitterness are melting in the burning heat of your reclaimed clarity, strength, and personal power. And—woowee—your liver is much much better too.

FIONA   I've been drinking far less alcohol and I'm eating healthier foods. I fasted for two days earlier this week.

D   Excellent. Your gallbladder is clearing too. That dark chamber has been sealed tight for a long, long time. It's been congested with extremely potent resentment: the toxic residue of your teenage years at your mother's mercy.

Five minutes later:

That's it, Fiona. Both you and your teenage self are clearing out of that house. *My hands rest on Fiona's thighs for a few minutes.* You are walking straight out of the dense forest of past betrayals and pain. You are setting yourself free.

FIONA   I'm even looking at other women in their forties and fifties differently. I feel firmly rooted in the earth as an empowered woman and see the wisdom and growth that lies ahead.

....

Dear Reader,

I was lying on Dany's table (as usual, with my ears full of my own tears and a disoriented feeling). A pulsating energy flowed through the top of my head and down through my feet into the ground. I felt pink, scrubbed, newborn, and clean. I felt my feet suddenly become comically enormous, fifteen feet long and heavy, and they thumped heavily on the ground, I had the sensation of them flopping over and yanking me up with them. Suddenly, instead of being buried under the mire, I was standing on the earth and able to look about and see the beautiful world around me for the first time in my life. A sentence screamed itself into my head: "Find the middle ground." Perhaps nothing earth-shattering, but the best advice I have ever given myself. Stepping onto the path I was meant to be on did not change my life dramatically, but it was the beginning.

Fiona

JUNE

Fiona at age forty-seven

FIONA   I have two ribs broken in six places: ribs four and nine.

D   Hmmm … One on top of the liver and the other below the liver. That's one hell of a summer solstice you've got happening here.

FIONA   I fell off a ladder.

D   OK—let's settle you in.

FIONA   OUCH … No no … Oooh … *Six pillows and three blankets later.* OK, I think I can manage.

D   Whoa—painful.

FIONA   I've been on morphine and just about every other painkiller on the planet for the past week. My goal is to stop the meds after today's session. My liver has never been more toxic.

D   Hmmm … Your sixth and seventh chakras are wide open and humming. Your access to the sun is more potent than last night's morphine hallucinations, that's for sure. Your energy field is sparkling with light. What happened in India?

FIONA   Oh, you're going to love this. In the last week of my trip, I was literally pulled off a very busy street by a holy man. He told me that I was not living my life's purpose. "You should be a teacher," he said. "When you return, you must accept the first teaching opportunity that is offered to you."

D   This encounter was a blessing. Your entire field vibrates with this man's wisdom and connection to the earth and the sun. His third eye shines on you. He is your spiritual guide and teacher and you are his student, whether your ego likes it or not. His karma and yours intersect.

FIONA   When I got back, I started practising yoga in my neighbourhood. After a few months, the studio owner pulled me aside and recommended I take the teacher training program. "We would love to have you as a teacher," he said. I did not hesitate; I said yes. And now I'm in the program and I'm planning on going back to India in the fall.

D   OK, this is all good, but you're clearly off-kilter somewhere. What else has been happening?

FIONA   I was laid off at work a couple months ago.

D   OK, so the decision was made for you. You were pushed out of your attachment to security and your busy-busy mode. But what else happened?

FIONA   Then the rib accident happened.

D   How did it happen?

FIONA   I was having one of my typical days: happily doing ten things at once with stuff strewn all over the yard. I climbed up a stepladder to trim a bush. I lost my balance and I landed on my chest on a lawn ornament.

D   Talk about bull's eye and all the way from India! He's good! You're being told in no uncertain terms that you are not on track with your life's purpose. Yoga training or no yoga training, job or no job, you are told in no uncertain terms to slow the fuck down now. In fact, don't just slow down, stop. You are being told to stop and listen.

FIONA   Moving always hurts.

D   I'm so sure it does. The brutal "accident" meets your stubborn refusal to slow down and listen. It had to be serious enough to obstruct the energy you were exerting to run away from the silence. It's time to stop to breathe and meditate.

FIONA   That's the only thing that is working. It's the only time I get relief.

D   I'm so sure it is. He's good, remember! He signed you up for a crash course in breathing (pardon the pun). You'll work on learning that foremost tool of rejuvenation and spiritual liberation. Your ribs are literally broken so that you can expand your chest and heart consciousness. You are given the opportunity to really go to another level of awareness and mindfulness with your ribs and breathing guiding you.

Fifteen minutes later:

Plus, it's going to be rather hard for you to hold on to the old hard-done-by narrative when you, in fact, have been blessed … in India … on the trip of your dreams. To be blessed in India, isn't that what everyone dreams of? You are given the tools to forge a conscious relationship with your Sacred Tree. That's where you wanted to be all along anyway. The path is now clear.

FIONA   Really?

D   Really. This is the best thing that has ever happened to you.

Dear Reader,

That accident was one of the best things that ever happened to me. I spent a summer laying in my garden writing a book in my head. As I recovered that winter, I got it down on paper, and now I am working on getting it published. I finished my yoga training and now teach. I engage in beneficial relationships and walk away, calmly no less, from destructive ones. My navel chakra, which was like a lump of lead in my belly, is more open all the time, and I feel less and less shame about the life I live. I feel I have the right to act on my own behalf and to make my own decisions. I no longer hide my art in shame but sell it in stores. I am finally an active member in the society of humankind, on the path I was meant to walk.

Thank you, Reiki.

Thank you, Dany.

Fiona

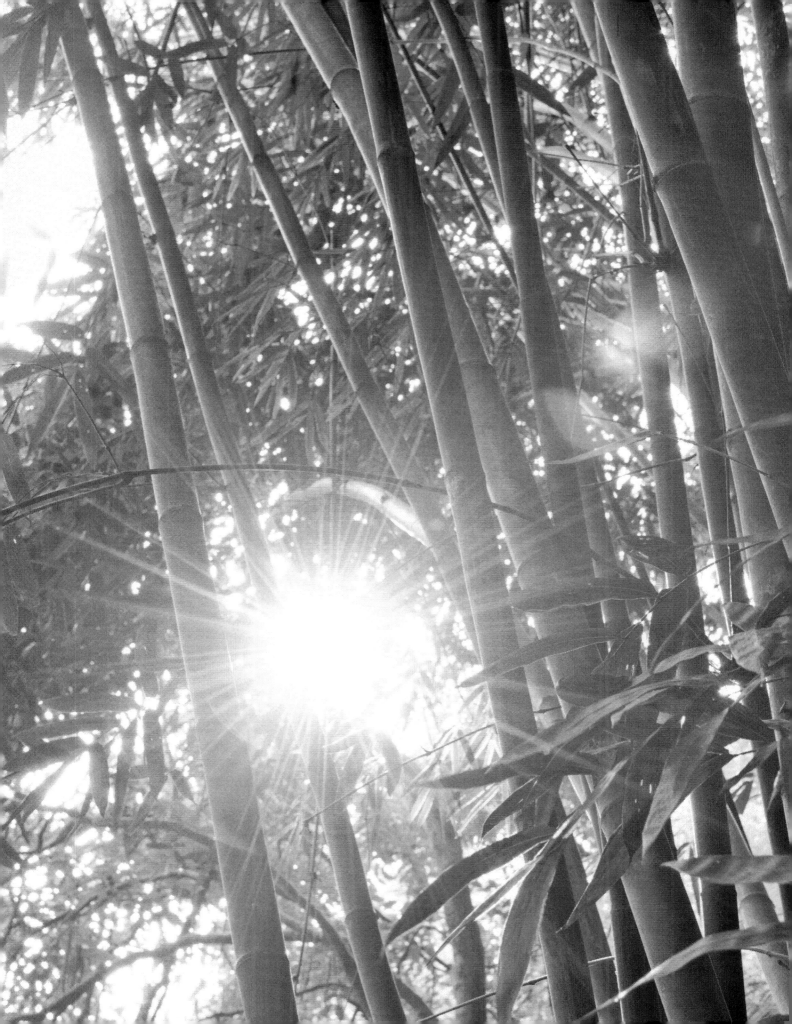

OM
SHANTI
SHANTI
SHANTI

PEACE
PEACE
PEACE

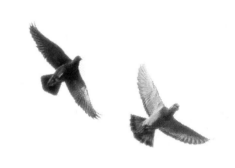

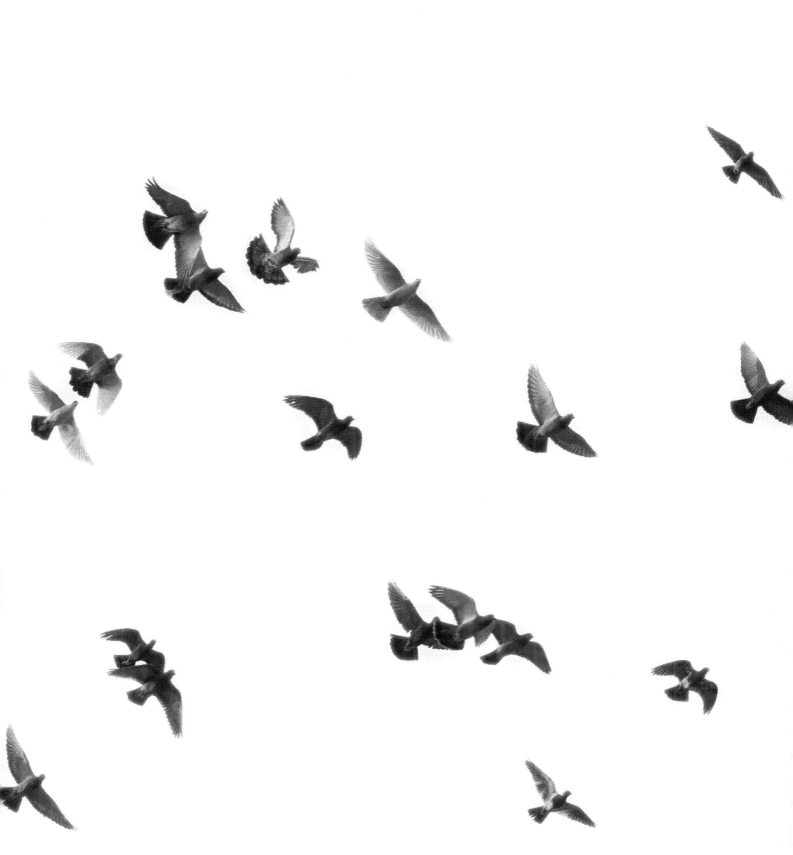

REIKI

ANATOMY OF THE SPIRIT: The Seven Stages of Power and Healing
Caroline Myss
Three Rivers Press, 1996

CORE LIGHT HEALING: My Personal Journey and Advanced Healing Concepts for Creating the Life You Long to Live
Barbara Ann Brennan
Hay House, Inc., 2017

EASTERN BODY, WESTERN MIND: Psychology and the Chakra System as Path to the Self
Anodea Judith
Celestial Arts, 2004

ESSENTIAL REIKI: A Complete Guide to an Ancient Healing Art
Diane Stein
Crossing Press Inc., 1995

HANDS OF LIGHT: A Guide to Healing Through the Human Energy Field
Barbara Ann Brennan
Bantam Books, 1988

NETTER'S ANATOMY FLASH CARDS (Netter Basic Science)
John T. Hansen
Elsevier Inc., 2019, 2014, 2011, 2007, 2002

THE ORIGINAL REIKI HANDBOOK OF DR. MIKAO USUI: The Traditional Usui Reiki Ryoho Treatment Positions and Numerous Reiki Techniques for Health and Well-Being
Dr. Mikao Usui and Frank Arjava Petter
Foreword by William Lee Rand, Translated by Christine M. Grimm
Lotus Press, 2007

THE SPIRIT OF REIKI: The Complete Handbook of the Reiki System
Walter Lübeck, Frank Arjava Petter, and William Lee Rand
Lotus Press, 2001

THE SUBTLE BODY: An Encyclopedia of Your Energetic Anatomy
Cyndi Dale
Sounds True, 2009

SURFACE ANATOMY: The Anatomical Basis of Clinical Examination
John S. P. Lumley
Churchill Livingstone / Elsevier, 2008

HEALING

THE ARTIST'S WAY: A Spiritual Path to Higher Creativity (25th Anniversary Edition)
Julia Cameron
TarcherPerigree / Penguin Random House, 2016

THE COURAGE TO HEAL: A Guide for Women Survivors of Child Sexual Abuse
Ellen Bass and Laura Davis
Harper Perennial, 1994

INA MAY'S GUIDE TO CHILDBIRTH
Ina May Gaskin
Bantam Books, 2003

INA MAY'S GUIDE TO BREASTFEEDING
Ina May Gaskin
Bantam Books, 2009

IN THE REALM OF HUNGRY GHOSTS: Close Encounters with Addiction
Gabor Maté, M.D.
Alfred A. Knopf Canada, 2008
Vintage Canada, 2009

I THOUGHT IT WAS JUST ME (but it isn't): Making the Journey from "What Will People Think?" to "I Am Enough"
Brené Brown
Penguin Group, 2007

NONVIOLENT COMMUNICATION: A Language of Life
Marshall B. Rosenberg. Ph.D.
Foreword by Deepak Chopra
PuddleDancer Press, 2015

ON DEATH AND DYING: What the Dying Have to Teach Doctors, Nurses, Clergy and Their Own Families
Elizabeth Kübler-Ross, M.D.
Scribner, 1969, 2014

POST TRAUMATIC SLAVE SYNDROME: America's Legacy of Enduring Injury and Healing
Dr. Joy DeGruy Leary, Ph.D.
Uptone Press, 2005

RAISING CHILDREN COMPASSIONATELY: Parenting the Nonviolent Communication Way
Marshall B. Rosenberg. Ph.D.
PuddleDancer Press, 2005

WAKING THE TIGER: Healing Trauma
Peter A. Levine, with Ann Frederick
North Atlantic Books, 1997

THE WAR OF ART: Break Through the Blocks and Win Your Inner Creative Battles
Stephen Pressfield
Black Irish Entertainment, 2012

WHEN THE BODY SAYS NO: The Cost of Hidden Stress
Gabor Maté, M.D.
Vintage Canada, 2004

WOMEN FOOD AND GOD: An Unexpected Path to Almost Everything
Geneen Roth
Scribner, 2011

WOMEN'S BODIES, WOMEN'S WISDOM: Creating Physical and Emotional Health and Healing
Christiane Northrup, M.D.
Bantam Books, 1994

VAGINA: A Cultural History
Naomi Wolf
HarperCollins Canada, 2012

INNER PEACE

ANIMAL SPIRIT GUIDES: An Easy-to-Use Handbook for Identifying and Understanding Your Power Animals and Animal Spirit Helpers
Steven D. Farmer, Ph.D.
Hay House Inc., 2006

AWAKENING SHAKTI: The Transformative Power of the Goddesses of Yoga
Sally Kempton
Sounds True, 2013

THE BOOK OF FORGIVING: The Fourfold Path for Healing Ourselves and Our World
Desmond Tutu and Mpho Tutu
HarperOne, 2014

INSIGHT YOGA: An Innovative Synthesis of Traditional Yoga, Meditation, and Eastern Approaches to Healing and Well-Being
Sarah Powers
Shambhala, 2008

MEDITATION FOR THE LOVE OF IT: Enjoying Your Own Deepest Experience
Sally Kempton
Foreword by Elizabeth Gilbert
Sounds True, 2011

THE TIBETAN BOOK OF LIVING AND DYING
Sogyol Rinpoche
HarperOne, 2002

THE UNTETHERED SOUL: The Journey Beyond Yourself
Michael A. Singer
New Harbinger Publications, Inc., 2007

THE WAY OF LIBERATION: A Practical Guide to Spiritual Enlightenment
Adyashanti
Open Gate Sangha, 2012

YOGA IS UNION: The Yoga of Amma Sri Karunamayi
Darin Somma
SMVA Trust, 2013

MEMOIRS

AUTOBIOGRAPHY OF A YOGI
Paramahansa Yogananda
Self-Realization Fellowship, 1971

THE AUTOBIOGRAPHY OF MALCOLM X: As Told to Alex Haley
Malcolm X
Ballantine Books, 1987

DYING TO BE ME: My Journey from Cancer, to Near Death, to True Healing
Anita Moorjani
Hay House Inc., 2012

THE ELEPHANT WHISPERER: The Extraordinary Story of One Man's Battle to Save His Herd
Lawrence Anthony, with Graham Spence
Pan Macmillan, 2009

GIRL WALKS OUT OF BAR: A Memoir
Lisa F. Smith
SelectBooks, 2016

GIRLS LIKE US: Carole King, Joni Mitchell, Carly Simon — and the Journey of a Generation
Sheila Weller
Washington Square Press, 2008

IN THE BODY OF THE WORLD: A Memoir of Cancer and Connection
Eve Ensler
Metropolitan Books / Henry Holt, 2013

LEFT TO TELL: Discovering God Amidst the Rwandan Holocaust
Immaculée Ilibagiza
Hay House, Inc., 2006

LONG WALK TO FREEDOM: The Autobiography of Nelson Mandela
Nelson Mandela
Little Brown & Co., 1994

RED HOT AND HOLY: A Heretic's Love Story
Sera Beak
Sounds True, 2013

SOMETHING FIERCE: Memoirs of a Revolutionary Daughter
Carmen Aguirre
Douglas & McIntyre, 2011
Vintage Canada, 2014

THE WHEEL OF LIFE: A Memoir of Living and Dying
Elisabeth Kübler-Ross, M.D.
Touchstone, 1998

WHY BE HAPPY WHEN YOU COULD BE NORMAL?
Jeannette Winterson
Grove Press, 2012

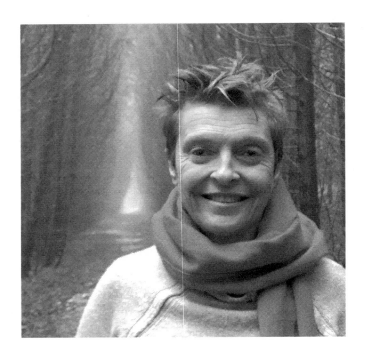

Dany Lyne uses the embodiment of high-frequency energy to activate full human potential. Her method ignites a new approach to living in creative genius and personal freedom through capturing and enhancing Loving Kindness and compassion in the four bodies: physical, emotional, mental, and spiritual. She draws from her experience as a trauma intuitive, Reiki practitioner, CranioSacral therapist, and studies with indigenous healers in Africa and Central America, insights during meditation, and her personal passion for stimulating her clients' connection to the life force. Her greatest joy is sharing her discoveries with others.

DANYLYNE.COM